THINNER LEANER STRONGER

The Simple Science of Building
the Ultimate Female Body

THIRD EDITION

By Michael Matthews

www.muscleforlife.com

oculus

Thinner Leaner Stronger

The Simple Science of Building the Ultimate Female Body

Third Edition

By Michael Matthews

www.muscleforlife.com

Cover designed by Damonza (www.damonza.com)

Book designed by Sarah Beaudin (www.cestbeaudesigns.com)

Edited by Armistead Legge, Christina Roth (www.christinarotheditorial.com), and Matthew Gartland (www.winningedits.com)

Published by Oculus Publishers, Inc. (www.oculuspublishers.com)

PRAISE FOR *THINNER LEANER STRONGER*

"If you want to use strength training for aesthetics, Mike is your source. Read this book, and read mine too, and come away with what you need to know. The rest will be up to you."
—Mark Rippetoe, author of *Starting Strength: Basic Barbell Training* and *Practical Programming for Strength Training*

"Nobody cuts through the fitness and nutrition confusion and clutter like Mike Matthews. And in *Thinner Leaner Stronger*, he draws on a powerful combination of time in the trenches and hard-core research to give you the straight talk about what actually works.

"This book is easy to read and incredibly effective. I highly recommend."
—Ben Greenfield, CEO of Kion & *New York Times* bestselling author of *Beyond Training: Mastering Endurance, Health & Life*

"Mike has written the encyclopedia of body recomposition for the twentieth century. A great book and a must-buy for beginners looking to get their feet wet."
—Martin Berkhan, fitness coach, pioneer, and author of *The Leangains Method*

"Mike Matthews stands alone in the fitness space. His books are based on scientific research and real-world results. *Thinner Leaner Stronger* can change your life."
—Strauss Zelnick, "America's fittest CEO" and author of *Becoming Ageless: The Four Secrets to Looking and Feeling Younger Than Ever*

"In *Thinner Leaner Stronger*, Mike takes us back to the fundamentals of losing fat and building muscle—time-tested and science-backed strategies that have been obscured by a rising tide of popular hype and pseudoscience.

"The good news: it doesn't have to be that hard!"
—Alex Hutchinson, author of the *New York Times* bestseller *Endure: Mind, Body, and the Curiously Elastic Limits of Human Performance*

"Matthews has masterfully distilled many years of research into the essence of what makes people fit—and fast.

"His training methods have worked better than anything else I've tried for improving my strength and physique. Get this book right now."
—Stephen Guise, international bestselling author of *Mini Habits*

"Mike Matthews has done it again. Great information backed by science, and complicated knowledge transformed into practical, applicable strategies.

"I loved *Thinner Leaner Stronger*. A must-read."

—Adam Schafer, co-host of top-ranked fitness and health podcast *Mind Pump*

"I haven't been this excited about a fitness book in years. It's required reading for all gals who want to get—and stay—in the best shape of their lives. A true classic in the making."

—Sal Di Stefano, co-host of top-ranked fitness and health podcast *Mind Pump*

"Would you rather spend a month of your life hoping the latest flavor of diet and exercise plan will work . . . or spend thirty days knowing your hard work will provide results you can not only see, but feel?

"Give me guaranteed results any day, and that's what *Thinner Leaner Stronger* provides—all the knowledge and motivation you need to get results for years to come."

—Jeff Haden, Inc. Magazine contributing editor and author of *The Motivation Myth: How High Achievers Really Set Themselves Up to Win*

"*Thinner Leaner Stronger* gives you everything you need to know for achieving the body you want. Full stop. No hype and no gimmicks, just solid info backed by solid science. An outstanding book."

—James Krieger, MS, founder of Weightology (www.weightology.net)

"As a clinical practitioner who specializes in obesity medicine, I truly appreciate *Thinner Leaner Stronger*. It's simple, science-based, and most importantly, it works, and that's why I recommend it to many of my patients.

"Drop whatever you're doing and read this book. It can change your life."

—Dr. Spencer Nadolsky, board-certified family and obesity medicine physician and founder of RP Health

"A highly actionable book that translates the latest science into a simple plan for strength. In a world filled with noise, Mike Matthews provides the clarity and practical strategies you need to get results."

—James Clear, author of *Atomic Habits: An Easy & Proven Way to Build Good Habits & Break Bad Ones*

CONTENTS

To all the women who have supported me and my work and made this third edition possible. Thank you for the feedback, love, and encouragement to make this edition the best one yet!

This is for you.

And to be honest, I hope that after reading it, you'll say it's the best fitness book for women ever written. If nothing else, it's the absolute best fitness book for women I'm currently capable of writing.

FREE BONUS MATERIAL

Thank you for reading *Thinner Leaner Stronger*.

I hope you find it insightful, inspiring, and practical, and I hope it helps you build that lean, sculpted, and strong body you really desire.

I want to make sure that you get as much value from this book as possible, so I've put together a number of additional free resources to help you, including:

- A savable, shareable, printable reference guide with all of this book's key takeaways, checklists, and action items.

- Links to form demonstration videos for all *Thinner Leaner Stronger* exercises.

- An entire year's worth of *Thinner Leaner Stronger* workouts neatly laid out and provided in several formats, including PDF, Excel, and Google Sheets.

- If you'd prefer the workouts in a digital or hardcopy book, check out *The Year One Challenge for Women* (www.thinnerleanerstronger.com/challenge).

- 10 *Thinner Leaner Stronger* meal plans that make losing fat and gaining lean muscle as simple as possible.

- A list of my favorite tools for getting and staying motivated and on track inside and outside of the gym.

- And more.

To get instant access to all of those free bonuses (plus a few additional surprise gifts), go here now:

www.thinnerleanerstronger.com/bonus

Also, if you have any questions or run into any difficulties, just shoot me an e-mail at mike@muscleforlife.com and I'll do my best to help!

FOREWORD

Mike and I have been doing podcasts together for a while now, and we've gotten to be buddies despite the fact that he's too skinny and has too many abs.

I keep telling him he'd make a great lifter at 275 pounds, but he plays golf, and you know how those people can be.

Nonetheless, I have a great deal of respect for anyone who insists on telling the truth in this ridiculous industry, the home of charlatans, frauds, liars, and fools all over the world. Mike and I agree about far more than we disagree, and we learn from each other.

More importantly, Mike is his own guy—he works for himself, thinks for himself, and writes for himself. And you are the beneficiary. He sells no useless quasi-pharmaceuticals, no silly devices, no "breakthrough" programming, and no bullshit. He gets no money from sponsors, and he is owned by no one.

Mike may be mistaken (as may I), but he doesn't lie to you. He tells you the truth, and you should listen.

If you want to use strength training for aesthetics, Mike is your source. He understands the importance of getting strong. He knows that muscle determines the shape and appearance of the human body, and that muscles grow when they are stressed by heavy loads. He knows that hard work is the only effective use of your training time. He understands the science of nutrition, and he can explain it to you—and even to me.

I'm an old hardheaded strength coach, but I have enough sense to know that most people are primarily interested in their appearance. So read this book, and read mine too, and come away with what you need to know. The rest will be up to you.

Mark Rippetoe

Author of *Starting Strength: Basic Barbell Training* and *Practical Programming for Strength Training*

PART 1

WHAT'S IN THIS FOR YOU

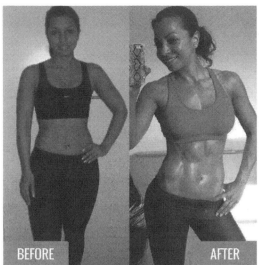

BEFORE　　　AFTER

"I liked that it gave me
direction and motivation
every time I went to the gym."

YVONNE A.

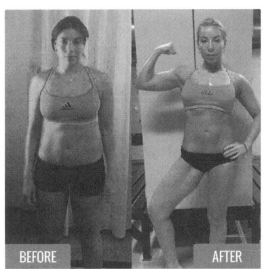

BEFORE　　　AFTER

"I lost 10 pounds of fat and
gained 6 pounds of muscle in
7 months!"

MARSHA M.

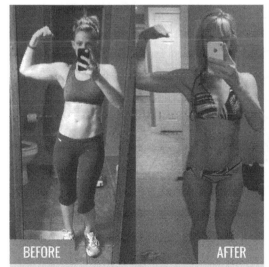

BEFORE　　　AFTER

"It was the perfect book to
educate and guide me."

CHRISSIE R.

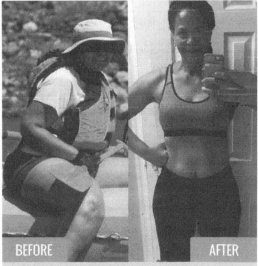

BEFORE　　　AFTER

"I have more energy, discipline,
and have gained more
confidence!"

SUSIE G.

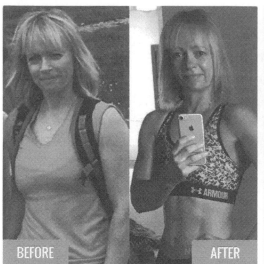

BEFORE   AFTER

"I am happier about myself, more confident, and I get compliments about my fitness which makes me smile!"

LOUISE C.

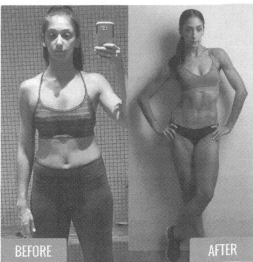

BEFORE   AFTER

"Eating the correct balance of macros has given me more consistent energy and I no longer have crashes."

KATHY V.

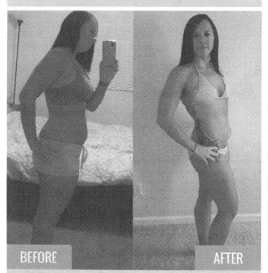

BEFORE   AFTER

"I never expected that I'd be able to get as fit and healthy as I am today."

ALI P.

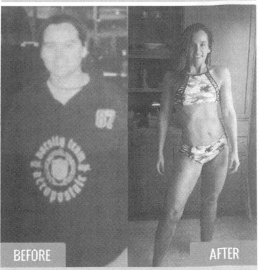

BEFORE   AFTER

"I have more energy and confidence, and as a whole am a completely different person."

JILL A.

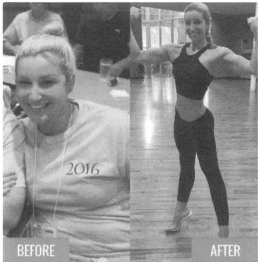

"For the first time in my life, I feel comfortable in my own skin."

ALICE S.

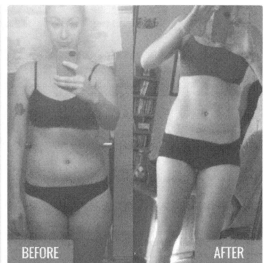

"I think I could write a book about how this program has changed my life."

ALEXIS E.

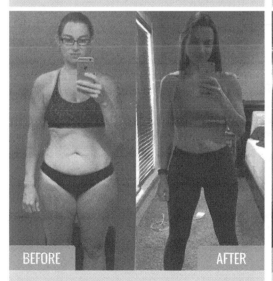

"It sounds cliche, but this has honestly changed my life. I have become happier and a better mother to my children."

RACHEL M.

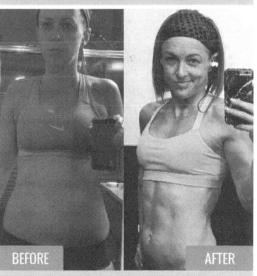

"This book helped me take control of my life. Trust the process and just keep going."

LIZ T.

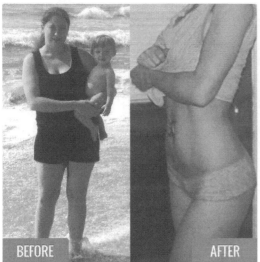

BEFORE AFTER

I lost 50 lbs in 7 months following Mike's books!

KELLY O.

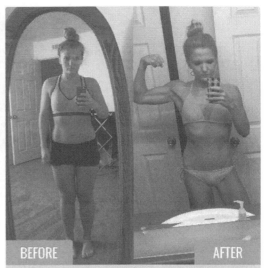

BEFORE AFTER

"I have never truly been this healthy in my life. I feel strong and sexy and finally have the confidence I have always wanted."

SHAY B.

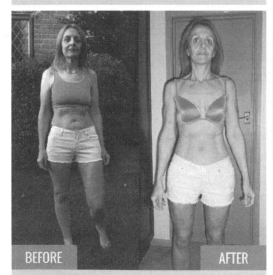

BEFORE AFTER

"I've lost 8kg (17lbs) so far!"

LAURA M.

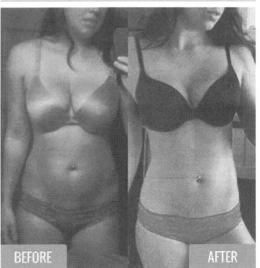

BEFORE AFTER

"I'm a beast. I lost 23 pounds and feel like a solid human made of meat not fat."

TARA Z.

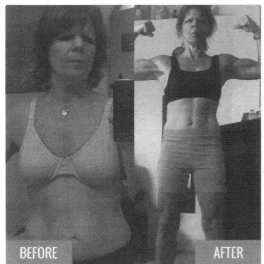

BEFORE   AFTER

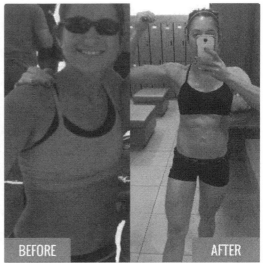

BEFORE   AFTER

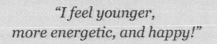

*"I feel younger,
more energetic, and happy!"*

ANGELA A.

*"It's so amazing how my
body has transformed in the
last few weeks!"*

KATIE T.

IT WORKS

ORDINARY WOMEN, EXTRAORDINARY RESULTS. WILL YOU BE NEXT?

The women you just saw are just like you.

They're in their 30s, 40s, and 50s, and they come from all walks of life and levels of fitness. Some were once fit, others were always overweight, some had tried many diet and exercise routines before and failed, others were brand new to it all, some had a lot of time and energy for working out, and others had very little.

What they all have in common, though, is they've all used the diet and exercise principles and programs you're about to learn to get into the best shape of their lives.

Every one of these women has dropped pounds of unwanted fat, added lean muscle in all the right places, and dramatically reduced their risk of disease and dysfunction.

And they did it eating the foods they love, doing workouts they enjoy, and taking few, if any, supplements.

I want to introduce you to several of them whose stories have inspired and touched me, and who are definitive proof that with the right know-how and guidance, anyone can build a body they can be proud of.

If they can do it, why not you?

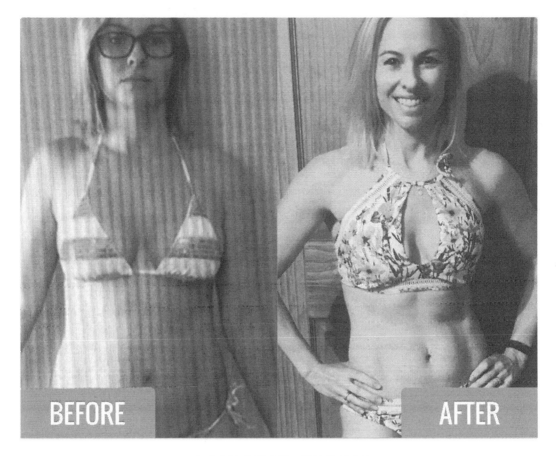

AMBER'S STORY

I really never struggled with weight until after my third baby. In the two years after she was born, I ran a half marathon and I did other weightlifting programs to no avail.

I was completely defeated and almost resigned to the fact that maybe it was just my age or stage of life.

When I couldn't drop the weight, I felt terrible about myself. I was constantly beating myself up because I had never struggled the way I was struggling.

Then I started the *Thinner Leaner Stronger* program, and I was shocked at how quickly the weight started to fall off. Results were quick for me because I started being honest with myself about what I was eating and not doing.

After starting the program, I dieted for eight weeks and lost 14 pounds, and I haven't gained any weight for a year.

I'm most proud of the amount of weight I can lift. I'm a little person by bone structure, but I feel SO STRONG! My squat increased by 45 pounds, my deadlift increased by 65 pounds, and my leg press increased by 110 pounds!

This program is superior to any program out there. It wasn't just about dropping weight, either—it was about taking time for myself as a mom and finding just one way to put myself first.

I'm most proud of my strength and that my kids ask me to flex on the daily—especially my girls.

Ninety-nine percent of the time after my workouts, I'm happy, energized, and ready to conquer my two jobs, kids, home life, and everything else on my plate.

The thing I've repeated to myself over and over is "trust the process." I trust Mike Matthews and his no-nonsense, "this is science" approach. Read the book, apply it, and you WILL see results.

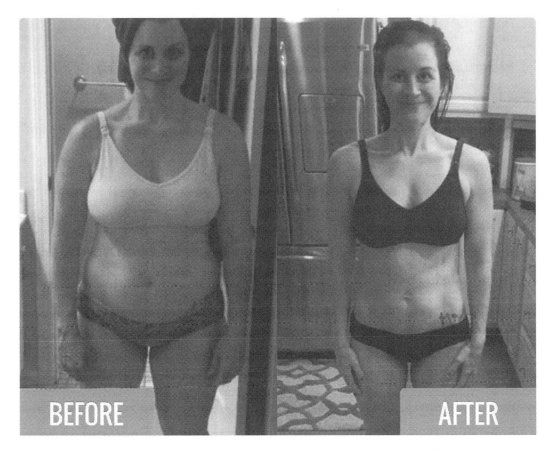

BEFORE · AFTER

JENNA'S STORY

I was sick of spending hours in the gym doing CARDIO, CARDIO, CARDIO and not getting results.

It worked okay for me when I was younger, but after having several children along with getting older, it just wasn't working, and I felt stuck at a certain number on the scale.

Since starting *Thinner Leaner Stronger*, I've lost 35 pounds in six months! I've also noticed that my energy levels have increased, my mood is better, and I don't fight unhealthy cravings the way I used to.

Overall, I just feel so much better.

I increased my bench press by 40 pounds, my squat by 60 pounds, my deadlift by 45 pounds, and my leg press by 240 pounds. In the past I would just do cycling, running, or elliptical—I had never lifted weights before. I relied mainly on counting calories and cardio to stay at my ideal weight.

This program is truly a lifestyle and is completely sustainable. I'm not quite at the maintenance stage yet, but I know it'll be even more flexible once I get to that point.

I have so much more to learn and new goals to set, but I'm genuinely enjoying the process. I really appreciate the self-discipline this program has taught me.

By following *Thinner Leaner Stronger*, you're building the body you want for the rest of your life, and it takes time, consistency, and patience. But it's worth it. Watching your body change is an amazing thing and very empowering.

I've managed to follow this program faithfully with three children under the age of four—one who is seven months old and exclusively breastfed. If I can do it under these circumstances, anyone can do it!

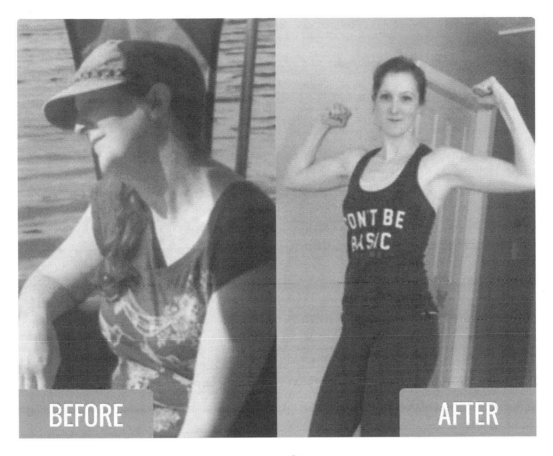

BEFORE   AFTER

GENEVIEVE'S STORY

My friend and long-distance fitness coach told me that if I followed the *Thinner Leaner Stronger* program, I'd be extremely happy with the results.

He said it wasn't complicated but that I had to have the motivation and willingness to work hard. He was right.

In one year and nine months, I lost 34 pounds and 8 percent body fat. I also added 55 pounds to my deadlift, 45 pounds to my squat, and got my bench press up to 50 pounds!

It took me some time to get into the rhythm of things. Once I realized how badly I wanted to lose weight and gain core strength, I noticed my body changing fast. (After having two children, my core strength was nonexistent.)

I saw results immediately, and that made me push harder to achieve my goals and make new ones.

When it comes to the workouts, the heavy weightlifting made me feel good, and I liked how Mike broke down proper form for every exercise. On the nutrition side of things, once I calculated a few breakfast, lunch, and dinner options, it wasn't so hard.

I'm definitely more confident now, too. I'm able to show my daughters that staying healthy and being strong is important in more ways than one. I have more energy, which is great for work, and I'm able to keep up with my kids after work.

I even had the courage to sign up for a Spartan Race this summer!

I'd recommend *Thinner Leaner Stronger* to anyone who's skeptical about working out. I've never been a gym person, and Mike Matthews made it accessible and fun for me.

Read the book, then reread it and take notes. Create a list of simple goals you'd like to achieve. Then set more goals once you've achieved those.

. . .

I hope you enjoyed those success stories as much as I did and are inspired to follow in the footsteps of the outstanding women you just met.

Who knows, maybe people will be reading about *your* transformation story one day?

Anything is possible if you want it enough. And in this book, I'm going to show you the way.

1

THE PROMISE

No matter how old you are, no matter how bad you might think
your genetics are, and no matter how lost you might feel after trying
and abandoning past diets and workout programs . . .

. . . you absolutely, positively can have the lean,
sexy body that you dream about.

What if I could show you how to dramatically transform your body and health faster than you ever thought possible?

What if I gave you a science-based, doctor-approved formula of eating and exercise that makes melting 10 to 15 pounds of fat while also adding just the right amount of lean muscle a breeze . . . and what if you could see dramatic results in the mirror in just the first 30 days?

What if I showed you how to get a toned, defined physique by investing no more than 5 *percent* of your time each day?

And what if I promised to be at your side the entire way, helping you discover what you're truly capable of, helping you overcome obstacles and setbacks and avoid pitfalls, and basically doing everything I can to see you achieve your fitness goals as quickly and painlessly as possible?

What if I promised to show you how to build that hot bikini body without having your life revolve around it?

What if you didn't have to starve yourself, put in long hours at the gym, or do grueling cardio workouts that turn your stomach? What if I even showed you how to get leaner and stronger while still indulging in the "bad" foods that you love, like chocolate, pizza, and ice cream?

Imagine waking up every morning, looking in the mirror, and feeling downright *excited* by your reflection. Imagine being able to proudly wear the clothes you really want to wear and take them off with confidence.

Imagine, just 12 weeks from now, being constantly complimented on how you look, having dawn-till-dusk energy to do all the things you want to do, and feeling up to getting other parts of your life under control and into the fast lane.

Well, you can have all these things, and it's not nearly as difficult or complicated as you probably think.

It doesn't matter whether you're 21 or 41 or whether you're in shape or not. No matter who you are, I promise that you have the power to transform your body and life.

Just ask the thousands of women whose lives have been changed by my work. They accepted my help, and now they look and feel better than ever before. They are the proof that this book can help you look and feel your best, too.

So, would you like my help?

If you answered "Yes!" then you've taken a *leap*, not a step, toward the new you—the leaner, stronger, healthier, and happier you who loves her body, inside and out.

Your journey begins as soon as you turn to the next page.

2

WHO IS MIKE MATTHEWS
AND WHY SHOULD I CARE?

"Opportunity is missed by most people, because it is dressed
in overalls and looks like work."

—UNKNOWN

I'm Mike, and I believe that every person can achieve the body of their dreams.

My mission is to give everyone that opportunity by providing time-proven, evidence-based advice on how to build muscle, lose fat, and get and stay healthy.

I've been training for more than a decade now. In that time, I've read thousands of pages of scientific literature and tried just about every type of workout program, diet regimen, and supplement you can imagine. At this point, I can confidently say that while I don't know everything, I know what works and what doesn't.

Like most people who get into weightlifting, I had no clue what I was doing when I started out. I turned to fitness magazines for help, which told me to spend a couple of hours in the gym every day and hundreds of dollars on pills and powders every month. This went on for years, and I jumped from diet to diet, workout program to workout program, and supplement to supplement, only to make mediocre progress and eventually get stuck in a rut.

I then turned to personal trainers for guidance, but they had me do more of the same. After spending many thousands of dollars with them, I still hadn't gained any more muscle or strength to speak of, and I still had no idea what to do with my diet and training to reach my goals. I liked working out too much to quit, but I wasn't happy with my body and didn't know what I was doing wrong.

I finally decided that something had to change, and I knew that I needed to start with learning the actual physiology of muscle growth and fat loss. So I threw the magazines away, fired the trainers, got off the internet forums, and searched out the work of top strength and bodybuilding coaches, talked to scores of natural bodybuilders, and started reading scientific papers.

Several months later, a clear picture was beginning to emerge.

The real science of getting into incredible shape is very simple—much simpler than the fitness industry wants us to believe. It flies in the face of a lot of the stuff we see on TV, Instagram, and YouTube and read in books, articles, and magazines.

For example:

- You don't need supplements to build a great physique.

- You don't need to constantly change up your workout routine to "confuse" your muscles.

- You don't need to "eat clean" to get and stay lean.

- You don't need to stop eating carbs and sugars to lose weight.

- You don't need to eat small meals every few hours to "boost your metabolism."

- You don't need to grind out hours and hours of boring cardio every week to get a ripped core.

- You don't need to be in the gym hours per day and sacrifice your relationships with your friends and loved ones.

As a result of what I had learned, I completely changed my approach to eating and exercising, and my body responded in ways I couldn't believe. My strength skyrocketed. My muscles started growing again. My energy levels went through the roof. And here's the kicker: I was spending less time in the gym, doing less cardio, and eating foods I actually liked.

Along the way, my friends and family noticed how my physique was improving and began asking for advice. I became their coach. I took "hardgainers" and put 30 pounds on them in a year, took people who were absolutely baffled as to why they couldn't lose weight and stripped away piles of fat, and took people in their 40s, 50s, and 60s who believed their hormones and metabolisms were beyond repair and helped them get into the best shape of their lives.

A couple of years later, these people started urging me to write a book. I dismissed the idea at first, but eventually I began to warm up to it. "What if I'd had such a book when I started training?" I thought. It would have saved me who knows how much time, money, and frustration, and I would have built the body of my dreams a lot faster. I also enjoyed helping people with what I had learned, and if I were to write a book and it became popular, what if I could help thousands or even hundreds of thousands of people?

That gave me a wild hair, and so I wrote *Bigger Leaner Stronger* and published it in January 2012. It sold maybe 20 copies in the first month, but within a couple of months, sales were growing, and I began receiving emails from readers with high praise. I was ecstatic. I started making notes on how I could improve the book based on feedback, and I outlined ideas for several other books that I could write.

Fast-forward to today, and I've now published a number of books, including this book for women and a "flexible dieting" cookbook (*The Shredded Chef*). Altogether, my books have sold over a million copies, and my work has been featured in a number of publications like *Women's Health*, *Muscle & Strength*, *Elle*, *Esquire*, and more.

More importantly, every day I get scores of emails and social media messages from readers who are thankful for my work and blown away by the results they're seeing. They're just as shocked as I was years ago when I first discovered just how straightforward and enjoyable getting fit and healthy can really be.

This is why I continue to write books and articles, record podcasts and YouTube videos, and generally do everything I can to be as helpful to as many people as I can. It's motivating to see the impact I'm having on people's lives, and I'm incredibly inspired by the dedication and determination of so many of my readers and followers. You guys and gals rock.

I also have bigger ambitions that I want to realize.

First, I want to help a million people get fit and healthy. "Help a million people" just has a sexy ring to it, don't you think? It's a big goal, but I think I can do it.

This goes beyond merely making people look hotter too.

I want to make a dent in some of the alarming downward trends we're seeing here in the West—in particular, the decline of people's physical and mental health and performance, which has significant and negative downstream effects in their family lives, careers, and personal happiness and satisfaction. I think helping people get strong and fit is a great way to do something about this.

Second, I want to lead the fight against mainstream health and fitness pseudoscience and BS.

Unfortunately, this space is full of misinformation, disinformation, idiots, liars, and hucksters, and I want to help change the status quo. I'd like to become known as the go-to guy for practical, easy-to-understand advice grounded in real science and results.

Third, I want to help reform the sport supplements industry.

The pill and powder pushers use all types of scams to foist their junk products on unwitting consumers. They use fancy-sounding-but-worthless ingredients; they cut their products with junk fillers like flour and useless amino acids; they use tiny, ineffective doses of otherwise good ingredients ("pixie dusting") and hide it with the notorious "proprietary blend"; and they rely on fake science, overhyped marketing claims, and steroid-fueled meatheads to convince people they have the "secret sauce."

So, that's me. From this point on, it's all going to be about you.

I hope you enjoy this book, and I hope it helps you reach your health and fitness goals faster.

Mike Matthews

Vienna, Virginia

May 20, 2018

P.S. If you're on social media, come say hi! Here's where you can find me:

- Facebook: www.facebook.com/muscleforlifefitness
- Instagram: www.instagram.com/muscleforlifefitness
- YouTube: www.youtube.com/muscleforlifefitness
- Twitter: www.twitter.com/muscleforlife

3

WHY THINNER LEANER STRONGER IS DIFFERENT

"A small daily task, if it be really daily,
will beat the labours of a spasmodic Hercules."

—ANTHONY TROLLOPE

I'm going to tell you something that the kings and queens of the multibillion-dollar health and fitness industry don't want you to know:

Getting toned, fit, and sexy isn't nearly as complicated or difficult as they want you to believe.

You don't need to starve yourself with very-low-calorie diets to lose stubborn hip, belly, and thigh fat and keep it off. In fact, this is how you slow your metabolism down and almost guarantee that you'll regain everything you lose.

You don't need to obsess over "clean eating" to get and stay lean, defined, and energized, and you don't have to completely abstain from carbs or the "cheat" foods you love most.

You don't need to constantly change up your workout routine to get sculpted muscles. All you'll really accomplish with "muscle confusion" is, well, mental confusion.

You don't need to toil away in the gym for a couple of hours per day doing tons of exercises and sets. As a matter of fact, this is a great way to stunt your gains and get nowhere.

You don't need to grind out hours and hours of boring cardio every week to get a tight, defined core. (How many flabby treadmillers have you seen over the years?)

You don't need to spend hundreds of dollars per month on worthless supplements, "cleanses," or fat loss pills. Supplements don't build great butts and bodies, and most don't do anything but drain your bank account.

Those are just a few examples of the harmful lies and myths that keep women from ever achieving the lean, toned, strong, and healthy bodies they truly desire. And this failure often undermines their self-confidence and self-esteem, sours their social lives and relationships, and discourages any future attempts at self-improvement.

Where did all this misinformation come from, and why are long-debunked lies still propped up by mainstream celebrities, social media "influencers," authors, and gurus?

Well, the long story short is this:

When millions of people are strongly motivated to solve a problem and willing to spend large amounts of money to do it, there will always be an abundance of things to buy and brilliant marketers to sell them.

It's pretty simple, really. Where do most people go for diet and exercise advice? TV, online and offline articles, friends, and personal trainers, right?

Most of what people learn from these sources is virtually useless.

How can I make such a bold claim?

Well, let's start with the mainstream fitness publications like magazines, websites, and books, which reach many millions of people every year. Their editors and publishers aren't diabolical scum, but they do have to grapple with a couple of dilemmas.

The first is this: publications of all kinds are in the business of selling information, and they need to keep people buying and subscribing. What's the best marketing button to push to accomplish this?

New.

The easiest way to keep people hooked is to continually give new advice—new training methodologies, diet "tricks," research "breakthroughs," and the like.

New information isn't bad per se. Health and fitness are vast subjects with myriad trails, tunnels, and caverns to explore. Most of it won't sell books, magazines, and website subscriptions though. Your average guy or gal isn't nearly as interested in the nuances of training periodization as how to finally lose that belly fat.

Which do you think will make a better magazine cover splash: how to understand your body weight set point, or how to build bigger biceps?

This is why *Men's Health* stopped writing new cover lines years ago.[1] They know their target market wants, more than anything else, abs, bigger arms and a bigger chest, and more sex, money, confidence, intelligence, and health. Hence, the endless repetition of cover lines like "Six-Pack Abs!" "Dress for More Sex!" and "Build Wealth Fast!" and the endless supply of rehashed … er, *reimagined* … articles to go with them.

The truth, however, is that it doesn't take 13 different articles to teach someone how to get six-pack abs or bigger arms or better glutes. If magazines told the simple truth, they would have maybe 25 articles that they could reprint, verbatim, over and over. The articles wouldn't sound terribly exciting, either. They might have titles like:

Ladies! How to Build 10 Pounds of Lean Muscle in Your First Year

Move More, Eat Less—The "Secret" to Faster Weight Loss

Why the Most Popular Fat Loss Supplements Do Absolutely Nothing

That is, these articles would teach you "inconvenient truths" like you can't get muscle definition as fast as you'd like, you can't target just belly fat for elimination, and you'll need more than 12 50-word tips to build the body of your dreams.

And that's a horrible business plan for a publishing company.

As you'll learn in this book, most of what you want to achieve with your body boils down to diligent and consistent application of the fundamentals. It also takes time. Not an interminable amount of time, but more than "they" want you to believe. The sooner you accept these realities, the sooner you can start making real progress.

The second problem most publications face is the nature of their revenue: advertising.

For example, many of the fitness magazines you see on the shelves of your local bookstore are little more than mouthpieces for supplement companies, which either own the magazines outright or buy the lion's share of their very pricey advertising space.

If these magazines are to stay in business, they must provide their advertisers with a strong return on investment, and they've gotten really good at it. They feature flashy ads that promise far more than any pill or powder can deliver, cleverly written "advertorials" that suck you in with education and conclude with product recommendations, and long-form pieces on various aspects of diet, nutrition, and exercise that contain convincing supplement tie-ins.

Therefore, much of what you're "learning" in these magazines (and their online counterparts) is geared toward selling you products, not helping you achieve your goals as efficiently and effectively as possible. And as long as these magazines and websites keep attracting eyeballs, supplement companies will keep paying, and all will be right in the world (of convincing people to pay to be lied to).

Let's move on and talk trainers. As a coach and trainer myself, I hate to say this, but most of my kind are a waste of money. Their hearts are often in the right place, but very few personal trainers have the know-how required to get their clients into great shape. Even worse, many who *do* have the know-how intentionally drag the process out to make life easier for them (new client acquisition is the toughest part of the gig).

This is why you see so many people paying anywhere from $50 to hundreds of dollars per hour to do the same types of silly, ineffective workout routines, and why so many of these poor people have so little to show for their efforts.

You've probably also noticed that many trainers aren't even in good shape themselves. How can you honestly sell yourself as a fitness expert when you're a skinny-fat weakling? Why should anyone believe you? For some reason, these people get business all the time, and their clients almost always stay flabby and out of shape too.

Compounding the disservice is the fact that most trainers don't give their clients proper diet and nutrition plans, which almost guarantees failure. How you look and feel is just as much a reflection of how you eat as it is of how you exercise, so no matter how many hours you put in at the gym, you won't see major improvements if you're not also managing your diet properly.

Eat incorrectly, and you'll be overweight no matter how much cardio you do. Eat incorrectly, and you'll be weak and "shapeless" no matter how much you struggle with resistance training. Eat correctly, however, and you can unlock everything that exercise has to offer, including rapid fat loss, effortless weight maintenance, and sexy whole-body muscle definition that you can be proud of and that your partner will love.

You probably know that though. In fact, you might be dreading the inevitable "diet" talk, and for good reason. Nobody wants to be told to starve themselves, give up all the foods they like, or follow strange, complicated, or downright annoying eating regimens.

Well, I have good news: you can rest easy because when I say "eating correctly," I mean something very different from what you probably expect. As you'll soon learn, you can actually enjoy "being on a diet." Yes, you read that right. You can lose fat and gain lean muscle while eating plenty of foods you like, including delicious carbs (and even, *gasp*, sugar), and without ever feeling denied or deprived.

But we'll get into all of that later. Let's get back to trainers.

You might be wondering why so many trainers know so little about the art and science of building lean, muscular, healthy bodies. These are certified professionals, right?

Yes, they are.

Unfortunately, you don't have to be a true expert who can get results to pass a PT certification test. You just have to memorize and regurgitate some basic information about nutrition, anatomy, and exercise. You can even do it all online, where test answers are just a Google search away. To make matters worse, a shocking amount of the information you learn when you're getting certified is outdated and even plain wrong. So in many ways, trainers are being set up to fail.

Another problem personal trainers have to live with is baked into the business. If you want to keep clients coming back, you need to keep them convinced that you're needed, and that they couldn't do just as well on their own.

While some people are happy to pay for the accountability alone, most want to feel like they're getting more for their money. An easy way to give them this feeling is to tell them what to do and how, but not *why*, and then regularly change up their routine according to various "sophisticated" training principles.

Personal training isn't all gloom and doom, though. There absolutely are great trainers out there who are in awesome shape themselves, who do know how to quickly and effectively get results in others, and who do care about their clients and deliver what they promise. If you're one of them, I applaud you because you're carrying the weight of the entire profession on your shoulders.

Aside from trainers, we should also discuss another popular but hit-or-miss (and mostly miss) resource people turn to for help: friends.

I've worked with thousands of people, and here's how it usually goes: someone reads an article online or offline, or chats with a trainer or jacked guy or gal in the gym, and passes along what they learned to their fitness-minded friends.

Such word of mouth is great in principle—my work thrives on it—but the results it produces depends entirely on the accuracy and validity of the information being accepted and relayed. And unfortunately, as you now know, much of that information is flawed or even misleading.

This book and everything you're going to learn in it is different because I have very different incentives and payoffs. I'm a self-published author, so my work and livelihood is not beholden to mainstream publishers, advertisers, or trends. Instead, my lifeblood comes directly from you, based entirely on how well I serve you and your interests.

Because of this, *Thinner Leaner Stronger* can go against the grain and recommend science-based diet, exercise, and wellness methods that make editors and marketers yawn. This is why a lot of what you're going to learn in this book is quite different from most of the diet and exercise advice peddled to unsuspecting women every day.

For example, I'm going to let you eat plenty of carbs while stripping fat and adding lean muscle to your frame, I'm going to have you lift heavy weights to make you strong and toned (and no, this won't make you "bulky"—more on this later), and I'm going to have you do as little cardio as possible while building your best body ever.

Sound too good to be true? It's not. It's unconventional, but it *works*, and as far as "truth" goes, what else really matters?

I can understand if you're skeptical. I was when I first came across the scientific research and practical strategies I'm going to share with you in this book. Take heart though because I'm not going to ask you to make a big leap of faith. Most of what you're going to learn has been around for decades, but nobody has put it all together in the way I'm going to for you.

Furthermore, *Thinner Leaner Stronger* is all about getting results, and *fast*. That means you're going to see real, tangible improvements in your body within the first 30 days of starting this program.

Your weight is going to start moving in the right direction, your clothes are going to start fitting a little better, and you're going to start seeing muscle definition peek through where there was none before. I promise.

And if, for whatever reason, you're *not* seeing these types of results within your first 30 days, I still have good news for you. It's not because *Thinner Leaner Stronger* is just another overhyped sell that can't deliver. It just means you need some help with the implementation, and I'd be happy to give it. Simply email me at mike@muscleforlife.com.

Remember too that over 300,000 women have read this book, and tens of thousands (that I know of) have applied its teachings and now have beautiful new bodies to show for it. So you're in good company.

You should also know that a lot of what you're going to learn in this book constitutes the "hush-hush secrets" of Hollywood superstars and A-list models, like the Victoria's Secret Angels. While some of these gals love to pretend that their bodies come effortlessly ("thanks, Mom!"), don't fall for it. These women work incredibly hard to maintain their photoshoot-ready physiques.

Many of these women spend a lot of time doing the same types of training that guys do. Namely, they do a lot of heavy (by most female standards at least) resistance training. They do cardio workouts as well, but many of the biggest stars rely primarily on resistance training to look the way they do.

For example, Miranda Kerr, an Australian supermodel, lifts weights several days per week and focuses on exercises like the barbell squat, barbell lunge, and barbell reverse lunge to lift her butt and tone her legs. Chanel Iman, an American fashion model, told *Shape* magazine that she has trouble toning her body and relies on "a lot of squats and weight lifting" to stay in runway shape.[2] Alessandra Ambrosio, a Brazilian model and actress, squats, lunges, and deadlifts for her famous gams and derriere.

In other words, these women take their resistance training seriously. A lot more seriously than even a lot of the guys you see in the gym every day.

The reason for this is simple: you need a fair amount of muscle in the right places if you want to have relatively low body fat levels *and* toned arms, defined legs, and perky glutes.

So trust me. You have nothing to fear from weightlifting. In the next few months, you're going to use it along with the rest of the information in this book to lose up to 15 pounds of fat and gain a considerable amount of strength and muscle definition.

Or maybe you're starting out skinny and looking to gain muscle tone and shape? Perfect. *Thinner Leaner Stronger* is going to work for you, too.

If you follow my advice, you can gain up to 5 pounds of lean muscle in your first few months, and up to 10 to 15 pounds in your first year. This is going to work wonders for your physique (think smooth, sexy curves and cuts) and boost your mental health, happiness, and self-confidence to new heights.

So, if you're ready to begin, here's the first step: forget what you think you know about getting fit.

That might sound a little harsh, but it's for your own good. Just let it all go, suspend your disbelief for the next few days, and approach *Thinner Leaner Stronger* with an open mind.

Along the way, you'll discover that some of the things you've been doing are right and others are wrong, and that's okay. I've made just about every mistake you can possibly make, so don't be discouraged.

Just follow this program exactly as I lay it out, and the results will speak for themselves.

Good luck. Have fun. And enjoy the body- and life-changing transformation that awaits you.

PART 2

KEY THINGS "THEY" AREN'T TELLING YOU

4

THE HIDDEN BARRIER

"The beginning of wisdom is the definition of terms."
—SOCRATES

Have you ever wondered why so many people find diet and exercise so confusing?

Why it's so rife with unworkable, conflicting, and illogical advice and opinions?

You know, nonsense like:

- "Counting calories doesn't work."
- "Exercise doesn't help you lose weight."
- "Broccoli has more protein than chicken."
- "Foods that spike insulin levels make you fat."
- "Eating a lot of 'healthy' dietary fat helps you stay lean."

These examples are but a few of the many false diet and exercise mantras that have maintained currency despite decades of scientific and anecdotal evidence to the contrary.

Why are people so susceptible to inaccuracies, lies, and oddball theories like these?

While that question might sound like it has a deep, complex answer, the reality is a lot of it can be chalked up to the simplest of things: misunderstood words.

You can experience this firsthand. The next time you hear someone declare that "calories in versus calories out is obsolete," ask them this simple question: What is a calorie?

Dollars to doughnuts your challenge will be met with an empty stare or foolish burbling, because they don't have a clue what the word means, let alone what "calories in versus calories out" really means or how that metabolic process could possibly work.

Chances are your experience with such a misinformed individual will be something like when Jimmy Kimmel asked random people in Los Angeles to define *gluten*. The best response any of them could muster was, "It's like a grain, right?" and my personal favorite response was, "It's a flour derivative of wheat . . ."

(And in case you're wondering, gluten is a mixture of two proteins present in many grains, which is responsible for the elastic texture of dough.)

Calorie and *gluten* are only the very top of the tip of the proverbial iceberg. What is protein? What is carbohydrate? What is sugar? What is body fat? What is muscle? What is metabolism? What is insulin? What is a hormone?

Very few people can answer these questions simply and accurately, so of course they spin around in circles, believing nearly anything they're told. How can you possibly gain a full and proper understanding of a subject when you don't understand the most basic words used to discuss its most important concepts?

That's why learning the precise meanings of key words is the first major hurdle you have to clear when you're trying to learn something new if you're going to have any hope of gaining a deep and practical understanding of it.

If you don't really understand many of the words you read or hear, how are you supposed to fully understand the ideas being communicated? You can't, of course. And instead, you'll reach your own distorted conclusions.

For example, if I were to tell you, "The children have to leave in the gloaming," you might wonder what I'm talking about because you don't understand the meaning of the word *gloaming*. The sentence doesn't give you any hints, as it could mean early, midday, late, or something else altogether.

In school, most of us were taught to guess at the meanings of words by looking at the surrounding context or by comparing them to other words in our vocabularies. The context in my example only reveals that gloaming might be a time of the day. You can then analyze the word itself, but that doesn't offer any clues, either. "Well, *gloaming* sounds like *glowing*," you might think, "and the sun glows, so I guess it could mean 'in the morning'?"

This is a highly unreliable way to learn and communicate. Without a precise, standard, and agreed-upon lexicon, we can never really know if we're understanding others correctly or are being understood correctly ourselves. It's like trying to play a game with others without first agreeing on the rules.

So, what is *gloaming*? It means the time of the day when the sun is just below the horizon, especially the period between sunset and dark. In other words, twilight. The sentence I shared earlier is now crystal clear, isn't it?

This is why the humble dictionary is an unsung hero of culture and civilization. It forms the intellectual bedrock upon which all ideas are formed and disseminated.

This is also why the first part of *Thinner Leaner Stronger* is going to be something you don't see in many books. We're going to review the exact dictionary definitions of a number of the most important words related to the main topics we'll be discussing throughout this book.

I know that reading the definitions of words is dry and unsexy, but it won't take long, it'll ensure we're on the same page on the fundamentals, and it may even set off some sparks in your brain. Chances are you're going to sort out at least a few long-standing misconceptions you've had and connect some dots in new and interesting ways.

And ironically, by perusing the meanings of these keywords, you'll know more about health, nutrition, and fitness than most women ever will. Seriously. If you don't believe me, go ask every trainer in your gym to define the word *calorie*.

What's more, this first, crucial step will go far in inoculating you against the constant and overwhelming barrage of false information hitting people's eyeballs and eardrums every day. Once you understand the ideas that form the underpinning of health, fitness, and wellness, you become a lot better at detecting and discarding BS.

So, let's get started with the first list of keywords, shall we?

5

WHAT MOST WOMEN WILL NEVER KNOW ABOUT GETTING FIT — PART 1

In this first keyword list, we're going to review basic physiological terms that you must understand to grasp the most important concepts in *Thinner Leaner Stronger* and achieve the best possible results.

(Physiology, by the way, is the scientific study of the normal functions of living organisms and their parts.)

Most women (and men for that matter) will never learn what these critical terms really mean, and their bodies will suffer for it. And therefore even their lives, in some cases. Don't underestimate the destructive power of misunderstanding the basics of something you're trying to learn and apply. It alone can be the difference between success and failure.

And in case you're wondering, every definition in this chapter (and the next one) comes directly from, or is a combination of definitions from, one of the following dictionaries:

- *New Oxford American Dictionary*, Third Edition (my personal favorite dictionary)
- *Webster's Third New International Dictionary*, Unabridged
- *Random House Unabridged Dictionary*

I highly recommend that you purchase one of these dictionaries, or all three (great for cross-checking definitions), and start using it to clarify the meanings of words you don't understand. Consider the money and time an invaluable life investment. I do.

All right, let's get started with the keywords.

. . .

ENERGY

1. Energy is the power received from electricity, fuel, food, and other sources to do work or produce motion.

2. Energy is the physical or mental strength of a person that can be directed toward some activity.

MATTER

1. Matter is a physical substance, as distinct from the mind and spirit.

2. In physics (the branch of science concerned with matter and energy), matter is that which occupies space and can be moved with force, especially as distinct from energy.

CHEMISTRY

Chemistry is the branch of science concerned with the substances of which matter is composed of, the investigation of their properties and reactions, and the use of such reactions to form new substances.

CHEMICAL

1. Chemical means having to do with chemistry, or the interactions of substances as studied in chemistry.

2. A chemical is any substance that can undergo a chemical process or change.

When people refer to chemicals, they're usually talking about manmade substances, but the definition isn't limited to just this meaning.

ORGANISM

An organism is a single living thing, such as a person, animal, or plant.

CELL

A cell is the basic unit of all living organisms.

Some living organisms exist only as a single cell, and according to the most recent research, your body is made of approximately 37.2 trillion cells."[1]

Cells produce energy, exchange information, multiply, and eventually die when their time has come.

TISSUE

Tissue is a group of cells in animals and plants that forms a definite kind of structural material with a specific function.

MUSCLE

Muscle is a tissue in the body, often attached to bones, that can tighten and relax to produce motion.

SKELETAL MUSCLE

Skeletal muscle is muscle tissue connected to the skeleton to form part of the system that moves the limbs and other parts of the body.

MUSCLE FIBER

A muscle fiber, also called a muscle cell or *myocyte*, is a collection of long, threadlike strands called *myofibrils* that contract, along with other structural elements that you find in other cells in the human body.

FAT

1. Fat is an oily or greasy substance found in animal bodies, especially when deposited as a layer under the skin or around certain organs.

2. Fat is a substance of this type derived from animals and plants that is solid or liquid in form, and often used in cooking.

ORGAN

An organ is a group of tissues that work together to perform a specific function in an organism, like the heart, skin, and lungs.

Skeletal muscle is not an organ because it contains just one type of tissue.

GRAM

A gram is a unit of weight in the metric system. One pound is about 454 grams.

KILOGRAM

A kilogram is a unit of weight in the metric system equal to 1,000 grams, or 2.2 pounds.

CELSIUS

Celsius is a scale of temperature on which water freezes at 0 degrees and boils at 100 degrees.

In the Fahrenheit scale used in the United States, water freezes at 32 degrees and boils at 212 degrees.

CALORIE

A calorie is the energy needed to raise the temperature of 1 kilogram of water by 1 degree Celsius.

This is also called a kilocalorie or large calorie, and is used to represent the energy value of food.

ELEMENT

An element (also called a chemical element) is a substance that can't be broken down into smaller parts by a chemical reaction.

There are more than 100 elements, and they are the primary building blocks of matter.

COMPOUND

A compound is a substance made up of two or more different elements.

MOLECULE

A molecule is the smallest particle of any compound that still exists as that substance.

If you were to break a molecule down any further, it would separate into the elements that make it up (meaning it would no longer exist as that original substance).

ACID

An acid is a chemical substance that can react with and sometimes dissolve other materials.

AMINO ACID

An amino acid is a naturally occurring compound found in proteins.

PROTEIN

A protein is a naturally occurring compound that's composed of one or more long chains of amino acids.

Proteins are an essential part of all organisms and are used to create body tissues such as muscle, hair, and skin, as well as various chemicals vital to life.

ESSENTIAL AMINO ACID

An essential amino acid is an amino acid needed by the body to maintain growth and health that must be obtained from food.

GAS

A gas is a substance that is in an air-like form (not solid or liquid).

CARBON

Carbon is a nonmetallic element found in all life and much of the matter on earth.

OXYGEN

Oxygen is a colorless, odorless gas that is necessary for most living things to survive.

HYDROGEN

Hydrogen is a colorless, odorless, flammable gas that is the simplest and most abundant element in the universe.

CARBOHYDRATE

A carbohydrate is a molecule composed of carbon, oxygen, and hydrogen that can be broken down in the body to release energy.

DIGESTION

Digestion is the process of breaking down food so it can be used by the body.

ENZYME

An enzyme is a substance produced by organisms that causes specific chemical reactions.

METABOLISM

Metabolism is the series of physical and chemical processes that occur in an organism in order to maintain life.

Metabolism involves the production of energy as well as the creation, maintenance, and destruction of cells and tissues.

ANABOLISM

Anabolism is a metabolic process in an organism by which energy is used to make more complex substances (such as tissue) from simpler ones (such as proteins).

This is also known as constructive metabolism.

CATABOLISM

Catabolism is the metabolic process by which more complex substances (such as proteins) are broken down into simpler ones (such as amino acids), together with the release of energy.

This is also known as destructive metabolism.

. . .

That's it for the first round of keywords! Great job!

Feel free to go over these words again to ensure everything is completely clear, because in the next chapter, we're going to build on the concepts you've just learned.

6

WHAT MOST WOMEN WILL NEVER KNOW
ABOUT GETTING FIT
— PART 2

In this second keyword list, we're going to build on the work we did in the last chapter and review basic terms that you need to know to successfully navigate the treacherous waters of diet, nutrition, and supplementation.

Just as before, these terms shipwreck more fitness-minded people than you would care to know. All it takes is a few core misconceptions to make entire categories of knowledge seemingly incomprehensible.

Is this stuff confusing? It can be. But it doesn't have to be. Let's dig in and master these words.

. . .

HEALTHY

1. If a body is healthy, it has good strength and high energy levels and is free from pain, illness, damage, and dysfunction.

2. If something is healthy, it's beneficial to one's physical, mental, or emotional state.

NUTRIENT

A nutrient is a substance an organism needs to live and grow.

FOOD

Food is material taken into the body to provide it with the nutrients it needs for energy and growth.

NOURISH

To nourish is to provide with the food or other substances needed for growth, health, and good condition.

NUTRITION

Nutrition is the process of getting nourishment, especially the process of getting food and nutrients and using them to grow bigger, build and replace tissues, and stay healthy.

MACRONUTRIENT

A macronutrient is any of the nutritional components of the diet required in relatively large amounts.

Specifically, these are protein, carbohydrate, fat, and minerals, such as calcium, zinc, iron, magnesium, and phosphorous.

VITAMIN

A vitamin is a substance that an organism needs for cells to function, grow, and develop correctly.

HORMONE

A hormone is a chemical that's transported by the blood or other bodily fluids to cells and organs, where it causes some action or has some specific effect.

MINERAL

A mineral is a carbonless substance that forms naturally in the earth.

Humans need various minerals, such as sodium, potassium, calcium, and zinc, for many different physiological functions, including building bones, making hormones, and regulating the heartbeat.

DIET

1. A diet is the food and drink that a person usually consumes.

2. A diet is a special course of controlled or restricted intake of food or drink for a particular purpose, such as weight loss, exercise support, or maintenance therapy (a treatment designed to help another primary treatment to succeed).

SUGAR

Sugar is a class of sweet-tasting carbohydrate that comes from various plants, fruits, grains, and other sources.

GLUCOSE

Glucose is a sugar that occurs widely in nature and is an important energy source in organisms.

Glucose is a component of many carbohydrates.

MILLIGRAM

A milligram is a unit of weight in the metric system equal to one-thousandth of a gram.

MILLILITER

A milliliter is a unit of capacity in the metric system equal to one-thousandth of a liter, which is equal to about 4.2 cups in the United States customary system.

BLOOD SUGAR

1. Blood sugar is glucose in your blood.

2. Blood sugar refers to the concentration of glucose in your blood, measured in milligrams of glucose per 100 milliliters of blood.

SUCROSE

Sucrose is a sugar that occurs naturally in most plants and is obtained commercially especially from sugarcane or sugar beets.

Sucrose is commonly known as table sugar.

FRUCTOSE

Fructose is a very sweet sugar found in many fruits and honey, as well as sucrose and high-fructose corn syrup, both of which are about 50 percent fructose and 50 percent glucose.

Fructose is converted into glucose by the liver and then released into the blood for use.

GALACTOSE

Galactose is a type of sugar found in dairy products that is metabolized similarly to fructose.

LACTOSE

Lactose is a type of sugar present in milk that contains glucose and galactose.

GLYCOGEN

Glycogen is a form of carbohydrate found primarily in the liver and muscle tissue.

Glycogen is stored energy and can be readily converted to glucose to satisfy the body's energy needs.

SIMPLE CARBOHYDRATE

A simple carbohydrate is a form of carbohydrate that breaks down quickly into glucose in the body.

Fructose, lactose, and sucrose are simple carbohydrates.

COMPLEX CARBOHYDRATE

A complex carbohydrate is a form of carbohydrate consisting of a chain of simple carbohydrates linked together. Because of this structure, a complex carbohydrate takes longer to break down into glucose in the body.

The sugars found in whole grains, beans, and vegetables are complex carbohydrates.

STARCH

Starch is a complex carbohydrate found naturally in many fruits and vegetables and added to certain foods to thicken them.

INSULIN

Insulin is a hormone made in the pancreas and released into the blood when you eat food.

Insulin causes muscles, organs, and fat tissue to absorb and use or store the nutrients from food.

INDEX

An index is a system of listing information in an order that allows one to compare it easily to other information.

GLYCEMIC INDEX

The glycemic index (GI) is a numeric system that ranks how quickly the body converts various foods into glucose. Foods are ranked on a scale of 0 to 100 depending on how they affect blood sugar levels once eaten.

A GI rating of 55 and under is considered low on the index, while a rating of 56 to 69 is medium, and a rating of 70 or above is high.

Simple carbohydrates are converted into glucose quickly and thus have high GI ratings. For example, sucrose's rating is 65, white bread's is 71, white rice's is 89, and white potato's is 82.

Complex carbohydrates are converted into glucose more slowly and thus have lower GI ratings. For example, apples' rating is 39, black beans' is 30, peanuts' is 7, and whole-grain pasta's is 42.

FIBER

Fiber is a mostly indigestible type of carbohydrate found in many types of foods, including fruits, vegetables, legumes, and grains.

FATTY ACID

A fatty acid is an acid found in the fats and oils of animals and plants.

ESSENTIAL FATTY ACID

An essential fatty acid is a fatty acid that's vital for proper bodily function and must be obtained from food.

SATURATED FAT

Saturated fat is a type of fat that's solid at room temperature and found in many animal and some plant sources, including meat, cream, cheese, butter, lard, coconut oil, cottonseed oil, and palm kernel oil.

UNSATURATED FAT

Unsaturated fat is a type of fat that's liquid at room temperature and found in many plant and some animal sources, including avocado, nuts, vegetable oils, and fish.

TRANS FATTY ACID

A trans fatty acid is a type of unsaturated fatty acid that's uncommon in nature and usually created artificially.

"Trans fats" are often found in highly processed foods like cereals, baked goods, fast food, ice cream, and frozen dinners. Anything that contains "partially hydrogenated oil" contains trans fatty acids.

CHOLESTEROL

Cholesterol is a soft, waxy substance found in most body tissues.

Cholesterol is an important part of the structure of cells and is used to create different hormones.

. . .

That's it for the keywords!

I hope you've found these definitions as helpful and enlightening as I did when I first learned them.

I remember how surprised I was to discover how many of these fundamental words and concepts I had wrong, and how simply clarifying these misunderstood ideas helped me begin to see health and fitness through a different, more rational and focused lens.

And speaking of surprises, there's a lot more to come, because in the next chapter we're going to learn the truth about ten of the absolute worst fat loss myths peddled by some of the biggest health and fitness authorities out there.

7

THE 10 ABSOLUTE WORST FAT LOSS MYTHS AND MISTAKES

"The road to nowhere is paved with excuses."
—MARK BELL

For thousands of years, a lean, toned, athletic body has been the gold standard of physical status and attractiveness. It was a hallmark of the ancient heroes, gods, and goddesses, and we still idolize it today.

With obesity rates over 35 percent here in America (and steadily rising), it would appear that achieving this type of physique and becoming one of the "physical elite" must require top-shelf genetics or a level of knowledge, discipline, and sacrifice far beyond what most people are capable of.

This isn't true. Your genetics can't stop you from getting superfit; the knowledge is easy enough to acquire—you're going to learn everything you need to know in this book—and it doesn't require nearly as much willpower as you might think. While you won't be able to eat large pizzas every day and get by on only a few workouts here and there, you *will* be able to build lean muscle and lose fat eating foods you love and doing workouts you enjoy.

That's what I want for you. That's why I wrote this book. Together I want us to upgrade not just your body, but your life.

Fat loss is a major component of this vision. If we're going to make it a reality, you're going to have to finally break free of fad diets, yo-yo dieting, and all the nutritional nonsense that keeps women overweight and frustrated. To master your body, you're going to need to know how to easily and consistently lose fat and keep it off.

To help you develop that ability, I want to start with debunking 10 of the worst fat loss myths and mistakes. Chances are you've heard or even bought into at least several of them, and if we don't address this first, you might be skeptical of or even reject the core tenets of the *Thinner Leaner Stronger* method of dieting.

So, let's dispel these harmful fallacies and errors once and for all so they can never again block your progress toward the body you want.

MYTH #1

"CALORIES IN VERSUS CALORIES OUT IS BAD SCIENCE"

"Calorie counting doesn't work," the overweight MD says in his latest bestselling book.

"It's a relic of our ignorant dietary past," the pretty woman who has been skinny her entire life tells Oprah.

"It's time we moved on and realized dieting is all about food quality, not calories," the former triathlete turned guru says on his blockbuster blog.

The sales pitch sounds sexy. Eat the right foods and you can "unclog and supercharge" your hormones and metabolism, and your body will take care of the rest. This is music to many people's ears who want to believe they can get lean and fit without ever having to restrict or even pay attention to *how much* they eat, only *what*.

This is malarkey. In fact, it's worse than that. It's a blatant lie because, as far as your body weight is concerned, how much you eat is *far* more important than what you eat.

Don't believe me?

Just ask Kansas State University Professor Mark Haub, who lost 27 pounds in 10 weeks eating Hostess cupcakes, Doritos, Oreos, and whey protein shakes.[1] Or a science teacher, John Cisna, who lost 56 pounds in six months eating nothing but McDonald's.[2] Or Kai Sedgwick, a fitness enthusiast who got into the best shape of his life following a rigorous workout routine and eating McDonald's every day for a month.[3]

I don't recommend you follow in their footsteps (the nutritional value of your diet does matter), but they prove an indisputable point: you *can* lose fat and gain muscle while eating copious amounts of junk food.

The key to understanding how this works—and to understanding what really drives weight loss and gain—is *energy balance*, which is the relationship between energy intake (calories eaten) and output (calories burned).

Various foods contain varying numbers of calories. For example, nuts are very energy dense, containing about 6.5 calories per gram, on average. Celery, on the other hand, contains very little stored energy, with just 0.15 calories per gram.

If you add up the calories of all the food you eat in a day and then compare that number to how many calories you burn in the same period, you'd notice one of three things:

1. You ate more calories than you burned. (Do this often enough and you'll gain weight.)

2. You ate fewer calories than you burned. (Do this often enough and you'll lose weight.)

3. You ate more or less the same number of calories as you burned. (Do this often enough and you'll maintain your weight.)

Your checking account is a good metaphor for how this process works.

If you "put" (eat) more calories into the account than you "spend" (burn), you create a *positive energy balance*, and your body will "save" (store) a portion of the surplus energy as body fat.

If you put fewer calories into the account than you spend, however, you create a *negative energy balance*, and your body will turn to its "energy savings" (body fat, mostly) to make up for the deficit and obtain the energy it needs to keep functioning.

Remember that our bodies require a constant supply of energy to stay alive, and if they didn't have these handy energy deposits to tap into (body fat), we would have to provide that energy through a carefully regulated feeding schedule. If we missed a meal, the energy would run out and we would die. The only reason we don't have to live like that is our bodies can break down body fat (and other tissues when necessary) and burn it for energy when food energy isn't available.

What do you think happens to your body fat stores, then, if you eat considerably fewer calories than you burn for weeks or months on end? That's right—they get whittled down to lower and lower levels, and you look leaner and leaner.

These aren't hypotheses or debunked theories, either. This is the first law of thermodynamics at work, which states that energy in a system can't be created or destroyed but can only change form. This applies to all physical energy systems, including the human metabolism. When we eat food, its stored energy is transformed by our muscles into mechanical energy (movement), by our digestive systems into chemical energy (body fat), and by our organs into thermal energy (heat).

This alone explains why every single controlled weight loss study conducted in the last 100 years has concluded that meaningful weight loss requires energy expenditure to exceed energy intake.[4]

This is also why bodybuilders dating back just as far, from the "father of modern bodybuilding" Eugen Sandow to the sword-and-sandal superstar Steve Reeves to the iconic Arnold Schwarzenegger, have been using this knowledge to systematically and routinely reduce and increase body fat levels as desired.

So, the bottom line is: A century of metabolic research has proven, beyond the shadow of a doubt, that energy balance is the basic mechanism that regulates weight gain and loss.[5]

All that evidence, however, doesn't mean you have to count calories to lose weight, but it does mean you have to understand how calorie intake and expenditure influences your body weight and then regulate your intake according to your goals.

MYTH #2

"CARBS AND SUGARS MAKE YOU FAT"

People love simple explanations and compelling conspiracies, and these two quirks explain the popularity of most mainstream diet trends.

The formula for a fad diet is simple:

1. "It's not your fault you're overweight and unhealthy."
"Jerks keep saying it's because you eat too much junk and food in general and move too little, but they're wrong. You're not lazy and undisciplined. You're a victim of bad science and worse food."

2. "New research shows you what to blame."
"And we've strung it up like a pinata for you to bludgeon into ribbons. Strike it down with all your hatred and your journey to the dark … er, light … side will be complete."

3. "Avoid this thing at all costs and you'll live happily ever after."
"Celibacy is the only way to escape this bogeyman's wrath. Renounce it and take charge of your destiny."

These emotion-based tactics are how marketers sold us on low-fat dieting a decade ago and how they sell us on low-carb and low-sugar dieting today. Cut the heinous carbohydrate and sugar molecules out of your life, they say, and the pounds will just melt away.

It all sounds so neat and tidy until someone like me comes along and points out the glitches in the matrix, like the professor and science teacher I introduced you to earlier in this chapter, or the well-designed and well-executed studies that have found no difference in weight loss whatsoever between low- and high-carb and low- and high-sugar diets.

For instance:

- Scientists at Arizona State University found no difference in weight or fat loss between people consuming 5 and 40 percent of their calories from carbohydrate for 10 weeks.[5]

- Scientists at the Medical College of Wisconsin found no difference in weight or fat loss between people consuming 4 and 30 percent of their calories from carbohydrate for six weeks.[6]

- Scientists at the Harvard School of Public Health found no difference in weight loss between people consuming 65, 45, and 35 percent of their calories from carbohydrate for two years.[7]

- Scientists at Stanford School of Medicine found no difference in weight or fat loss between people who consumed 50 and 25 percent of their calories from carbohydrate for one year.[8]

- Scientists at Duke University found no difference in weight or fat loss between people consuming 4 and 43 percent of their calories from sugar for six weeks.[9]

- Scientists at Queen Margaret University College found no difference in weight loss between people consuming 5 and 10 percent of their calories from sugar for eight weeks.[10]

Later in this book, we'll talk more about why carbs and sugars aren't nearly as dangerous or fattening as you've been told, but for now, know this:

If you consistently consume fewer calories than you burn, you'll lose weight, regardless of how much carbohydrate or sugar you eat.

There's a corollary here, too:

No individual food can make you fatter. Only overeating can.

If you consistently consume more calories than you burn, you'll gain weight, even if those calories come from the "healthiest" food on earth.

Look around for easy proof of this one. How many people do you know who are overweight despite their obsession with "clean eating"? Well, now you know why.

MYTH #3

"SOME PEOPLE JUST 'MYSTERIOUSLY' CAN'T LOSE WEIGHT"

The number one reason most people "inexplicably" can't lose weight is they're eating too much.

Seriously. That's the climax. The big reveal. The way out of the haunted house. The rub, however, is they often don't realize it.

For starters, studies show that most people are really bad at estimating the actual number of calories they eat.[11] They underestimate portion sizes, assume foods contain fewer calories than they do, measure intake inaccurately, and, in some cases, simply lie to themselves about how much they're actually eating.

A particularly egregious example can be found in a study conducted by scientists at Columbia University.[12] They found that obese people who claimed to have been eating 800 to 1,200 calories per day for years were underestimating their true daily calorie intake by a whopping 2,000 calories, on average.

That's right, on average, these people were eating about 3,000 calories per day while claiming to have been eating just 800 to 1,200 calories per day.

This inability to estimate calorie intake accurately is why so many people fail with diets that deal in rules and restrictions instead of hard numbers. You can lose weight without counting calories but it's a bit of a crapshoot, and it becomes less and less viable as you get leaner and leaner.

There are plenty of ways to screw up calorie counting too.

If you eat a lot of prepackaged and prepared foods, it's fairly easy to accidentally overeat because the calorie counts we're given for various restaurant and packaged foods are often inaccurate.[13] In fact, food manufacturers can underreport calories by 20 percent and pass FDA inspection, and you'd better believe many are unscrupulous enough to use this to their advantage.[14] Maybe those "low-calorie" cookies aren't so low-calorie after all?

People who know this and stick to foods they cook and prepare themselves are often no better in the end because they don't measure their foods properly. Here's an all-too-common scenario:

It's mealtime and you break out the oatmeal, peanut butter, blueberries, and yogurt, and the measuring cups and spoons. You measure out one cup of oatmeal, one tablespoon of peanut butter, and half a cup each of blueberries and yogurt. You cook it all up, scarf it all down, and move on with your day. Unfortunately, you've just eaten a couple hundred more calories than you thought.

How did this happen?

Well, that (slightly heaping) cup of oatmeal that you scooped out contained 100 grams of dry oats and 379 calories. The "cup" on the label, however, contains only 307 calories because it assumes 81 grams of dry oats. That's 72 more calories than you thought. And your tablespoon of peanut butter? You packed in 21 grams for a count of 123 calories, but your app's tablespoon assumes just 16 grams and 94 calories. There's another 29 "hidden" calories.

Make these types of errors meal after meal, food after food, day after day, and this alone can be the reason you "mysteriously" can't lose weight.

MYTH #4

"YOU CAN EAT AND DRINK WHATEVER YOU WANT IN YOUR 'CHEAT MEALS'"

"Cheat" meals are a staple of many weight loss diets, and they usually entail eating more or less whatever your hungry little heart desires.

There's merit in this idea, and as you'll learn later in this book, *Thinner Leaner Stronger* also allows for "cheat" or "normal" meals, mostly as a way to relieve psychological stress and cravings.

There are, however, right and wrong ways to "cheat" on your diet, and many people who struggle to lose weight do it very wrong.

For instance, they often cheat too frequently. To understand why this is a problem, we only have to look back to the big picture of calories and weight loss. If you moderately overeat just a few days per month, your overall results aren't going to be much affected. If you do it a few times per week, however, you're going to slow down your weight loss considerably.

Another common mistake is indulging in no-holds-barred cheat *days*. If you let loose for just one meal, you can only do so much damage. Your stomach is probably going to be begging for mercy by the 2,000-calorie mark. Eat everything in sight for an entire day, however, and you can easily put down many thousands of calories and erase your weight loss progress for the last several days, if not the entire week.

Yet another way to screw up individual cheat meals is eating too many calories and dietary fat in particular. I know I just said you can only do so much damage in one meal, but if you're of the hearty eating type, it can be enough to noticeably impact your weight loss.

The worst type of cheat meal is one that is very high in both calories and dietary fat, which is chemically similar to body fat and thus requires very little energy for conversion into body fat (between 0 and 2 percent of the energy it contains).[15]

Protein and carbohydrate, on the other hand, are chemically dissimilar to body fat, cost quite a bit more energy to process (25 and 7 percent of the energy they contain, respectively), and are rarely converted to body fat under normal conditions.[16]

This is why research shows that high-fat meals cause more immediate fat gain than high-protein or high-carbohydrate meals.[17]

This information is particularly relevant when you're lean and wanting to get even leaner. You simply can't afford to be in a large calorie surplus very often, especially not when the surplus is primarily from dietary fat.

Drinking alcohol while cheating is also generally a bad idea. While alcohol itself basically can't be stored as body fat, it blunts fat burning, which accelerates the rate at which your body stores dietary fat as body fat, and it increases the conversion of carbohydrate into body fat.[18]

In short, it's not the calories from alcohol that can make you fatter, but all the delicious food most people eat with it, which is hard to resist when you're hammered.

MYTH #5

"YOU CAN BURN THE FAT COVERING YOUR [BODY PART]"

Pick up just about any fitness magazine and you'll find workouts for getting ab definition, slimming the thighs, eliminating back and arm fat, and the like.

If only it were that simple.

While research shows that training a specific muscle increases blood flow and lipolysis (the breakdown of fat cells into usable energy) in the area, the effects are far too small to matter.[19] Training your muscles burns calories and can result in muscle growth, both of which certainly can aid in fat loss, but it doesn't directly burn the fat covering them to any significant degree.[20]

Instead, fat loss occurs in a whole-body fashion. You create the proper environment (a calorie deficit) through diet and exercise, and your body reduces fat stores all over, with certain areas leaning out faster than others (more on why this occurs later).

This is why studies show you can do all the crunches you want, but you'll never have defined abs until you've adequately reduced your body fat levels.[21]

MYTH #6

"DIETING CAN 'DAMAGE' YOUR METABOLISM"

According to most theories, "metabolic damage" refers to a condition where various physiological systems have been disrupted, and as a result, your metabolism burns less energy than it should.

In other words, it's a hypothetical state wherein you burn fewer calories than you should based on your body weight and activity levels. Furthermore, the story goes, once you've "damaged" your metabolism, it can remain hamstrung for weeks, months, and even years.

It's called "metabolic damage" because the idea is your metabolism is literally "broken" to one degree or another and requires "fixing."

The common causes of metabolic damage are believed to be remaining in a calorie deficit for too long, starvation dieting, and doing too much cardio. Therefore, when you're restricting your calories and stop losing weight for no apparent reason, or when you're struggling to stop gaining weight after a period of dieting, some people will say that you probably have metabolic damage that needs repairing.

The evidence to support this hypothesis is almost always stories. Stories of people failing to lose weight on a measly few hundred calories per day, and even worse, stories of people gaining weight on very low-calorie diets and intense exercise routines.

And so people everywhere have become convinced that dieting has screwed up their bodies—maybe even irreversibly—and that their only hope for returning to normalcy is special dietary measures.

What does science have to say on the matter?

Well, several studies have shown that the metabolic decline associated with dieting, including long periods of very low-calorie dieting, ranges from less than 5 to about 15 percent.[22]

Furthermore, it took about a 10 percent reduction in body weight to produce the larger, double-digit drops, and most of the research on the matter was conducted with people who made the cardinal diet mistakes of eating too few calories and too little protein and doing no resistance training.

We also know that while these metabolic adaptations can persist long after weight loss has stopped, they can also be easily reversed by raising your calories, lifting weights, and eating a high-protein diet.[23]

And that's true even for people who have already gone to extreme measures to drop pounds in the past. No matter what they've done, it can only produce a relatively small metabolic dip that can be easily reversed with proper diet and training.

Even more encouraging is research on what happens to your metabolism over time when you do things correctly, which we'll discuss later in this book.

MYTH #7

"DIETING CAN SEND YOUR BODY INTO 'STARVATION MODE'"

The idea behind "starvation mode" is similar to metabolic damage.

It goes like this: if you're too aggressive with your calorie restriction, then your metabolism will slow to a crawl, making it more or less impossible to continue losing weight without eating like a runway model.

The way most people describe it, starvation mode and metabolic damage work together to stymie your progress in a process that looks like this:

1. You eat too little and lose weight too fast.

2. You plunge your body into starvation mode, and weight loss stops.

3. You eat even less and move even more, which further aggravates the problem and causes metabolic damage.

4. The longer you remain in starvation mode, the less and less weight you'll lose regardless of what you do, and the more and more damaged your metabolism will become.

One of the only ways to avoid this metabolic carnage, we're told, is losing weight slowly through very mild calorie restriction. If we get greedy, they say, we'll pay for it later.

There's a shade of truth here, but like many of the things that "everybody knows" in the fitness space, it's more wrong than right.

Your body responds to calorie restriction with countermeasures meant to stall weight loss, but there's no "mode" it enters or physiological switch that flips to magically block weight loss.

A striking example of this is one of the most extreme studies on the human metabolism ever conducted: the Minnesota Starvation Experiment.[24]

This experiment started in 1944 as the end of World War II was approaching to discover the healthiest way to help the millions of starving people in Europe return to a normal body weight.

As you can guess, this study involved intentionally starving people. And by "starving," I truly mean *starving*. Scientists took 36 volunteers who had the choice of shipping off to the front lines or offering their metabolisms to science, and subjected them to the conditions of your average POW camp. These volunteers had to do several hours of manual labor every day and march 22 miles per week on a diet that provided about 50 percent of their average daily energy expenditure (or about 1,500 calories per day). For six freaking months.

As you can imagine, things got pretty grim. By the end of the study, the men were rawboned, some had almost starved to death, and one even cut off several of his fingers to wash out.

What about their metabolisms, though? Were they as devastated as proponents of starvation mode and metabolic damage would predict?

Nope.

After losing about 25 percent of their body weight on average, their metabolisms were about 20 percent lower than scientists predicted based on their new, lower body weights. In other words, their metabolisms were "underperforming" by just 20 percent on average after enduring six months of the most extreme weight loss regimen you could ever devise.

Then, in the next phase of the study, the same people were put on a "recovery diet" to allow them to regain most of the weight they lost.

After 12 weeks of this recovery diet, their metabolisms were assessed again. This time, average metabolic performance was only about 10 percent lower than it should have been, and for some individuals, everything was already back to normal, as if their severe weight loss had never happened.

Moreover, according to a recent study conducted by my friend and researcher Menno Henselmans, when you analyze the data beyond the first 12 weeks of recovery, you find that everything eventually returned to normal in every volunteer.[25] Some just took longer to recover than others.

This groundbreaking experiment also provided another nail to drive into the coffin of the starvation mode myth: every volunteer continued to lose weight until the very end. The rate of weight loss slowed, of course, but it never came to a complete standstill.

It's safe to assume, then, that if people can eat about 1,500 calories per day and do many hours of moderately intense exercise every week and still lose weight steadily—for six months—then we have nothing to worry about with our comparatively ho-hum diet and exercise routines.

MYTH #8

"EATING MORE SMALLER MEALS IS BETTER FOR WEIGHT LOSS THAN FEWER LARGER ONES"

Raise your hand if you've heard this one before: you should eat many small meals when trying to lose weight to "stoke the metabolic fire," accelerate fat loss, and better control your appetite.

The theory here is simple: When you eat, your metabolism speeds up as your body processes the food. Thus, if you eat every few hours, your metabolism will remain in a constantly elevated state, right? And nibbling on food throughout the day should help with appetite control, right?

While this may seem plausible, it doesn't pan out in scientific research.

In an extensive review of diet literature, scientists at the French National Institute of Health and Medical Research looked at scores of studies comparing the metabolic effects of a wide variety of eating patterns, ranging from 1 to 17 meals per day.[26]

They found no meaningful difference between nibbling and gorging, because small meals caused small, short metabolic increases, while large meals caused larger, longer increases. Therefore, when viewed in terms of 24-hour energy expenditure, eating pattern had no significant effect.

Further evidence of this conclusion can be found in a study conducted by scientists at the University of Ottawa, which split subjects into two dietary groups:[27]

1. Group one ate three meals per day.
2. Group two ate three meals plus three snacks per day.

Both groups maintained the same calorie deficit, and after eight weeks, scientists found no significant difference in weight, fat, or muscle loss.

And what about the appetitive effects of meal frequency? This can go both ways.

For example, a study conducted by scientists at the University of Missouri found that after 12 weeks of dieting to lose weight, increasing protein intake improved appetite control, but meal frequency (three versus six meals per day) had no effect.[28]

Scientists at the University of Kansas conducted a similar experiment, investigating the effects of meal frequency and protein intake on perceived appetite, satiety (fullness), and hormones.[29]

They also found that higher protein intake led to greater feelings of fullness, but surprisingly, six meals resulted in generally lower levels of satiety than three.

On the other hand, you can find studies wherein subjects were less satiated on three meals per day than more, and where increasing meal frequency also increased general feelings of fullness and made it easier for people to stick to their diets.[30]

In some ways, the best dietary protocol is the one you can stick to, and that's very true in the case of meal frequency. Most people I work with enjoy eating four to six meals per day (I'm the same way), but some enjoy eating just two or three meals per day, and that's totally fine.

MYTH #9

"YOU HAVE TO EXERCISE TO LOSE WEIGHT"

If you're willing to eat very little food every day, you can create a large calorie deficit without doing any exercise.

You can lose plenty of weight this way, but you'll probably also lose at least a fair amount of muscle, which is undesirable for a number of reasons, not the least of which being vanity.[31]

This is one of the main reasons you should exercise when you're dieting to lose weight and you shouldn't do just any exercise, either. The best kind of exercise to do while in a calorie deficit is resistance training, which is a form of exercise that improves muscular strength and endurance.

A good example of the effectiveness of resistance training while dieting is found in a study conducted by scientists at West Virginia University, which split 20 men and women into two groups:[32]

1. Group one did one hour of cardio four times per week.

2. Group two lifted weights three times per week.

Both groups followed the same diet, and after 12 weeks, everyone lost about the same amount of fat, but the cardio group also lost nine pounds of lean body mass, whereas the weightlifting group didn't lose any.

A number of other studies have echoed that finding: if you want to lose fat quickly and not muscle, then you want to include resistance training in your weight loss regimen.[33]

MYTH #10

"CARDIO IS BETTER FOR FAT LOSS THAN WEIGHTLIFTING"

This one is a natural follow-up to the previous myth.

When most people start exercising to lose weight, they choose some form of cardio, like jogging, swimming, or biking.

This is all well and good, but unfortunately, simply doing cardio guarantees little in the way of weight loss.[34] In fact, studies show many people wind up even heavier than when they began their cardiovascular exercise routines.[35]

Hence the crowds of overweight people addicted to burning calories instead of getting fit.

There are two primary reasons why cardio alone doesn't always produce significant weight loss:

1. It's too easy to eat the calories you burn.

Guess how much energy 30 minutes of vigorous running burns? For someone who weighs 150 pounds, about 400 calories. And guess how easy it is to eat that right back? A handful of nuts, a bit of yogurt, and an apple does the trick. Or if you're the more indulgent type, a measly chocolate chip cookie with a cup of milk.

2. My point isn't that you shouldn't eat nuts, yogurt, apples, or cookies when you want to lose weight, of course, but that cardiovascular exercise just doesn't burn as much energy as we wish it did.

The energy you do burn during cardio does support your weight loss efforts, of course, but your goal isn't to just burn calories, it's to reduce body fat levels. And if you're eating too much, no amount of cardio is going to get you there.

Your body adapts to the exercise to reduce calorie expenditure.

Research shows that when in a calorie deficit, the body strives to increase energy efficiency.[36] This means that, as time goes on, less and less energy is needed to continue doing the same types of workouts. This also means that you're no longer burning as much energy as you think you are when performing the same exercise under the same conditions, which increases the likelihood of overeating and stalling out in your weight loss efforts.

Many people who experience this try to beat it with more cardio, which may raise energy expenditure enough to get the needle moving again but can also accelerate muscle loss and metabolic slowdown.

And what about weightlifting?

Well, research clearly shows that it's an effective way to lose fat, so why is it generally associated with "bulking up" and not "slimming down"?[37]

The answer is simple. Weightlifting isn't a popular way to lose weight because it's a bad way to lose weight, but it is a fantastic way to speed up fat loss and preserve muscle.

A study conducted by scientists at Duke University illustrates this point perfectly.[38] Researchers recruited 196 obese or overweight men and women ranging from 18 to 70 years old and split them into three groups:

1. Group one did three one-hour resistance training workouts per week.

2. Group two jogged three days per week at a moderate intensity for about 45 minutes per session.

3. Group three did both the resistance training and cardio workouts.

After eight months, guess which group lost the most weight?

No, it wasn't groups one or three. It was number two, the cardio-only group. BUT! That was also the only group that lost muscle as well. And guess who lost the most fat while also gaining muscle? That's right, group number three—the resistance training and cardio group.

In other words, adding resistance training to the cardio workouts resulted in less *weight* loss due to muscle gain but more *fat* loss due to various physiological factors that we'll talk more about later in this book.

. . .

I'm genuinely excited for you right now, because in reading this one chapter, you've taken your fitness knowledge to a whole new level—a level very few people, including many doctors, athletes, and even scientists, rarely achieve. And we're just getting warmed up!

In the next chapter, we're going to analyze muscle building in the same way as we just examined fat loss.

That means it's time to discuss the 10 absolute worst muscle-building myths and mistakes that keep women from ever getting that lean, athletic body that looks as good as it performs.

KEY TAKEAWAYS

- Energy balance is the relationship between energy intake (calories eaten) and output (calories burned).

- Energy balance is the basic mechanism that regulates weight gain and loss.

- If you consistently consume fewer calories than you burn, you'll lose weight, regardless of how much carbohydrate or sugar you eat.

- If you consistently consume more calories than you burn, you'll gain weight, even if those calories come from the "healthiest" food on earth.

- No individual food can make you fatter. Only overeating can.

- The number one reason most people "inexplicably" can't lose weight is they're eating too much.

- The inability to estimate calorie intake accurately is why so many people fail with diets that deal in rules and restrictions instead of hard numbers.

- There are right and wrong ways to "cheat" on your diet, and many people who struggle to lose weight do it very wrong.

- The worst type of cheat meal is one that is very high in both calories and dietary fat, which is chemically similar to body fat and thus requires very little energy for conversion into body fat (between 0 and 2 percent of the energy it contains).

- Research shows that high-fat meals cause more immediate fat gain than high-protein or high-carbohydrate meals.

- While alcohol itself basically can't be stored as body fat, it blunts fat burning, which accelerates the rate at which your body stores dietary fat as body fat, and it increases the conversion of carbohydrate into body fat.

- Training your muscles burns calories and can result in muscle growth, both of which certainly can aid in fat loss, but it doesn't directly burn the fat covering them to any significant degree.

- The metabolic decline associated with dieting, including long periods of very low-calorie dieting, ranges from less than 5 to about 15 percent

- Metabolic adaptations can persist long after weight loss has stopped, but they can also be easily reversed by raising your calories, lifting weights, and eating a high-protein diet.

- Your body responds to calorie restriction with countermeasures meant to stall weight loss, but there's no "mode" it enters or physiological switch that flips to magically block weight loss.

• Meal frequency has no significant effects on total daily energy expenditure or weight loss.

• If you want to lose fat quickly and not muscle, then you want to include resistance training in your weight loss regimen.

8

THE 10 ABSOLUTE WORST MUSCLE BUILDING MYTHS AND MISTAKES

"If you don't risk anything, you risk even more."
—ERICA JONG

Nine out of ten people you see in the gym don't train correctly.

I could write an entire chapter cataloguing their mistakes, but here are some of the more common ones:

- They spend too much time on the wrong exercises.
- They undertrain and overtrain various muscle groups.
- They use poor form, especially on the more technical exercises.
- They use too light or too heavy weights.
- They rest too little or too much in between sets.

In fact, what most people do in the gym doesn't even qualify as training but is merely *exercise*.

What's the difference?

Well, exercise is physical activity done for its own sake—to burn calories or improve energy levels or mood—whereas training is a systematic method of exercising done to achieve a specific, longer-term goal, like increased strength, muscle definition, or athleticism.

There's nothing inherently wrong with exercise (it beats sitting on your keister), but only training can give you the type of lean, toned physique that most women really want.

Exercise can make you healthier, but it guarantees nothing in the way of fat loss or muscle gain, the two biggest physiological levers you need to know how to work to build the body of your dreams.

Unfortunately, most gymgoers don't understand this, and that's why days, weeks, months, and even years can go by with them doing the same old exercises, lifting the same old weights, and looking at the same old bodies.

In the last chapter, you learned why so many women struggle to lose fat, and in this chapter, you're going to learn why building lean muscle is far more difficult for most women than it should be.

Let's get to it, starting with myth number one.

MYTH #1

"YOU CAN 'TONE,' 'SHAPE,' AND 'SCULPT' YOUR MUSCLES"

Tone those arms!

Shape that butt!

Sculpt those abs!

It sounds so nice and feminine. Nothing like the brutish gym talk about "gaining size" or "adding mass."

Phrases like these make for snazzy marketing, but they're often used to sell nonsense.

You can't "lengthen" and "tighten" your muscles, fundamentally change how they're shaped, or selectively strip fat away so they look more defined.

You can, however, add muscle to your frame and remove body fat. Nothing more or less. If you do that right, you get the right amount of muscle definition, curves, and lines in all the right places.

The claims that certain forms of exercise produce "long, lean" muscles, like a dancer's body, while others produce "bulky, ugly" muscles, like a bodybuilder's, are bogus.

Whether you do Pilates, yoga, or heavy weightlifting to strengthen and build your muscles, their shape will come out the same. The only difference is the rate at which they will grow.

What this means is that while you can absolutely have a great butt, shapely legs, and sexy arms, you can't necessarily have the same butt, legs, or arms as your favorite model or celebrity because their muscles are structurally different from yours. Who knows though, maybe you'll like yours even more!

The exercise advice generally given for "toning," "sculpting," and "shaping" is also hogwash.

The key, so many women are told, is a lot of high-repetition, low-weight resistance training. This is about as wrong as can be because you should do the exact opposite if you want a toned, defined body as quickly as possible—a lot of lower-repetition, higher-weight resistance training.

"But wait," you might be thinking, "won't that make me 'bulky'?"

Yeah, about that …

MYTH #2

"HEAVY WEIGHTLIFTING MAKES WOMEN 'BULKY'"

If there's one mainstream misconception that causes more harm to women's physiques than any other, it's this one.

At first glance, it sounds plausible. Heavy weights are for the boys who want bulging biceps, right? Why would women, who want sexy, defined, feminine muscles, train in the same way?

Apparent proof of this myth can be found at any local CrossFit gym, where you'll see at least a few women with figures that would make an NFL linebacker jealous.

Here's what you don't see, however: it's very hard for women to build a big, bulky body. It doesn't happen by accident or overnight. It takes elite muscle-building genetics and years of concerted effort in the gym and kitchen. Anabolic steroids are often involved as well, and especially in the case of professional athletes.

That said, there are still enough women in gyms everywhere who hit the weights regularly and look "bulky" enough to give you pause. And that's why you need to know what really gives women that look: too much body fat.

Harsh, I know, but let me explain.

Take an athletic woman with an enviable body. You know, toned legs, curvy butt, tight arms, and flat stomach. Now add 15 pounds of fat to her frame, and you might be surprised how "blocky" she looks.

This is because fat accumulates inside and on top of muscle, and the more fat and muscle you have, the larger and more amorphous your body looks. Your legs turn into logs. Your butt gets too big for your britches. Your arms fill up like sausages.

Reduce your body fat levels, however, and everything changes. The muscle you've built is able to shine. Instead of looking large and fluffy, you look lean and toned. Your butt becomes round and perky. Your legs have sleek curves. Your arms look cut.

Thus, a rule of thumb for women who want to be lean, toned, and defined: the more muscle you have, the less body fat you must have to avoid looking bulky.

For example, a woman with little muscle might feel scrawny at 18 percent body fat—the percentage of body weight that is fat—and comfortable at 25 percent, whereas a woman with a significant amount of muscle will probably love how she looks at 18 percent but feel a bit roly-poly at 25 percent.

This is why most women I've worked with are happiest when they've gained 10 to 15 pounds of muscle and dropped their body fat percentage to about 20 percent.

If you're not sure what that looks like, think Evangeline Lilly in *Ant-Man and the Wasp*.

Want to see what different body fat percentages look like?
Go to www.thinnerleanerstronger.com/bodyfat.

My observation about most fitness-minded women's preferred look has been borne out in scientific research as well.

In a study conducted by female scientists at the University of Missouri-Kansas City, pictures were gathered of scantily clad "fitspiration" women from Pinterest, Instagram, and Tumblr with varying degrees of muscularity and thinness.[1]

Then, the researchers digitally modified the pictures to make the women look even thinner but less toned and defined.

Next, they showed both the original and modified pictures to a group of 30 female undergraduate students and asked them to rate the women in terms of muscularity, thinness, and attractiveness.

65 percent of the women surveyed thought the fitter (unmodified) women looked more attractive than the thinner but less athletic (modified) women.

In the same study, the scientists did an analysis of the last 15 winners of the Miss USA beauty pageant. They found that the winners in 2013 were about 10 percent more muscular and 20 percent leaner than the winners in 1999.

In the final analysis, the researchers concluded that "although they [women] continue to find a thin female figure to be attractive, they prefer the appearance of a thin and toned female body."

All that isn't to say that you can't be attractive if you aren't sporting an extra 10 to 15 pounds of muscle, of course, but it does indicate that most women nowadays think this will make you look better, not worse.

MYTH #3

"HEAVY WEIGHTLIFTING IS DANGEROUS"

Many people think weightlifting, especially heavy weightlifting, is inherently dangerous, and I understand why.

When you compare deadlifting, squatting, and bench pressing large amounts of weight to other forms of exercise, like jogging, cycling, or calisthenics, weightlifting looks more like a death wish than a discipline.

Poke around on internet forums and you'll find plenty to feed your anxiety. Personal stories range from the tame—mild joint and muscle aches and the like—to the downright horrific, with some long-time bodybuilders so incapacitated that they can't even tie their shoes until the ibuprofen kicks in.

And so weightlifting, and strength training in particular, has been saddled with a bum rap for decades now. Thankfully, the tides are turning and strength training is gaining more and more mainstream popularity, but many people still think that its dangers far exceed the benefits.

While weightlifting does have its risks, they're not nearly as bad as many people think. Ironically, research shows that when done properly, it's actually one of the safest kinds of athletic activities you can do.

For instance, in one review of 20 studies conducted by scientists at Bond University, it was found that bodybuilding produced an average of just one injury for every 1,000 hours of training.[2]

To put that in perspective, if you spend five hours per week weightlifting, you could go almost four years without experiencing any kind of injury whatsoever.

Researchers also noted that most of the injuries tended to be minor aches and pains that didn't require any type of special treatment or recovery protocols. In most cases, a bit of extra R & R won the day.

As you'd expect, more intense and technical types of weightlifting, like CrossFit, Olympic weightlifting, and powerlifting, result in more injuries, but fewer than you might think. These activities produced just two to four injuries per 1,000 hours of training.

For comparison, studies show that sports like ice hockey, football, soccer, and rugby have injury rates ranging from 6 to 260 per 1,000 hours, and long-distance runners can expect about 10 injuries per 1,000 hours of pavement pounding.[3]

In other words, you're about 6 to 10 times more likely to get hurt playing everyday sports than hitting the gym for some heavy weightlifting.

The payoff for weightlifting is also tremendous. It delivers a number of health and fitness benefits that you simply can't get from other types of sports and exercise.

Here's a short list of what a well-designed weightlifting routine can do for you:

- Stronger, healthier joints[4]
- More muscle mass[5]
- Better heart health[6]
- Improved brain health[7]
- Greater longevity and quality of life[8]
- More bone density[9]
- Lower risk of fracture[10]
- Faster metabolism[11]
- Improved flexibility[12]

When you compare all that to the rather negligible risk of injury, and the generally mild nature of the injuries that do occur, the choice is clear: choosing to lift weights is far better than choosing not to out of fear of getting hurt.

If you're adamant about experiencing no physical injuries whatsoever, then your only surefire option is to never leave your bed (and even then you'll have to contend with bedsores!). Remember that every time you step into your car, take the stairs instead of the elevator, or, heck, type on a computer, you're flirting with one kind of injury or another.

Dealing with risk is just part of life. All we can do is weigh the probabilities and potential upsides and downsides, make choices that are most likely to play out in our favor over time, and do everything we can to create positive outcomes.

MYTH #4

"WOMEN CAN'T GAIN MUCH MUSCLE"

You may have heard that women don't have the physiology to gain muscle effectively, and that they should stick to Zumba and stretching instead.

A reason commonly cited for this is the well-known (and immediately obvious) fact that women produce a lot less testosterone than men—about 15 to 20 times less, to be exact.[13]

Testosterone is the primary hormonal driver of muscle growth, so it's fair to assume that a body with very little testosterone flowing through its veins won't be able to build much muscle, right?

Wrong.

While women's low testosterone does put them at a hormonal disadvantage for gaining muscle, testosterone isn't the only hormone heavily involved in muscle building.

Another major player is estrogen, which women produce much more of than men, and which provides several muscle-building benefits, including stimulating growth hormone production, which significantly aids in postworkout recovery, and preventing muscle breakdown.[14]

Women also produce more growth hormone throughout the day than men, which further helps with muscle gain.[15]

This is why research shows that women can gain muscle more or less as effectively as men, and why many elite female athletes have about 85 percent as much muscle as their male counterparts.[16]

Why, then, do you rarely see women who are anywhere near as jacked as many guys?

Because women start out with about half as much total muscle as men and can't gain as much whole-body muscle, thanks mainly to differences in hormones and anatomy.

In other words, it isn't so much that we men have far superior muscle-building machinery as it is we have a huge head start.

MYTH #5

"IF YOU DO THE SAME EXERCISES TOO OFTEN, YOU'LL GET STUCK IN A RUT"

How many times have you heard that you need to constantly change your workout routine to continue making progress?

That you have to "confuse" and "shock" your muscles into growth by regularly subjecting them to new exercises and workouts?

This sounds sensible. If we want to improve something, whether a skill or a muscle, we have to continually push the envelope and challenge ourselves in new ways, right? And what better way to challenge our muscles than subject them to new types of physical demands again and again?

While it's true that doing the *exact same* workouts every week will eventually result in stagnation, the "muscle confusion" theory misses the forest for the trees.

Your muscles have no cognitive abilities. They're not trying to guess what workout you're going to do today and can't be "confused" by fancy workout programming. Muscle tissue is purely mechanical. It can contract and relax. Nothing more.

That said, there's validity to the basic premise that for your muscles to keep growing in both size and strength, they must be continually challenged. Where muscle confusion goes astray, however, is with the *type* of challenge it emphasizes.

You can change up your workout routine every week—heck, every day—and hit a plateau because "change" doesn't stimulate muscle growth.

Progressive overload does, and more so than any other single training factor.[17]

Progressive overload refers to increasing the amount of tension your muscles produce over time, and the most effective way to do this is by progressively increasing the amount of weight that you're lifting.

In other words, the key to gaining muscle and strength isn't merely changing the types of stimuli your muscles are exposed to—it's *making your muscles work harder*. And this is exactly what you do when you force your muscles to handle heavier and heavier weights.

This is why your number one goal as a weightlifter should be to increase your whole-body strength over time, and why that is one of the primary goals of my *Thinner Leaner Stronger* program.

MYTH #6

"YOU MUST USE BANDS, MACHINES, AND OTHER CONTRAPTIONS"

You've just learned a major part of my plan for you: I want to make you as strong as possible.

To do that, I'm going to have you train very differently from most of the women—and men, for that matter—in the gym.

Instead of telling you to work with big rubber bands, superset every machine in the gym, or play around with the Bosu ball or other toys, I'm going to have you focus on just a few basic things:

1. Pushing
2. Pulling
3. Squatting

Not only that, but I'm going to have you spend most of your time in the gym with a barbell or pair of dumbbells in your hands, because free weights give you the most muscle-building bang for your buck.

Some people would disagree with that statement, pointing to studies that have shown that machines and free weights are equally effective for gaining muscle and strength.

You can't take such research at face value. You have to look deeper to get the whole picture.

For instance, in almost all cases, the subjects in these studies—at least all the ones I've seen—are untrained individuals, meaning they're brand new to resistance training.

This is important because your body and muscles are hyperresponsive to resistance training in the beginning. This "newbie gains" or "honeymoon" phase generally lasts three to six months in most people, which means that for a little while, you can do just about anything in the gym and see progress and results.

Once that mojo runs out, however, it's gone forever, and what has been working can suddenly stop producing any change whatsoever.

Furthermore, a number of studies have demonstrated that free weights are superior to machines for gaining muscle and strength. For example:

- In a study conducted by scientists at the University of Saskatchewan, the free weight squat produced 43 percent more leg muscle activation than the Smith machine squat.[18]

- In a study conducted by scientists at California State University, the free weight bench press produced 50 percent more shoulder muscle activation than the Smith machine bench press.[19]

- In a study conducted by scientists at Duke University Medical Center, the free weight squat produced 20 to 60 percent more quadriceps activation and 90 to 225 percent more hamstring activation than the leg press.[20]

Anecdotal evidence agrees here as well.

For decades now, the most successful bodybuilders have almost always emphasized free weights over machines, and I'll bet that the strongest people in your gym do the same.

MYTH #7

"YOU SHOULD SPEND MOST OF YOUR TIME ON ISOLATION EXERCISES"

If you want to gain muscle and strength as quickly as possible, it's not enough to just do any type of free weight exercises.

You have to do the *right* free weight exercises, and for our purposes, the best ones we can do are known as *compound exercises*.

A compound exercise involves multiple joints and muscles. For example, the squat involves moving the knees, ankles, and hips and requires a whole-body co-ordinated effort, with the quadriceps, hamstrings, and glutes bearing the brunt of the load.

On the other hand, an exercise like the Nordic hamstring curl involves moving the knees and focuses on strengthening the hamstrings and glutes.

That's why the Nordic hamstring curl isn't considered a compound exercise. It's an *isolation exercise*, which involves just one joint and a limited number of muscles.

The biceps curl is another example of an isolation exercise because the only joint involved is the elbow, and the biceps muscles do more or less all the work.

One of the biggest fitness mistakes people make is underestimating the impor-tance of compound exercises. They deserve a lot of your time and effort for several reasons:

1. They train many muscles at once.

    The more muscles you can effectively train in a given exercise, the more muscle you can gain as a result.
    This also makes for more time efficiency. One compound exercise can do the work of several isolation exercises.

2. They allow you to lift heavier weights.

    The best compound exercises put dozens of muscles and multiple joints through large ranges of motion. Consequently, they enable you to move more weight than isolation exercises and thus better progressively over-load your muscles. This means faster muscle growth.

3. They significantly raise testosterone and growth hormone levels.

    The magnitude of postworkout elevations in anabolic hormones is influ-enced by the total amount of muscle involved in the workout. This is why research shows that compound exercises produce larger increases in both testosterone and growth hormone than isolation exercises.[21]

    These effects don't influence muscle gain as much as some people would have you believe, but they do have other benefits as well.

I attribute much of my success with my physique to the fact that, after learning about the power of compound exercises, I've made them 70 to 80 percent of the work I do in the gym. And I'm going to have you do the same.

MYTH #8

"PROGRESSIVE OVERLOAD ISN'T THAT IMPORTANT"

If I could go back in time and share just one bit of workout advice with 17-year-old me, it would be this: whatever you do, make sure you progressively overload your muscles.

And I would have gotten bigger muscles a lot faster (*single tear*).

We recall that progressive overload refers to increasing the amount of tension your muscles produce over time, and that it's the primary mechanical driver of muscle growth.

This sounds simple enough, but how do you actually accomplish it?

Most people don't. Instead, they go through more or less the same motions for weeks and months on end and wonder why they have so little to show for it.

You must do three things if you don't want to be one of these people:

1. Follow a proven progression model.
2. Track your workouts.
3. Adjust your diet and training as needed.

And later in this book, you're going to learn how to do each of these things correctly, and when you start *Thinner Leaner Stronger*, you're going to experience their transformative power firsthand.

MYTH #9

"YOU DON'T NEED TO EAT A LOT OF PROTEIN"

I'm not sure if I've ever met a woman not into working out who ate a high-protein diet. Heck, many women I meet who *are* into working out don't eat a high-protein diet.

As muscle tissue is made mostly of protein, it's no surprise that scores of studies have shown that a high-protein diet is better for gaining muscle and strength than a low-protein one.[22]

For example, research conducted by scientists at McMaster University, the Nestlé Research Centre, and Kent State University found that women need to eat at least 0.6 to 0.8 grams of protein per pound of body weight per day to maximize muscle gain.[23]

To put that in perspective, that's 70 to 100 grams of protein per day for a 120-pound woman, which, in my experience, is far more than most 120-pound women eat. I haven't seen any research on the matter, but anecdotally speaking, I'd guess the average woman eats just 30 to 50 grams of protein per day.

Thus, it's no surprise that so many women struggle to develop strong, defined muscles despite regular resistance training. In fact, a number of women I've worked with saw immediate improvements in muscle tone by simply increasing protein intake.

MYTH #10

"YOU HAVE TO DO CARDIO TO HAVE A GREAT PHYSIQUE"

You've probably heard that you must sacrifice inordinate amounts of time to the treadmill or StairMaster to look good.

Allow me to disabuse you of such nonsense.

When it comes to improving your body composition (how much muscle and fat you have on your bones), cardio is a double-edged sword.

It burns energy and thus contributes to your fat loss efforts, but it can burn up muscle too. This detracts from your ultimate goal of building a lean, toned physique, because that requires gaining a fair amount of muscle.

Furthermore, if you want to gain muscle and strength as quickly as possible, then you want to limit your cardio for two reasons:

1. In the short term, cardio can interfere with strength and muscle gain by making you more generally fatigued, which makes it harder to progress in your weightlifting workouts.[24]

2. In the long term, cardio can interfere with strength and muscle gain by disrupting cell signaling related to muscle growth.[25]

That doesn't mean you should completely shun cardio, though.

It does have significant health benefits—some of which you don't get from resistance training—and it can help you burn more energy, which means faster fat loss and easier weight maintenance.

You just need to know how to do cardio correctly. More on that soon.

You've just learned some of the most important lessons about how to effectively gain muscle and strength: free weights, compound exercises, and progressive overload are at least half the game.

. . .

You've also learned the biggest reasons why so many women wallow in muscle-building misery: they waste too much time with the Barbie weights and oversized rubber bands and spend too many hours on the treadmills.

Later in this book, you're going to learn how to turn all this newfound knowledge into a simple, practical system for transforming your body, but first, let's return to fat loss and learn exactly how to do it right.

KEY TAKEAWAYS

- Exercise can make you healthier, but it guarantees nothing in the way of fat loss or muscle gain, the two biggest physiological levers you need to know how to work to build the body of your dreams.

- You can't "lengthen" and "tighten" your muscles, fundamentally change how they're shaped, or selectively strip fat away so they look more defined.

- You can add muscle to your frame and remove body fat—nothing more or less.

- The claims that certain forms of exercise produce "long, lean" muscles, like a dancer's body, while others produce "bulky, ugly" muscles, like a bodybuilder's, are bogus.

- It's very hard for women to build a big, bulky body. The real reason some women look "bulky" is they're carrying too much body fat.

- The more muscle you have, the less body fat you must have to avoid looking bulky.

- Most women I've worked with are happiest when they've gained 10 to 15 pounds of muscle and dropped their body fat percentage to about 20 percent.

- When done properly, weightlifting is one of the safest kinds of athletic activities you can do.

- Weightlifting delivers a number of health and fitness benefits that you simply can't get from other types of sports and exercise.

- Women can build muscle more or less as effectively as men due in part to higher levels of estrogen and growth hormone, which promote muscle growth.

• Progressive overload refers to increasing the amount of tension your muscles produce over time, and the most effective way to do this is by progressively increasing the amount of weight that you're lifting.

• The key to gaining muscle and strength isn't merely changing the types of stimuli your muscles are exposed to—it's making your muscles work harder.

• Your number one goal as a weightlifter should be to increase your whole-body strength over time.

• Free weights give you the most muscle-building bang for your buck— far more than machines, bands, and other contraptions in the gym.

• Compound exercises are superior to isolation exercises for gaining muscle and strength because they train many muscles at once, allow you to lift heavier weights, and significantly raise testosterone and growth hormone levels.

• As muscle tissue is made mostly of protein, it's no surprise that a high-protein diet is better for gaining muscle and strength than a low-protein one.

• Women need to eat around 0.6 to 0.8 grams of protein per pound of body weight per day to maximize muscle gain.

• If you want to gain muscle and strength as quickly as possible, then you want to limit your cardio because it can interfere with strength and muscle gain by making you more generally fatigued and disrupting cell signaling related to muscle growth.

• Cardio does have significant health benefits—some of which you don't get from resistance training—and it can help you burn more energy, which means faster fat loss and easier weight maintenance.

9

THE 3 LITTLE BIG THINGS
ABOUT RAPID FAT LOSS

"For me, life is continuously being hungry. The meaning of life is not simply to exist, to survive, but to move ahead, to go up, to achieve, to conquer."
—ARNOLD SCHWARZENEGGER

Most people view body fat as ugly, greasy flesh that must be ruthlessly exterminated, but it's actually vital for our survival.

Not only is it an organ that helps in the creation of various important hormones, but many thousands of years ago, it was all that kept our ancient ancestors alive.

They often journeyed for days without food. Starving, they would finally kill an animal and feast, and their bodies prepared for the next bout of starvation by storing excess energy as fat.

This genetic programming is still in us, and it explains in part why so many people are overweight.

For the first time in our history, we have an endless supply of delicious, calorie-dense foods literally at our fingertips—foods that are, in many cases, carefully engineered to be as satisfying and "addictive" as possible.

(Read Michael Moss's *Salt Sugar Fat: How the Food Giants Hooked Us* if you want to learn the truth about the "dark side" of food science.)

Fortunately, none of this determines our destinies. Although we can't "hack" or override this biological hardwiring, we can lose excess and unwanted body fat and maintain aesthetically pleasing (and healthy) body fat levels.

It's not complicated or difficult, either. As you'll learn in this chapter, you really only need to understand and abide by three rules to never again struggle to lose fat and keep it off.

RULE #1

ENERGY BALANCE IS KING

A couple of chapters ago, you learned how energy balance alone dictates your body weight.

Eat more energy than you burn for long enough, and you'll gain weight. Eat less, and you'll lose weight. Period.

Although that's all you really need to know to create a diet plan that gets the types of results that most people are after, it helps to understand how energy balance directly impacts fat storage and burning, so let's get into that here.

Scientifically speaking, when your body is digesting and absorbing food you've eaten, it's in the *postprandial state* (*post* means "after," and *prandial* means "having to do with a meal"). This is also called the "fed" state.

When in this state, the body uses a portion of the energy provided by the meal to increase its fat stores. Some people call this the body's "fat-storing mode."

Once your body has finished digesting, absorbing, and storing the food eaten, it enters the *postabsorptive* state ("after absorption"). This is also called the "fasted" state.

When in this state, the body must rely mostly on its fat stores for energy. Some people call this the body's "fat-burning mode."

Your body flips between these fed and fasted states every day, storing small amounts of fat after meals, and then burning small amounts after food energy runs out.

Here's a simple graph that shows this visually:

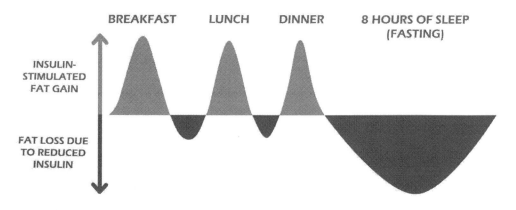

The lighter portions are the periods where you've eaten and provided your body with energy to use and store as fat. The darker portions are the periods where food energy has run out, and your body has to burn fat to stay alive.

You probably also noticed the mention of insulin in the graph, which, as you know, is a hormone that causes muscles, organs, and fat tissue to absorb and use or store nutrients like glucose and amino acids.

Lately, this vital hormone has been under vicious attack by health and diet "gurus," because it also inhibits the breakdown of fat cells and stimulates fat storage.[1]

That is, insulin tells the body to stop burning fat for energy, and to start using and storing the energy being provided by food.

This makes sense given what you've just learned about fed and fasted states. Insulin tells your body whether it has food to burn or must rely on fat for energy.

This also makes insulin an easy target and scapegoat. Here's how the story usually goes:

> High-carb diet = high insulin levels – burn less fat and store more = get fatter and fatter.

And then, as a corollary:

> Low-carb diet = low insulin levels = burn more fat and store less = stay lean.

This is wrong, and the "evidence" used to sell it is pseudoscience. Eating carbs does trigger insulin production, and insulin does trigger fat storage, but none of that makes you fatter. Only overeating does.

This is why a number of overfeeding studies have confirmed that the only way to cause meaningful weight gain is to eat a large surplus of calories, whether from protein, carbohydrate, or dietary fat.[2]

Without that energy surplus, no amount of insulin or insulin-producing foods can significantly increase body fat levels.

Another gaping hole in the great insulin conspiracy is the fact that high-protein, low-carb meals can result in higher insulin levels than high-carb meals.[3]

Research shows that whey protein raises insulin levels more than white bread, and that beef stimulates just as much insulin release as brown rice.[4]

Furthermore, studies show that both protein and carbohydrate generally produce the same type of insulin response—a rapid rise, followed by a rapid decline.[5]

Carbohydrate and insulin demonizers also often talk about an enzyme in your fat cells called *hormone-sensitive lipase* (HSL), which helps release fatty acids to be burned.

Insulin suppresses the activity of HSL and thus is believed to promote weight gain, but dietary fat—the current darling of the mainstream health and diet marketing machines—suppresses it as well.[6]

And thanks to an enzyme called *acylation stimulating protein*, your body doesn't need high levels of insulin to store dietary fat as body fat.[7]

At this point, you may want to believe what I'm telling you about energy balance, but are hung up on claims that it has been refuted by recent scientific research, or on people's personal stories about their own experiences that seem to defy my explanations.

Let's review a few of the more common allegations and anecdotes.

CLAIM #1

"I LOST WEIGHT ON [INSERT DIET HERE] AND NEVER COUNTED CALORIES."

It's easy to find people who've lost significant amounts of weight without ever paying attention to how many calories they were eating.

Maybe they went low-carb. Maybe they stopped eating meat, sugar, or animal products. Or maybe they just started eating "cleaner." And they sure lost weight.

What they don't realize, though, is that the root cause of their weight loss wasn't their food choices per se, but how those choices impacted their energy balance.

In other words, they lost weight because their diets kept them in a state of negative energy balance long enough for meaningful weight loss to occur, not because they ate the "right" foods and avoided the "wrong" ones.

Most weight loss diets revolve around food restriction. You have to limit or avoid foods or entire food groups, and this inevitably forces you to cut various higher-calorie fare out of your diet. Many of these higher-calorie foods also happen to be delicious and easy to overeat, like refined carbs and sugars.

Thus, when you stop eating these foods, your calorie intake naturally goes down, and the more it dips below your calorie output (expenditure), the more fat you lose.

What's more, many people who start dieting to lose weight also start exercising or exercising more, which bumps up energy expenditure and makes it easier to maintain the calorie deficit needed to get results.

CLAIM #2

"I STARVED MYSELF AND DIDN'T LOSE WEIGHT."

Every week, I hear from people who report no weight loss despite (allegedly) eating a small number of calories every day.

While their frustration is understandable, this doesn't mean their metabolisms work in fundamentally different ways from everyone else's.

What's actually happening is almost always nothing more than a matter of human error, just like we discussed in chapter seven: accidentally eating too much and "cheating" their progress away.

Water retention is another issue that can throw many dieters—and female dieters, in particular—for a loop.

When you restrict your calories to lose fat, especially when you do it aggressively, your body tends to retain more water. The reason for this is that calorie restriction increases production of the "stress hormone" cortisol, which in turn increases fluid retention.[8]

Depending on your physiology, this effect can be negligible and unnoticeable, or it can be so strong that it completely obscures several weeks of fat loss. In this way, people can lose fat for several weeks without losing weight and conclude that calorie counting "doesn't work."

Later in this book, you'll learn how to make sure you don't make the same mistake.

CLAIM #3

"IF YOU EAT CLEAN, CALORIES DON'T MATTER."

If all we're talking about is body weight, then a calorie is very much a calorie, and "clean" calories count just as much as "dirty" ones.

That said, it's accurate to say that "clean" or "healthy" foods are more *conducive* to weight loss and maintenance than "dirty" or "unhealthy" ones, because they're generally lower in calories and harder to overeat.

Think about it for a second. What's most likely to lead to excess calorie consumption, "dirty" foods like pizza, cheeseburgers, candy, and ice cream, or "clean" ones like chicken breast, broccoli, brown rice, and apples?

This is why getting the majority of your daily calories from "diet-friendly" foods makes for easier and more enjoyable weight loss and maintenance.

CLAIM #4

"THE HUMAN BODY ISN'T AN INORGANIC MACHINE. YOU CAN'T APPLY THE SAME RULES."

Some people say that the first law of thermodynamics doesn't apply to the human metabolism. They say our bodies are far more complicated than the simple engines that power our refrigerators and cars.

Their arguments can be convincing, too, chock-full of weasel words like *entropy*, *chaos theory*, and *metabolic advantage*, and tangents on the more esoteric aspects of our endocrine system.

This is all smoke and mirrors.

It's true that the human body is far more complex than a combustion engine, but as I mentioned earlier, there's a reason why every single controlled weight loss study conducted in the last century has concluded that meaningful weight loss requires "calories in" to be lower than "calories out." It works the same in the lean and obese, and even in the healthy and diseased.[9]

Energy balance is a first principle of the human metabolism, the "master key" to your body weight, and it simply can't be circumvented or ignored.

RULE #2

MACRONUTRIENT BALANCE IS QUEEN

You've heard me say that as important as energy balance is, it's not the whole story, especially not when the goal is to improve your body composition.

Well, it's time to hear the rest of the weight loss tale, and this is the final act.

Macronutrient balance refers to how the calories you eat break down into protein, carbohydrate, and dietary fat.

If you want to lose fat and not muscle, or gain muscle and not fat, then you need to pay close attention to both your energy *and* macronutrient balances.

In this context, a calorie is no longer a calorie because a calorie of protein does very different things in your body than a calorie of carbohydrate or dietary fat.

Let's take a closer look at each of these "macros" and discover how they fit into the fat loss puzzle.

MACRONUTRIENT #1

PROTEIN

While the scientific search for the "One True Diet" continues, there's one thing we know for certain: it's going to be high in protein.

Study after study has already confirmed that high-protein dieting is superior to low-protein dieting in just about every meaningful way.[10] Specifically, research shows that people who eat more protein:

- Lose fat faster[11]
- Gain more muscle[12]
- Burn more calories[13]
- Experience less hunger[14]
- Have stronger bones[15]
- Generally enjoy better moods[16]

Protein intake is even more important when you exercise regularly because this increases your body's demand for protein.[17]

It's also important when you restrict your calories to lose fat, because eating adequate protein plays a major role in preserving lean mass while dieting.[18]

Protein intake is important among sedentary folk as well. Studies show that such people lose muscle faster as they age if they don't eat enough protein, and the faster they lose muscle, the more likely they are to die from all causes.[19]

MACRONUTRIENT #2

CARBOHYDRATE

To really understand why carbs aren't your enemy, let's briefly discuss their chemical structure and what happens when you eat them.

There are four primary forms of carbohydrate that you need to know about:

- Monosaccharides
- Disaccharides
- Oligosaccharides
- Polysaccharides

Monosaccharides are often called *simple sugars* because they have a very simple structure. *Mono* means "one" and *saccharide* means "sugar," so "one sugar."

There are three monosaccharides: glucose, fructose, and galactose. You learned these words earlier in this book, but let's brush up on them quickly here.

- Glucose is a sugar that occurs widely in nature and is an important energy source in organisms, as well as a component of many carbohydrates.

- Fructose is a sugar found in many fruits and honey, as well as processed products like table sugar and high-fructose corn syrup.

- Fructose is converted into glucose by the liver and then released into the blood for use.

- Galactose is a sugar found in dairy products that's metabolized similarly to fructose.

Disaccharides, meaning "two sugars," are commonly found in nature as sucrose, lactose, and maltose. Again, a quick review of the two terms you're familiar with, and then the new, third term:

- Sucrose is a sugar that occurs naturally in most plants and is obtained commercially especially from sugarcane or sugar beets.

It's commonly known as table sugar.

- Lactose is a sugar present in milk that contains glucose and galactose.

- Maltose is a sugar that consists of two glucose molecules linked together.

It's uncommon in nature and is used in alcohol production.

Oligosaccharides are molecules that contain several monosaccharides linked together in chain-like structures. *Oligos* is Greek for "a few," so a "few sugars."

The fiber found in plants is partially made of oligosaccharides, and many vegetables also contain *fructooligosaccharides*, which are short chains of fructose molecules.

Another common form of oligosaccharide that we eat is *raffinose*, a chain of galactose, glucose, and fructose. This is found in a variety of foods like whole grains, beans, cabbage, Brussel sprouts, broccoli, asparagus, and other vegetables.

Galactooligosaccharides round out this list, and they're short chains of galactose molecules found in many of the same foods as raffinose. They're indigestible but play a role in stimulating healthy bacteria growth in the gut.

The last form of carbohydrate that we need to discuss is the polysaccharide, which is a long chain of monosaccharides, usually containing 10 or more of these sugars.

Starch (the energy stores of plants) and cellulose (a natural fiber found in many plants) are two examples of polysaccharides that we often eat. Our bodies easily break starches down into glucose, but cellulose passes through our digestive system intact.

Except for those that aren't digested, all these types of carbs have something very important in common: they all end up as glucose in the body.

Whether we're talking about the natural sugars found in fruit, the processed ones found in a candy bar, or the "healthy" ones found in green vegetables, they're all digested into glucose and shipped off in the blood for use.

The key difference between these forms of carbohydrate is the rate at which this conversion happens.

The candy bar turns into glucose rather quickly because it contains a large number of quickly digested monosaccharides, whereas the broccoli takes longer because it contains slower-burning oligosaccharides.

Some people say that makes *all* the difference—that the speed with which carbs are converted into glucose determines whether they're "healthy." These people are mostly wrong.

For instance, baked potato is rather high on the glycemic index (85) but packed with vital nutrients. Watermelon is up there on the index as well (72), and even oatmeal (58) is higher than a Snickers Bar (55).

Does that mean you can eat all the simple sugars you want, then? That so long as you keep your energy and macronutrients balanced, you can replace potato and oatmeal with soda and candy as often as you'd like?

Well, you *could*, but it would eventually catch up with you because our bodies need to get a lot more than calories and macros from the food we eat. They also need a long list of nutrients, like vitamins, minerals, and fiber, that simply aren't in Coca-Cola and Twizzlers.

This is one of the reasons why research shows there's an association between high *added sugar* intake—sugars like sucrose and fructose added to foods to sweeten them—and several metabolic abnormalities and health conditions, including obesity, as well as varying degrees of nutritional deficiency.[20]

There's simply no denying that eating too much added sugar can harm our health and that reducing intake is generally a good idea.

That doesn't mean we need to reduce or limit our consumption of all forms of carbohydrate, however. In fact, if you're healthy and physically active, particularly if you lift weights regularly, chances are that you'll do better with more carbs in your diet, not less.

You'll find out why in the next chapter.

MACRONUTRIENT #3

DIETARY FAT

Dietary fat doesn't deserve all the attention it's getting these days.

You should eat enough to stay healthy, but have no reason to follow a high-fat diet unless you really enjoy it. And even then you need to do so with caution.

To understand why, let's start at the top. There are two different types of fat found in food:

1. Triglycerides
2. Cholesterol

Triglycerides make up the bulk of our daily fat intake and are found in a wide variety of foods ranging from dairy to nuts, seeds, meat, and more.

They can be liquid (unsaturated) or solid (saturated), and they support health in many ways. They help absorb vitamins, they're used to create various hormones, they keep the skin and hair healthy, and much more.

We recall that saturated fat is a form of fat that's solid at room temperature and found in foods like meat, dairy, and eggs.

The long-held belief that saturated fat increases the risk of heart disease has been challenged by recent research, which claims "that there is no significant evidence for concluding that dietary saturated fat is associated with an increased risk of CHD or CVD [heart disease]."[21]

The fad diet industry has exploited this "revelation" marvelously with runaway hits like the paleo and ketogenic diets.

The problem, however, is that much of the scientific literature used to promote these diets has also been severely criticized by prominent nutrition and cardiology researchers for various flaws and omissions.[22]

These scientists maintain that there is a strong association between high intake of saturated fat and heart disease, and that we should follow the generally accepted dietary guidelines for saturated fat intake (less than 10 percent of daily calories) until we know more.

Given the current weight of the evidence, nobody can honestly claim that we can eat as much saturated fat as we want without any chance of negative consequences.

This is why I think it's much smarter to "play it safe" and wait for further research before joining in the mainstream saturated fat orgy.

Earlier in this book, you learned that unsaturated fat is a form of fat that's liquid at room temperature and found in foods like olive oil, avocado, and nuts. There are two distinct types of unsaturated fats:

1. Monounsaturated fat

2. Polyunsaturated fat

Monounsaturated fat is liquid at room temperature and starts to solidify when cooled. Foods high in monounsaturated fat include nuts, olive and peanut oil, and avocado.

Polyunsaturated fat is liquid at room temperature and remains so when cooled. Foods high in polyunsaturated fat include safflower, sesame, and sunflower seeds, corn, and many nuts and their oils.

Unlike saturated fat, there's no controversy over monounsaturated fat. Research shows that it can reduce the risk of heart disease, and it's also believed to be responsible for some of the health benefits associated with the Mediterranean diet, which involves eating a lot of olive oil.[23]

Polyunsaturated fat, on the other hand, isn't as cut-and-dried. The two primary polyunsaturated fats are *alpha-linolenic acid* (ALA) and *linolenic acid* (LA). ALA is what's known as an *omega-3 fatty acid* while LA is an *omega-6 fatty acid*. These designations refer to the structure of the molecules.

ALA and LA are the only types of fat that our bodies can't produce and that we must obtain from our diets. This is why they're referred to as *essential fatty acids*.

These two substances cause an enormous number of effects in the body. The chemistry is complex, but here's what you need to know for the purpose of our current discussion:

- LA is converted into several compounds in the body, including the anti-inflammatory *gamma-linolenic acid*, as well as the pro-inflammatory *arachidonic acid*.

- ALA can be converted into an omega-3 fatty acid known as *eicosapentaenoic acid* (EPA), which can be converted into another called *docosahexaenoic acid* (DHA).

A large amount of research has been done on EPA and DHA, and it appears that they bestow many, if not all, of the health benefits generally associated with ALA, including:

- Decreased inflammation[24]
- Improved mood[25]
- Faster muscle growth[26]
- Increased cognitive performance[27]
- Faster fat loss[28]

It's an oversimplification to say that the effects of LA (omega-6) are generally "bad," and the effects of ALA (omega-3) are generally "good," but it's more accurate than inaccurate.

That's why it has been hypothesized that a diet too high in omega-6 and too low in omega-3 fatty acids can cause a whole host of health problems.

Research conducted by scientists at the University of Illinois casts doubt on this, though.[29] There's no question that inadequate omega-3 intake is bad for your health, but ironically, studies have found that increasing omega-6 intake can decrease the risk of heart disease, not increase it.[30]

Thus, scientists suspect that the absolute amount of omega-3 fatty acids in the diet is more important than the ratio between omega-3 and omega-6 intakes. Hence the considerable amount of work that has been done to boost the omega-3 content of various foods like eggs and meat.

The key takeaway here is if you're like most people, you're getting enough omega-6 fatty acids in your diet, but probably not enough omega-3s (and EPA and DHA in particular). An easy way to fix this is with an omega-3 supplement, which we'll discuss later in this book.

Cholesterol is the other type of fat found in food. It's a waxy substance present in all cells in the body, and it's used to make hormones, vitamin D, and substances that help you digest your food.

Several decades ago, it was believed that foods that contained cholesterol, like eggs and meat, increased the risk of heart disease. We now know it's not that simple. Eggs, for instance, have been more or less exonerated, and studies show that *processed meat* is associated with high incidence of heart disease but red meat per se is not.[31]

One of the reasons the relationship between cholesterol and heart health is tricky is foods that contain cholesterol also often contain saturated fat, which can indeed increase the risk of heart disease.

Another reason has to do with how cholesterol travels throughout your body. It's delivered to cells by molecules known as *lipoproteins*, which are made out of fat and proteins. There are two kinds of lipoproteins:

1. Low-density lipoproteins (LDL)

2. High-density lipoproteins (HDL)

When people talk of "bad" cholesterol, they're referring to LDL because research shows that high levels of LDL in your blood can lead to an accumulation in your arteries, and increase the risk of heart disease.[32]

This is why foods that can raise LDL levels, such as fried and processed foods and foods high in saturated fat, are generally considered bad for your heart.[33]

HDL is often thought of as the "good" cholesterol because it carries cholesterol to your liver, where it's processed for various uses.

RULE #3

ADJUST YOUR FOOD INTAKE BASED ON HOW YOUR BODY IS RESPONDING

Tweaking your calories and macros up and down based on what's actually happening with your body is vitally important for two reasons:

1. Formulas for calculating your calories and macros may not work perfectly for you right out of the box.

2. What has been working can stop producing results.

To the first point, your metabolism may be naturally faster or slower than the formulas assume. You may engage in a lot of spontaneous activity throughout the day without realizing it, like walking around while on the phone, hopping to the bathroom, drumming your fingers while you read, or bobbing your legs while you think. Your job or hobbies may burn more energy than you realize (causing you to underestimate your energy expenditure), and you may burn more (or less) energy than average during exercise.

And to the second point, we recall that the body responds to calorie restriction with countermeasures meant to stall weight loss, including metabolic slowdown. This is the primary reason why a calorie intake that initially results in weight loss can eventually stop working.

Similarly, the body responds to a calorie surplus with countermeasures meant to stall weight gain, including metabolic speedup. This is mostly why a calorie intake that initially results in weight gain can also eventually stop working.

The good news is you don't have to try to account for all this before beginning your fat loss diet. Instead, you can start simple and adjust your calories and macros based on how your body is actually responding.

Here's the basic rule of thumb:

If you're trying to lose weight but aren't, you probably need to eat less or move more.

(And if you're trying to gain weight but aren't, you probably just need to eat more.)

We'll talk more about this, including what you should do when you stop losing weight, later in this book.

. . .

Phew, you made it.

You've just learned the biggest dietary "secrets" to building your best body ever. The material is dry, but so are most principles of most everything you could want to learn.

Remember that the value of information isn't determined by how it makes you feel but by how well you understand it and how workable it is.

You've also learned that losing fat quickly and healthily without losing muscle isn't complicated or even all that difficult, really.

It takes a bit of guidance and discipline, but once you know how to put everything you've just learned in this chapter into practice (and you will soon), you might be surprised at how smoothly it can go.

In fact, this "flexible" style of dieting will probably be the easiest you've ever tried, *and* the most effective and sustainable. Exciting, right?

KEY TAKEAWAYS

- When your body is digesting and absorbing food you've eaten, it's in the postprandial state. This is also called the "fed" state.

- Once your body has finished digesting, absorbing, and storing the food eaten, it enters the postabsorptive state. This is also called the "fasted" state.

- Your body flips between fed and fasted states every day, storing small amounts of fat after meals, and then burning small amounts when there's no food energy left.

- Without an energy surplus, no amount of insulin or insulin-producing foods can significantly increase body fat levels.

- When you restrict your calories to lose fat, especially when you restrict them aggressively, you tend to retain more water.

- If all we're talking about is body weight, then a calorie is very much a calorie, and "clean" calories count just as much as "dirty" ones.

- "Clean" or "healthy" foods are more conducive to weight loss than "dirty" or "unhealthy" ones because they're generally lower in calories and harder to overeat.

- Getting the majority of your daily calories from "diet-friendly" foods when dieting for fat loss makes for a much easier, more enjoyable dieting experience.

- Macronutrient balance refers to how the calories you eat break down into protein, carbohydrate, and dietary fat.

- If you want to lose fat and not muscle, or gain muscle and not fat, then you need to pay close attention to both your energy and macronutrient balances.

- People who eat more protein lose fat faster, gain more muscle, burn more calories, experience less hunger, have stronger bones, and generally enjoy better moods.

- Protein intake is even more important when you exercise regularly because this increases your body's demand for it.

- Whether we're talking about the natural sugars found in fruit, the processed ones found in a candy bar, or the "healthy" ones found in green vegetables, they're all digested into glucose and shipped off to the brain, muscles, and organs for use.

• There's no difference in weight loss between people whose diets contain a large amount of high-glycemic foods versus those that focus on low-glycemic foods.

• There's an association between high sugar intake and several metabolic abnormalities and adverse health conditions, including obesity, as well as varying levels of nutritional deficiencies.

• When dieting to lose fat, high-protein, high-carbohydrate dieting allows you to push harder in your workouts and maintain more muscle mass.

• We should eat at least enough dietary fat to support our health and only raise intake beyond that based on our goals, fitness, and preferences.

• Triglycerides make up the bulk of our daily fat intake and are found in a wide variety of foods ranging from dairy to nuts, seeds, meat, and more.

• Saturated fat is a form of fat that's solid at room temperature and found in foods like meat, dairy, and eggs.

• There's a strong association between high intake of saturated fat and heart disease, and we should follow the generally accepted dietary guidelines for saturated fat intake (less than 10 percent of daily calories) until we know more.

• Monounsaturated fat can reduce the risk of heart disease, and it's believed to be responsible for some of the health benefits associated with the Mediterranean diet, which involves eating a lot of olive oil.

• The absolute amount of omega-3 fatty acids in the diet is more important than the ratio between omega-3 and omega-6 intakes.

• If you're like most people, you're getting enough omega-6 fatty acids in your diet, but probably not enough omega-3s (EPA and DHA in particular).

• Cholesterol is the other type of fat found in food. It's a waxy substance present in all cells in the body, and it's used to make hormones, vitamin D, and substances that help you digest your food.

• Scientists used to believe that foods that contained cholesterol increased the risk of heart disease, but we now know that this isn't the case.

• When people talk of "bad" cholesterol, they're referring to LDL. High levels of LDL in your blood can lead to an accumulation in your arteries and increase the risk of heart disease.

• If you're trying to lose weight but aren't, you probably need to eat less or move more.

• If you're trying to gain weight but aren't, you probably just need to eat more.

10

THE 3 LITTLE BIG THINGS
ABOUT BUILDING LEAN MUSCLE

*"If you think taking care of yourself is selfish, change your mind.
If you don't, you're simply ducking your responsibilities."*
—ANN RICHARDS

If you've spent any amount of time in the fitness space, you've heard a lot of things about muscle building.

Things like:

- Muscles respond differently to different types of training.
- Muscles don't know weight. They only know tension.
- There are different types of muscle growth.
- Training with lighter weights and higher reps is best for muscle gain.
- Training with heavier weights and lower reps is best for muscle gain.
- Muscle building is mostly genetic, and how you train doesn't much matter.

And you've also probably heard that most of that is pseudoscientific nonsense, and that some other theory or model altogether is the real "secret" to gaining muscle quickly and effectively.

If this has left you confused and frustrated, unsure of what to believe (and do in the gym) and what to ignore, I understand. I've been there.

Fortunately, while the physiology of muscle growth is tremendously complex, the science of gaining muscle is far simpler. In fact, at least 80 percent of effective muscle building comes down to understanding and applying a handful of laws that are as certain, observable, and irrefutable as those of physics.

When you throw a ball in the air, it comes down. When you apply the three principles you're going to learn in this chapter, your muscles grow bigger and stronger.

It's that simple.

LAW #1

THERE ARE THREE WAYS TO STIMULATE MUSCLE GROWTH

The first thing you need to understand about the physiology of muscle building is there are three primary "triggers" or "pathways" for muscle growth:[1]

1. Mechanical tension
2. Muscle damage
3. Cellular fatigue

Mechanical tension refers to the amount of force produced in muscle fibers.

When you lift weights, you produce two types of mechanical tension in your muscles: "passive" and "active" tension. Passive tension occurs when your muscles are stretching, and active tension occurs when they're contracting.

Muscle damage refers to microscopic damage caused to the muscle fibers by high levels of tension.

This damage requires repair, and if the body is provided with proper nutrition and rest, it'll make the muscle fibers larger and stronger to better deal with future bouts of tension.

(It's still not entirely clear whether muscle damage directly stimulates muscle growth or whether it's just a side effect of mechanical tension, but as of now, it deserves a place on the list.)

Cellular fatigue refers to a host of chemical changes that occur inside and outside muscle fibers when they contract repeatedly.

When you repeat the same movement over and over again to the point of near failure, this causes high amounts of cellular fatigue.

Research conducted by scientists at Harvard Medical School shows that mechanical tension is the most important of these three pathways for muscle growth.[2] This has been confirmed in a number of other studies as well.[3]

In other words, mechanical tension produces a stronger muscle-building stimulus than muscle damage and cellular fatigue.

These three factors also relate to what scientists call the "strength-endurance continuum," which works like this:[4]

- Heavy, lower-rep weightlifting primarily increases muscle strength and results in higher amounts of mechanical tension and muscle damage, but less cellular fatigue.

- Lighter, higher-rep weightlifting primarily increases muscle endurance and results in lower amounts of mechanical tension and muscle damage, but more cellular fatigue.

Given what you just learned, which style of training do you think is more effective for gaining muscle over time? That's right—heavy, lower-rep work, because it produces more mechanical tension than lighter, higher-rep work.

This isn't just a theory of mine, either. It has good science on its side.

For instance, a meta-analysis (an in-depth examination of a number of studies) conducted by scientists at Lehman College and Victoria University reviewed 21 studies that compared training with heavier weights (60-plus percent of one-rep max) and lower reps versus lighter weights (less than 60 percent of one-rep max) and higher reps.[5]

The scientists found that both styles of training caused similar amounts of muscle growth, but training with heavier weights caused greater increases in strength.

One of the researchers, a friend and fellow author named James Krieger, also pointed out in an interview I did with him on my podcast (www.muscleforlifepod-cast.com) that training with lighter weights only resulted in significant muscle growth when sets were taken to or close to muscle failure (the point where you can no longer keep the weight moving).[6]

This can be done, of course, but it's extremely difficult. If you want to get a taste of what it's like, do a 20-rep set of barbell squats that ends a rep or two shy of muscle failure. And then imagine having to do a couple more sets, and then having to do it all again in a few days.

In other words, higher-rep training can be effective for muscle gain, but it requires a level of masochism that most of us just don't care to embrace.

Fortunately, we don't need to because we can simply train with heavier weights, which is equally (if not more) effective for muscle gain, and far less grueling.

This brings us back to your primary goal as a weightlifter: to get stronger, and especially on key whole-body exercises like the squat, deadlift, and bench press.

The more weight you can push, pull, and squat, the more muscle definition you're going to have.

That isn't to say that lighter weights and other training methods have no place in your workout routine, but if your goal is to gain muscle as quickly as possible, the best way to do this is to gain strength as quickly as possible.

LAW #2

MUSCLES DON'T GROW IN THE GYM

You might have heard this old bodybuilding adage before.

There's truth in it. Weightlifting alone doesn't make your muscles bigger and stronger. That's what happens after the workouts, when your body repairs the stress and damage they cause.

Every day, your body is constantly breaking down and rebuilding muscle proteins. This process is known as *protein turnover*, and when viewed on the whole, protein breakdown and synthesis (creation) rates generally balance each other out.[7]

This is why the average, non-exercising person doesn't gain or lose muscle at an accelerated rate.

Mechanically speaking, muscle growth is the result of protein synthesis rates exceeding breakdown rates over extended periods of time.

In other words, if your body is creating new muscle proteins faster than it's breaking them down, you're gaining muscle (and if it's breaking them down faster than it's creating them, you're losing muscle).

Therefore, if you want to gain muscle as effectively as possible, then you want to do everything you can to keep protein synthesis rates at or above breakdown rates. The more time your body spends in this anabolic state, the faster you gain muscle.

When you do resistance training or cardiovascular exercise, protein synthesis rates decline during the workouts.[8] Then, both protein synthesis and breakdown rates rise soon after you finish, with breakdown rates eventually overtaking synthesis rates.

In this way, exercise is a catabolic activity, especially with longer workouts, and repair, recovery, and growth can only occur after.

Unsurprisingly, sleep plays a vital role in this process, because much of what your body does to recuperate and rebuild happens in bed.[9] This is why studies show that sleep deprivation directly inhibits muscle growth (and fat loss) and can even cause muscle loss.[10]

Interestingly, these negative effects become even more pronounced when you're in a calorie deficit.[11]

Furthermore, research shows that even a single night of poor sleep can interfere with your performance in the gym, and two nights is enough to ruin it.[12] Multiple studies have also clearly demonstrated that athletes who get enough sleep perform the best.[13]

MUSCLES DON'T GROW UNLESS PROPERLY FED

Most people think that calories only count when you're talking weight loss.

What they don't realize, though, is that if you don't eat enough, your body can't do many things as effectively, including everything it needs to do to recover from your workouts.

This is why research shows that when you're in a calorie deficit, your body's ability to repair and grow muscle tissue is impaired.[14] This is also why workouts take a bigger toll on you when you're dieting, and why intermediate and advanced weightlifters have to accept slow or no muscle gain when dieting to lose fat.

Remember that calories are what fuel every process in your body, and the system for muscle building is metabolically expensive. Therefore, if you want to maximize muscle growth, then you need to make sure you aren't in a calorie deficit.

The best way to do this is to deliberately eat a bit more calories than you're burning every day. This ensures that your body has all the energy it needs to push hard in the gym and recover from your workouts.

Another vital aspect of "feeding your muscles" is eating enough protein. In fact, this is just as important as eating enough calories, if not more so.[15]

Carbohydrate also contributes to your muscle-building efforts. One of the substances that carbs are converted to in the body is *glycogen*, which is stored in the muscles and liver and is the primary source of fuel during intense exercise.

When you restrict your carb intake, your body's glycogen stores drop, and studies show that this inhibits genetic signaling related to postworkout muscle repair and growth.[16]

When you're exercising regularly, restricting your carbs also raises your cortisol and lowers your testosterone levels, which further hampers your body's ability to recover from your workouts.[17]

All this is why research shows that athletes who eat low-carb diets recover slower from their workouts and gain less muscle and strength than those who eat more carbs.[18]

It's also worth mentioning that eating a low-carb diet will reduce your strength and muscle endurance, which makes it harder to progressively overload your muscles in the gym and thereby maximally stimulate muscle growth.

And what about the final macronutrient, dietary fat?

Some people say a high-fat diet is conducive to muscle gain because of its effects on anabolic hormone production, testosterone production in particular.

When you dig into the research, however, you quickly realize that these effects are far too small to make a noticeable difference in the gym.[19]

Furthermore, the more dietary fat you eat, the less carbs you'll be able to eat, which will more than wipe out any potential muscle-building benefits from slight hormonal upticks.

. . .

You can spend hundreds of hours studying muscle growth and barely scratch the surface. It's extremely complex and involves scores of physiological functions and adaptations.

Fortunately, you don't need to be a scientist to have a working understanding of the research, and to be able to use it to gain whole-body strength and muscle tone.

You now have the foundation of this understanding. You overload, damage, and fatigue your muscles in your workouts, and then feed and repair them after.

This also brings us to the end of part two of this book, and I want to congratulate you on making it this far. You've digested a lot of information and gained a whole new perspective on fat burning and muscle building.

If you've been enjoying yourself, then you're going to absolutely love what I have in store for you next.

In the third part of this book, we're going to take a break from the physiology of fitness and dive into the psychology, because if you don't "get your mind right," you're probably never going to "get your body right."

KEY TAKEAWAYS

- There are three primary "triggers" or "pathways" for muscle growth: mechanical tension, muscle damage, and cellular fatigue.

- Mechanical tension refers to the force you apply to your muscles against a resistance.

- Muscle damage refers to microscopic damage caused to the muscle fibers by high levels of tension.

- Cellular fatigue refers to a host of chemical changes that occur inside and outside muscle fibers when they contract repeatedly.

- Mechanical tension is the most important of these three pathways for muscle growth.

- Heavy, lower-rep weightlifting primarily increases muscle strength and results in higher amounts of mechanical tension and muscle damage, but less cellular fatigue.

- Heavy, lower-rep work results in more muscle gain because it produces more mechanical tension than lighter, higher-rep work.

- Muscle growth is the result of protein synthesis rates exceeding breakdown rates over extended periods of time.

- Exercise is a catabolic activity, especially longer workouts, and repair, recovery, and growth can only occur after.

- Sleep deprivation directly inhibits muscle growth (and fat loss) and can even cause muscle loss.

- If you want to maximize muscle growth, you need to make sure you aren't in a calorie deficit.

- A vital aspect of "feeding your muscles" is eating enough protein, and this is just as important as eating enough calories, if not more so.

- One of the substances that carbs are converted to in the body is glycogen, which is stored in the muscles and liver and is the primary source of fuel during intense exercise.

- When you're exercising regularly, restricting your carbs raises your cortisol and lowers your testosterone levels, which hampers your body's ability to recover from your workouts.

- A low-carb diet will reduce your strength and muscle endurance, which makes it harder to progressively overload your muscles in the gym and thereby maximally stimulate muscle growth.

- The more dietary fat you eat, the less carbs you'll be able to eat, which will more than wipe out any potential muscle-building benefits from slight hormonal upticks.

PART 3

HOW TO WIN THE "INNER GAME" OF GETTING FIT

11

THE GREAT "INNER GAME" SECRET

"The discipline of desire is the background of character."
—JOHN LOCKE

In his timeless bestseller *The Inner Game of Tennis*, Tim Gallwey wrote the following:

> Every game is composed of two parts, an outer game and an inner game. The outer game is played against an external opponent to overcome external obstacles, and to reach an external goal. Mastering this game is the subject of many books offering instructions on how to swing a racket, club or bat, and how to position arms, legs or torso to achieve the best results. But for some reason most of us find these instructions easier to remember than to execute.

How fitting those words are to fitness.

Most books, magazines, trainers, and influencers focus exclusively on the outer game of losing fat and building muscle.

They talk about how to eat, exercise, supplement, and so forth, but they give little attention to the inner game, which is arguably more important, because simply knowing what to do is never enough.

You then have to be able to actually do it, and keep doing it every day, week, month, and year.

If you ask me, mastering the outer game of fitness is simple and straightforward. Half of it is knowing how to press the right physiological buttons to achieve your intended results, and the other half is just showing up every day and rolling up your sleeves.

Mastering the inner game can be much trickier, however. It's what sets the "fitness elite" apart from everyone else. Building and maintaining an outstanding physique requires a disciplined, orderly approach to not just your diet and exercise, but your life in general.

And for most women, this comes about as easily as shaving their legs with an axe.

Motivation and discipline are the biggest inner-game barriers, of course. Every week, guys and gals leap into fitness programs with full tanks of resolve and energy, but it doesn't take long for their enthusiasm to flag.

That new TV show is starting during their gym time, that extra hour of sleep would really hit the spot, skipping a few workouts isn't that big of a deal, another cheat meal shouldn't matter too much. So goes the skid down the slippery slope back toward the status quo of quiet desperation.

This loss of momentum is probably why many people seem to give up on their fitness aspirations around the three-month mark. I've seen it time and time again. Someone buys into some new fad diet or exercise regimen, follows it for three, maybe four, months, and then for one reason or another, throws in the towel.

Sometimes they get sick and never return, other times they take a week off and never come back, and other times they "stop caring" about getting in shape and go back to life as they knew it.

Maybe you've been there yourself. I know I have, which is why I wrote an entire book on getting and staying motivated called *The Little Black Book of Workout Motivation* (www.workoutmotivationbook.com). In that book, I share my personal, practical blueprint for radical transformation, inside and outside the gym.

The truth is that fitness is hard, and no matter how gritty you might be, if you're not seeing clear and consistent results and progress for all your work in the kitchen and gym, it's only natural for your drive to dry up.

I want to make sure this doesn't happen to you. I want to do everything I can to give you your best shot at success on my *Thinner Leaner Stronger* program.

In fact, if I'm being totally honest, I want this to be *the* program that finally makes all the difference in your life and delivers the goods. Heck, maybe even the last fitness program you ever need.

That's why I want to work with you to sharpen both your inner and outer game. I want to provide you with workable principles, strategies, and tools for winning in not just the physical realm of fitness, but the mental and emotional realms as well.

So, in this part of the book, we're going to learn how to develop a winning mindset that'll empower you to overcome the obstacles, resist the temptations, and surmount the setbacks that we all have to experience at one time or another in our fitness journeys.

Then, in the next part, we'll dig into the outer game in earnest and discover the nuts and bolts of my *Thinner Leaner Stronger* program.

12

THE ANATOMY OF WILLPOWER

"Would you have a great empire? Rule over yourself."
—PUBLILIUS SYRUS

According to a 2010 survey conducted by the American Psychological Association, the lack of willpower is the number one obstacle people face in achieving their goals.[1]

Many feel guilty about their lack of self-control, like they're letting themselves and others down. They feel like their lives are, in large part, not under their control, and that their actions are dictated by emotions, impulses, and cravings.

For many of these people, exerting self-discipline ultimately just leads to exhaustion.

And what about those with higher levels of willpower?

Research conducted by scientists at the University of Pennsylvania, Case Western Reserve University, and the University of Maryland shows that they do better in school, earn more money, make better leaders, and are generally happier, healthier, and less stressed.[2] They also have better social and romantic relationships (they can keep their mouths shut), and they even tend to live longer.[3]

Considering all this evidence, it's clear that no matter the circumstances, more willpower trumps less.

Regardless of where we generally fall on the willpower spectrum, we all have challenges to face, especially those of us who want to get and stay fit.

Some of these difficulties are biological—for example, the desire to eat greasy, sugary foods that our brains recognize as vital to our survival—and others are more uniquely ours. What we find tempting someone else might find repulsive. And their vices might be as appealing to us as airline food.

Whatever the details, the machinations are the same. Your excuse for skipping the gym—*again*—is remarkably similar to the foodie's justification for bingeing for the third day in a row. How you talk yourself into eating everything in sight is how someone else eases the guilt of giving in to her cravings for a cigarette.

My point is that the internal struggle of self-discipline is just part of being human. Why is it such a heavy burden for some people though? Why do they give up so easily on goals, and why do they blissfully indulge in so many self-sabotaging behaviors? And what can be done about it? How can they get themselves and their lives under control?

While I definitely don't have all the answers to those questions, I'm going to share the insights that have helped me understand the nature of the beast and how to better tame it.

As you'll see, the self-awareness that comes with gaining a deeper understanding of how we tick is incredibly empowering. By learning about what makes us likely to lose control and why, we can more skillfully manage our "willpower reserves" and avoid the pitfalls that drain them.

Let's start with a clear definition of what willpower really is.

I WILL, I WON'T, I WANT

What do we mean when we say someone has or lacks willpower?

We're usually referring to their ability or inability to say no. They're supposed to study for the exam but instead accept the invitation to the movies. They're trying to lose 10 pounds but just couldn't resist the apple pie. In short, they have trouble saying "I won't."

There are two other aspects to willpower, though: "I will" and "I want."

"I will" power is the other side of the "I won't" coin. It's the ability to do something when you don't want to, like crawling out of bed to grind through a workout, paying the overdue bill, or burning the midnight oil on that work project.

"I want" is the ability to remember the *why* when temptation strikes—the long-term goal or thing you really want more than the fast food or night on the couch.

Become the master of your won'ts, wills, and wants, and you become the master of your destiny. Procrastination can be licked. Your worst habits can be dismantled and replaced. Whiffs of temptation lose their sway over you.

Don't expect these abilities to come easily, though. "Reprogramming" yourself to favor the harder choices is uncomfortable. You might find it overwhelming at first. You're going to be drawn back to what's familiar.

Stay the course, however, and you'll find it progressively easier and easier to say no to the distractions and yes to the things you need to do.

Now that we've established what willpower consists of and what the stakes are, let's move on to the physiology of desire and why it can sometimes make it so hard to resist being "bad."

WHY GIVING IN FEELS SO GOOD

A real willpower challenge isn't a fleeting, "wouldn't that be nice" thought that disappears as quickly as it came. It's more like an all-consuming battle raging inside your skull between good and evil, virtue and sin, yin and yang. You feel it physically.

What's going on?

You're experiencing your brain fixating on a promise of reward. Once you catch sight of that cheeseburger, a chemical called *dopamine* floods your brain, and all of a sudden, all that matters in life is consuming that greasy, delicious pile of meat, cheese, and bun.[4]

To make matters even worse, your brain is now anticipating the imminent spike in insulin and energy, so it begins to lower your blood sugar levels. This makes you crave the burger even more, and before you can give it another thought, you're in line salivating.[5]

Once you become aware of an opportunity to score a reward of any kind, your brain squirts out dopamine to tell you that this indeed is the droid you're looking for (may the Force be with you). It plays up the sweet song of immediate gratification and plays down any chatter about negative consequences.[6]

This chemical is particularly devious, too, because it's not engineered to make you feel happy and content. Its role is to stimulate you to action, and it does this by arousing you, sharpening your focus, and revving up your drive to move toward the prize.[7]

Furthermore, when dopamine is released, it also triggers the release of stress hormones that make you feel anxious.[8] This is why the more you think about the thing you want, the more important it becomes to you and the more you think you have to have it *right now*.

What we don't realize, however, is that this stress we feel isn't caused by not having the apple pie, pair of shoes, or Candy Crush trophy. It's caused by the desire itself. It's an emotional stick to compel us to obey.

Our brain doesn't give a damn about the bigger picture, either. It cares nothing about how we're going to feel 30 pounds heavier or a few thousand dollars poorer. Its job is to identify promises of pleasure and then raise hell until we give in, even if pursuing those promises will entail risky, chaotic behavior likely to cause more problems than it's worth.

Ironically, the rewards can elude us every time, but even the slimmest possibility of payoff and the anxiety of giving up the quest can keep us hooked, sometimes to the point of obsession.

Anything we think will bring pleasure kicks this reward-seeking system into gear: the smell of the pizza, the Black Friday sale, the wink from the guy, or the advertisement for the handbag. Once dopamine has our brain in its grasp, obtaining the desirable object or doing the desirable thing can become a "do-or-die" proposition.

The dopamine problems don't end here, either.

Research shows that the dopamine release triggered by a promise of one type of reward can make us more likely to pursue others. For example, if a guy looks at pictures of naked women, he's more likely to make risky financial decisions.[9] If you dream about striking it rich, food can suddenly become very appetizing.[10]

This reward-seeking behavior is especially problematic in today's modern world, which in many ways is literally engineered to keep us always wanting more.

Netflix uses machine learning (artificial intelligence that learns and improves) to populate our home screens with the options we're most likely to want to watch.

Video game makers carefully craft experiences that can elevate dopamine to amphetamine-like levels, which explains a lot of the obsessive-compulsive behavior seen in gaming.[11]

Food scientists test hundreds of variations of products to find their "bliss points"— the precise amounts of key ingredients like sugar, salt, and fat needed to produce an explosion of flavor and delight in every bite.

Retailers design many aspects of our in-store experiences to entice us to buy more, from what we see when we enter to the way the aisles are arranged and shelves are stocked, to the scents pumped in the air, to the free samples offered, to the tempo of the music playing in the background, and more.

Just about everywhere we go, something screams "here's a reward!" to our brains. Constantly awash in dopamine, it's all too easy for us to feel like one big itch that always needs scratching.

When we consider how overtargeted and overstimulated our neurons really are, it's no surprise that the average person is an overweight procrastinator hooked on junk food, entertainment, and social media. It also means that it takes a rather dramatic shift away from "normal" behavior to escape from these traps.

If we're going to succeed in this brave new world (sorry, had to), we must learn to distinguish between the many toxic rewards dangled in front of us every day, and the genuine rewards that give us true fulfillment and meaning in our lives.

Let's return to the burger shop. Remember? You're in line, craving the thousand-calorie heap of fatty, cheesy bliss that you're about to consume in under two minutes (a new personal record).

Your mind clears for a moment, however, and you remember that you're on a diet. Losing the weight matters, too. You want to be fit, healthy, and happy. You swore on everything sacred (with a nod to everything slightly profane) that you would see it through this time.

When viewed in that context, the food you're about to eat poses a sort of threat to you. Your brain has a protocol for dealing with threats: fight or flight. Stress levels rise, but there's nothing to kill or escape from because this isn't a real threat. The cheeseburger can't force itself down your throat with a few handfuls of french fries in tow. It needs your cooperation. So in this way, you're the threat.

My point is we need protection from ourselves, not from diabolical ground beef and potato sticks, and that's what self-control is for. It's for relaxing the muscles, slowing the heart rate, elongating the breaths, and buying some time to think about what we really want to do next.

How do we get better at self-control, especially when it matters most?

A number of evidence-based strategies can help us, and in the next chapter, we're going to discuss the one that is arguably the most important.

KEY TAKEAWAYS

- Those with higher levels of willpower do better in school, earn more money, make better leaders, and are generally happier, healthier, and less stressed, have better social and romantic relationships, and tend to live longer.

- When we say someone has or lacks willpower, we're usually referring to their ability or inability to say no—they have trouble saying "I won't."

- "I will" power is the ability to do something when you don't want to, like crawling out of bed to grind through a workout, paying the overdue bill, or burning the midnight oil on that work project.

- "I want" is the ability to remember the why when temptation strikes—the long-term goal or thing you really want more than the fast food or night on the couch.

- Dopamine's role is to stimulate you to action, and it does this by arousing you, sharpening your focus, and revving up your drive to move toward the prize.

- Dopamine also triggers the release of stress hormones that make you feel anxious.

- The brain's job is to identify promises of pleasure and then raise hell until we give in, even if pursuing those promises will entail risky, chaotic behavior likely to cause more problems than it's worth.

- Anything we think will bring pleasure kicks this reward-seeking system into gear: the smell of the pizza, the Black Friday sale, the wink from the guy, or the advertisement for the handbag.

- The dopamine release triggered by a promise of one type of reward can make us more likely to pursue others.

- If we're going to succeed, we must learn to distinguish between the many toxic "rewards" dangled in front of us every day, and the genuine rewards that give us true fulfillment and meaning in our lives.

- Self-control is for relaxing the muscles, slowing the heart rate, elongating the breaths, and buying some time to think about what we really want to do next.

13

13 EASY WAYS TO BOOST YOUR WILLPOWER AND SELF-CONTROL

"Success consists of going from failure to failure without loss of enthusiasm."

—UNKNOWN

Nothing undermines willpower and self-control like the stresses of everyday living.[1]

The more stressed we generally feel, the more likely we are to overeat, overspend, and do the many other things we regret shortly thereafter.

Anything that causes stress, whether mental or physical, drains our supply of willpower and reduces our capacity for self-control. And anything we can do to reduce stress in our lives and improve mood improves our self-control.

How do most people try to cope with stress, though? What do they routinely turn to for consolation? Food, alcohol, video games, television, shopping, and surfing the internet are the usual suspects.[2]

Ironically, studies show that the same people using these strategies often rate them as ineffective for reducing stress levels.[3] In some cases, they rate them as stress inducing because indulging unhealthy and unproductive impulses leads to guilt, followed by more indulging, followed by more guilt, and so on.

Comfort food is particularly problematic because it spikes blood sugar levels to provide emotional reprieve, and then crashes them, which, like stress, is a precursor to willpower failures.[4] Research shows that when blood sugar levels are low, we're more likely to give up on difficult tasks, vent our anger, stereotype others, and even refuse to donate to charity.[5]

If we shouldn't turn to feel-good vices to feel better, what should we do instead?

An effective way to recover from the stresses of the "daily grind" is to deliberately relax. That's not surprising, of course, but it's not necessarily simple, either. For most people (myself included), it's a skill they have to learn.

A good way to measure stress levels in your body is to look at something called *heart rate variability*, which is how much your heartbeat speeds up and slows down as you breathe. The more stressed you are, the less variability there is in your heartbeat—the more it gets "stuck" at a faster rate.

This is why people who generally have a desirable amount of heart rate variability are also generally less stressed and display remarkably better self-control than those with less variability.[6]

For instance, a study conducted by scientists at the University of Kentucky found that people with more variability were more likely to resist temptations; less likely to develop heart disease, experience depression, and give up on difficult work; and better at dealing with trying situations.[7]

If you want to see this in action, the next time you face a willpower challenge, deliberately slow your breathing to about 10 to 15 seconds per breath, or four to six breaths per minute.

An easy way to do this is to exhale through your mouth slowly and fully with your lips pursed as if you were blowing lightly through a straw. By slowing down your breathing like this, you can increase your heart rate variability and instantaneously boost your willpower and ability to resist the effects of stress.[8]

Relaxation shouldn't be something you "turn on" only when you feel frazzled, however. Studies show that taking time to properly relax every day not only reduces stress hormones and increases willpower but helps preserve health as well.[9]

For many people, that means an evening of wine and Netflix, but a much better choice is an activity that elicits a specific type of physiological response.

When you're truly relaxed, your heart rate slows, your blood pressure drops, your muscles loosen, and your mind stops analyzing and planning. Everything just slows down.

Here are 13 simple and effective ways to enter this state.

1. YOU CAN ENJOY NICE SMELLS.

Aromatherapy is a couple-thousand-year-old method of reducing stress and promoting relaxation. It also has some modern scientific evidence on its side.

For instance, a study conducted by scientists at Asia University found that the scent of certain essential oils, like lavender, bergamot, chamomile, and geranium, can lower blood pressure, reduce anxiety, and improve sleep quality.[10]

The easiest way to incorporate this into a daily relaxation routine is to use a diffuser.

2. YOU CAN GIVE AND GET A MASSAGE.

I probably don't need to cite research to convince you that receiving a massage is a great way to relieve stress, but one rather interesting study conducted by scientists at the University of Oxford and ORYGEN Research Centre found that *giving* a massage has similar effects.[11]

That's right: make a deal with your significant other to trade massages before bed, and a whole lot of relaxation is probably going to occur.

The benefits of massage don't stop there, either. Studies show it also reduces pain, anxiety, and depression, and increases immunity as well.[12]

It doesn't take a lot to get the job done, either. Just 10 to 15 minutes of massage is enough to reap its many benefits.

3. YOU CAN HAVE MORE SEX.

If you're not having much sex these days, science says you should bump those rookie numbers up.

Why?

Because research shows that regular sex reduces anxiety, stress, and depression and improves mood, happiness, and resilience.

For example, a study conducted by scientists at Arizona State University had 58 middle-aged women record their sexual activity, physical affection, stressful events, and mood every morning for eight months.[13]

Researchers found that "physical affection or sexual behavior with a partner on one day significantly predicted lower negative mood and stress and higher positive mood on the following day."

A study conducted by scientists at Florida State University found that this "afterglow" effect of sex boosts mood and well-being for about 48 hours in most people.[14]

Sex can benefit you physiologically as well.

Research conducted by scientists at Michigan State University found that women who have more quality sex have a lower risk of heart disease, likely because of sex's positive effects on mood and stress.[15]

Interestingly, sex's many benefits seem to be greatest for couples who have been together the longest or are married, and mostly apply to traditional forms of intercourse.[16]

4. YOU CAN CHANGE YOUR PERCEPTION OF STRESS.

We know that high amounts of stress are associated with impaired mental and physical health and well-being, but there's a twist.

Research shows that our perception of stress as harmful is what really gives it teeth.[17] That is, getting overly stressed about stress is what really pushes us into the mud.

This is why a study conducted by scientists at the University of Denver found that if we can consciously reappraise stressful situations—choose to look at them differently—we can drain them of much of their destructive power.[18]

For instance, a frustrating situation doesn't have to be an excuse to rip your hair out. Instead, you can view it as an opportunity to exercise a virtue like patience, tolerance, or resilience. Similarly, a setback is also an opportunity for you to learn what doesn't work, and a painful situation can teach you that you're tougher than you thought.

This reappraisal strategy is far from new. Marcus Aurelius, one of Rome's most famous emperors, had it right a couple thousand years ago with his *Meditations*, which you need to read if you haven't already.

5. YOU CAN GET MORE SLEEP.

If you sleep too little too regularly, you'll find yourself more susceptible to stress and temptation and lacking the mental energy needed to keep your good habits in play and your bad ones at bay.

In fact, research shows that sleep deprivation causes symptoms similar to ADHD: distractibility, forgetfulness, impulsivity, poor planning, and hyperactivity.[19]

6. YOU CAN AVOID SCREENS BEFORE BEDTIME.

It's fairly well known these days that nighttime light exposure suppresses your body's production of *melatonin*, a hormone that induces sleepiness.[20] This not only makes it harder to fall asleep but also reduces the quality of the sleep you do get.

Melatonin suppression does more than just mess up your sleep, too. It has also been shown to impair immunity and increase the risk of cancer, type 2 diabetes, and heart disease.[21]

That said, completely eliminating all exposure to light once the sun goes down isn't exactly feasible. I doubt you're willing to "go dark" come 7 p.m. Fortunately, you don't have to.

First, light's melatonin-suppressing effects depend on intensity. The more intense the light, the more it suppresses melatonin levels.[22] Thus, a good rule of thumb is to keep light after dark as dim as possible, and sleep in complete darkness.

Second, the short-wavelength, "blue" light emitted by devices like televisions, computer screens, and smartphones is the real villain here because it suppresses melatonin production more than longer-wavelength, warmer light.[23]

Thus, reducing or eliminating your nighttime exposure to blue light is an effective way to preserve healthy levels of melatonin production.

How do you do this, though?

Banning the use of all electronics after sundown would work, of course, but again, that probably isn't going to happen. What you can do, however, is use free software like f.lux (www.justgetflux.com), which automatically adjusts the color of your device screens to the time of the day, eliminating blue light at night.

If you're using an iOS or Android device, you don't need special software for this—simply turn on the Night Shift (iOS) or Night Light (Android) feature.

And what about blue light exposure from other sources like ambient lighting or the television?

Research shows that amber-lensed glasses are great for dealing with this, and can result in improved mood and sleep.[24] A dorky solution, yes, but seriously useful for minimizing your exposure to blue light at night.

7. YOU CAN SPEND LESS TIME WITH TECH.

Staring at screens at night messes up your melatonin production, and it appears that staring at them too much in general can mess up your mind.

A number of studies have shown that the more people use and feel tied to their computers and cell phones, the more stressed they generally feel.[25]

In fact, a study conducted by scientists at the University of Gothenburg found that technology overuse is associated with a number of symptoms of poor mental health.[26] Here's a quick summary of their conclusions:

- People who used their cell phones heavily were more likely to complain of sleep disorders and depression.

- People constantly available on their cell phones were the most likely to experience mental health issues.

- People who regularly use the computer late at night were more likely to experience sleep disorders, stress, and depression.

- Frequent computer use without breaks increases the likelihood of stress, sleep problems, and depression.

Researchers aren't clear as to the causes just yet, but the relationship is unmistakable. The more time we spend with our devices, the worse our mental state will likely be.

8. YOU CAN LISTEN TO CLASSICAL MUSIC.

Next time you're stressed, put on some slow, quiet classical music, and before long, you'll be nestled in its soothing embrace.

(Some of my personal favorites are Max Richter, Ludovico Einaudi, Beethoven, and Bach.)

Mozart can do more than just chill you out, too. Several studies show that classical music can sharpen your mind, engage your emotions, lower blood pressure, lessen physical pain and depression, and help you sleep better.[27]

9. YOU CAN DRINK GREEN TEA.

I'm a big fan of tea and its many health benefits, and here's another reason to drink it regularly: it's a powerful stress buster.

Good evidence of this is a study conducted by scientists at the Tohoku University Graduate School of Medicine that found that regular green tea consumption is associated with lower levels of psychological distress.[28]

Researchers believe the primary way green tea accomplishes this is the high doses of the amino acid L-theanine and ascorbic acid, which have known anti-stress properties.[29]

10. YOU CAN GO FOR A WALK IN THE PARK.

When you review the daily routines of many of history's greatest thinkers and innovators, you'll quickly notice how many of them valued long walks in nature.

For example, Beethoven spent his afternoons walking in the Vienna Woods and found his best inspiration always came while walking. Tchaikovsky was equally adamant about his twice-a-day walks, which he felt were essential for his health and creativity. Thomas Jefferson advised his nephew that "there is no habit you will value so much as that of walking far without fatigue," and took regular walks around his Monticello estate well into old age.

Science shows they were onto something. In a study conducted by scientists at Heriot-Watt University, just 25 minutes of walking in an urban park was enough to noticeably reduce frustration and improve mood.[30]

11. YOU CAN TAKE A HOT BATH.

For thousands of years, hot baths have been used to ease pain, aid in relaxation, and ward off and treat disease.

In fact, the word *spa* comes from the Latin *sanus per aquam*—"health through water"—which was an ancient Roman remedy for battle-weary soldiers.

Modern medical research has confirmed that regular dips in hot water are indeed healthful and restorative.

For instance, a study conducted by scientists at Loughborough University found that an hour-long soak in a hot tub causes similar improvements in blood sugar control and other markers of metabolic health as an hour-long bike ride.[31]

(You can get even more relaxation from regular baths by adding essential oils!)

12. YOU CAN CONSUME LESS MEDIA.

This shouldn't come as a surprise to anyone, really, but research shows that exposing yourself to a constant barrage of bad news, scare tactics, and morbid reminders of your mortality increases the likelihood of overeating, overspending, and other willpower failures.[32]

If the world appears to be ripping apart at the seams, why should we care about keeping our own affairs in order?

By reducing our exposure to the daily dose of pessimism and fear-mongering, we can also reduce our stress levels.

13. YOU CAN EXERCISE REGULARLY.

Nothing seems to improve self-control in all aspects of our lives like exercise. If you want a willpower "quick fix," this is it.

Several studies show that regular exercise reduces cravings for both food and drugs, increases heart rate variability, makes us more resistant to stress and depression, and even optimizes overall brain function.[33]

Its effects are immediate, too, and it doesn't even take a lot to boost willpower. Studies show that just five minutes of low-intensity exercise outdoors is enough to improve your mental state.[34]

So the next time you're feeling too tired or short on time to work out, remember the bigger picture. Every workout you do replenishes your willpower and energy, even lighter ones like walks and bodyweight training.

Think of exercise as your "secret weapon" for staying on top of your game.

. . .

Most people think of stress as purely negative, assuming that it should be avoided at all costs. This is wrongheaded.

Like with exercise, our bodies were designed to handle stress. In fact, research shows that acute stress enhances immunity, which in turn accelerates recovery processes and increases resistance to infection.[35]

In many ways, regular bouts of stress are conducive to your overall health and well-being. Overdose on it, though, and the problems begin, because our bodies haven't learned how to effectively cope with *chronic* stress. This forces our body to remain on high alert, and causes us to age faster, become more susceptible to disease, and have increased levels of systemic inflammation.[36]

The solution, however, isn't to shy away from all forms of stress or numb ourselves to their effects, but to learn how to manage stress effectively. Rest and relaxation are powerful tools for this.

Like stress, their effects go deeper than most people realize, including altering genetic expression involved with inflammation, programmed cell death, and free radical neutralization.[37]

It's not a stretch to say that the overall quality and longevity of our lives is going to depend heavily on how well we can relax.

So let's get smart about how we relax.

Develop a relaxation routine that you follow like your diet and exercise regimens, and it probably won't take long for you to start noticing improvements in your happiness, productivity, emotional stability, and health.

Here's my personal routine:

1. A nightly hot bath with my wife.

We usually add essential oils and put on light classical music as well.

2. Sex at least two to three times per week.
I could pretend we're still going at it like crazed teenagers, but hey, this works for us.

In fact, research shows that sex just once per week is a sweet spot of sorts for happiness.[38] For most people, more frequent sex doesn't increase happiness, and less frequent sex results in less fulfillment.

3. In bed seven and a half to eight hours before my alarm.
My general sleep needs seem to be around six and a half hours per night, but since having kids, I don't sleep as well as I used to, so I have to give myself a buffer for one to three wakings.

4. Little to no "blue light" screens for at least one hour before bed.
This means minimal computer, tablet, TV, or smartphone use.
I do most of my reading on my phone, but when I read before bed, I use a Kindle Paperwhite, which doesn't emit blue light.

5. A pot of green tea every morning.
Genmaicha is my favorite.

6. Daily exercise.
I currently lift weights Monday through Friday and do about 30 minutes of biking on Saturdays and Sundays.

Think of stress management as the "nutritional" aspect of your willpower and self-control.

Minimizing the negative side effects of stress in your life not only helps you maintain a healthy level of self-possession but also opens the door to improvement through "exercising" your discipline.

And how do you do that—exercise and improve your resolve? Keep reading to find out!

KEY TAKEAWAYS

• Anything that causes stress, whether mental or physical, drains our supply of willpower and reduces our capacity for self-control. And anything we can do to reduce stress in our lives and improve mood, improves our self-control.

• The same people who use food, alcohol, television, shopping, and surfing the internet as coping strategies for stress often rate them as ineffective for reducing stress levels.

• The next time you face a willpower challenge, deliberately slow your breathing to about 10 to 15 seconds per breath, or four to six breaths per minute.

• Taking time to properly relax every day not only reduces stress hormones and increases willpower but helps preserve health as well.

• Aromatherapy is a couple-thousand-year-old method of reducing stress and promoting relaxation, and the easiest way to incorporate this into a daily relaxation routine is to use a diffuser.

• Both giving and receiving a massage can relieve stress, reduce pain, anxiety, and depression, and increase immunity.

• Regular sex reduces anxiety, stress, and depression and improves mood, happiness, and resilience.

• Our perception of stress as harmful is what really gives it teeth. That is, getting overly stressed about stress is what really pushes us into the mud.

• If you sleep too little too regularly, you'll find yourself more susceptible to stress and temptation and lacking the mental energy needed to keep your good habits in play and your bad ones at bay.

• Nighttime light exposure suppresses your body's production of melatonin, a hormone that induces sleepiness.

• A good rule of thumb is to keep light after dark as dim as possible, and sleep in complete darkness.

• Reducing or eliminating your nighttime exposure to blue light in particular is an effective way to preserve healthy levels of melatonin production.

• The more time we spend with our devices, the worse our mental state will likely be.

• Classical music can sharpen your mind, engage your emotions, lower blood pressure, lessen physical pain and depression, and help you sleep better.

- Green tea and walking—especially walking in nature—are powerful stress busters.

- Regular hot baths are healthful and restorative.

- Exposing yourself to a constant barrage of bad news, scare tactics, and morbid reminders of your mortality increases the likelihood of overeating, overspending, and other willpower failures.

- Regular exercise reduces cravings for both food and drugs, increases heart rate variability, increases resistance to stress and depression, and even optimizes overall brain function.

- In many ways, regular bouts of stress are conducive to your overall health and well-being.

- It's not a stretch to say that the overall quality and longevity of our lives is going to depend heavily on how well we can relax.

14

USE IT OR LOSE IT
HOW TO TRAIN YOUR WILLPOWER

"The greatest discovery of my generation is that you can change your circumstances by changing your attitudes of mind."

—WILLIAM JAMES

You've probably heard that willpower is like a muscle.

That it only has so much strength, and every time you "flex" it, it becomes a little bit weaker, until finally, it fails.

If that's true, it would also mean that you could train your "willpower muscle" like a physical one and make it stronger and more resistant to fatigue.

Scientists are still working to see how correct this hypothesis really is, but we all do seem to "run out" of self-control juice at some point, leaving us especially susceptible to temptation.[1]

This is one of the reasons why researchers have observed that, regardless of the types of tasks performed, people's self-control is at its highest in the morning and steadily declines as the day wears on.[2]

(You can use this knowledge to your advantage by doing your toughest and most unpalatable work and tasks, including working out, first thing in the day, when your will is strongest.)

There's also good evidence that we can indeed increase our overall willpower by "training" it with regular, small acts of self-control.

Studies show this can be accomplished in various ways, including eating fewer sweets, tracking spending, correcting our posture, refraining from swearing, squeezing a handgrip every day, and using our nondominant hand for various tasks.[3]

What we're really training here is what psychologists call the "pause-and-plan response," which involves pausing before we act, noticing what we're about to do, and choosing wisely.[4]

By doing this, we can better condition ourselves to successfully navigate the many irritating moments in life where we have to resist sweets, fight emotional impulses, ignore shiny distractions, compel ourselves to do things, and even make trivial purchase decisions, all of which seems to pull from the same willpower reserve.[5]

So, let's discuss several effective ways to consciously train our willpower and self-control in much the same way as we train our muscular and cardiovascular capacities.

DON'T FIGHT THE URGE, RIDE THE WAVE

You've just hit the couch after a long, tiring day, and your mind begins to wander.

Suddenly, a glowing pint of ice cream materializes, and your salivary glands snap to attention. *No*, you say to yourself, *anything but ice cream! Don't think about ice cream!*

The commands don't work, though. The harder you try to banish the vision of the cold, creamy dessert, the more it dominates your consciousness and nervous system. Finally, the only way to extinguish the desire is to spoon the stuff down your gullet.

The problem in this scenario isn't the fall into the quicksand, but rather the forceful attempt to escape. What should you have done instead?

Research shows that a willingness to think thoughts and feel feelings without having to act on them is an effective method of dealing with a wide variety of challenges, such as mood disorders, food cravings, and addiction.[6]

On the other hand, trying to suppress negative thoughts and feelings, like self-criticism, worries, sadness, or cravings, can lead to greater feelings of inadequacy, anxiety, and depression, and even overeating.[7]

In other words, instead of "fighting the urge," if you can "ride the wave" until it crests and peters out, cooler heads can prevail.

This isn't hard to do, either. When a disturbing thought or longing appears, face it calmly instead of trying to forcefully eject it from your mind. You don't have to contemplate its meaning or read into it. You just have to accept that it's there and play it down as something unimportant that will fade.

"Riding the wave" is particularly relevant to dieting, as research shows that the more you try to suppress thoughts about food, the more likely you are to struggle with cravings and binge eating.[8]

A much better strategy for dealing with hunger and cravings can be found in a study conducted by scientists at the University of Washington to help people smoke fewer cigarettes.[9]

The strategy starts with noticing and accepting the undesirable feelings. Then, remind yourself that while you may not always be able to control where your mind wanders, you can always control how you respond. Finally, before indulging in whatever has your eye, remember the goal that's at stake and why you committed to abstaining in the first place.

You can use this formula as a "surfboard" for riding out the waves of wish and want until they crash and dissolve.

A simple way to implement it in your life is to put a mandatory 10-minute wait time in place before you allow yourself to act on a craving or other impulsive urge to do something you know you shouldn't.

This may not seem like much time, but research conducted by scientists at Princeton University shows that it can make a big difference in how you perceive the situation.[10]

The wait not only gives you time to pause and reflect on the matter, but it also tarnishes the allure of immediate gratification. By pushing the reward just 10 minutes into the future, you can disarm its most effective weapon for undermining your intentions.

This strategy can be used to overcome "I will" challenges as well.

If you're dreading something you know you need to do, commit to doing it for 10 minutes and then decide whether to continue. Chances are, you'll find that once you're in motion, you'll want to keep going.

DO IT FOR (FUTURE) YOU

> "I want the works
> I want the whole works
> Presents and prizes and sweets and surprises
> Of all shapes and sizes
> And now
> Don't care how, I want it now
> Don't care how, I want it now"

Those words were sung by Veruca in *Willy Wonka and the Chocolate Factory*, and if you listen closely, you can hear millions of people softly singing along every day.

They want it all, and they want it now. Food, entertainment, money, love, abs, you name it. We live in the age of instant gratification, and it appears to be a race to the bottom.

The rub with rewards is this: the longer we have to wait for them, the less desirable they become. Economists refer to how much we "discount" a reward's value based on how long it will take to receive it as our *time preference*.

People with a high time preference discount heavily and care far more about immediate satisfaction than long-term rewards or consequences. Those with a low time preference, however, exhibit the opposite behaviors, caring more about future pleasure and foregoing immediate prizes to maximize it.

Some people discount the future more steeply than others, and studies show the higher someone's time preference is, the worse their self-control will be.[11] Because of this, they'll also be more likely to behave impulsively and have problems with addiction.

That helps explain why consumer credit card debt is soaring, why fast-food joints are far more profitable than gyms, and why millions of people still light up cigarettes every day. When it comes to the crunch, one bird   or Big Mac—in the hand is often worth many more in the bush.

Like most positive and meaningful things in life, fitness is very much an exercise (pun intended) in time preference.

How much discomfort are you willing to endure now to get that lean, toned, and sculpted body? How many immediate rewards are you willing to refuse in pursuit of larger, delayed ones? How well can you keep your eyes on the horizon?

One powerful way to lower our time preference and increase our chances for long-term success is to change how we view the nature of today's and tomorrow's rewards.

For example, if I gave you a $200 check postdated a couple of months from now and then tried to buy it back for $100 today, would you accept the deal? Probably not.

What if I gave you $100 now and tried to buy it back with a $200 postdated check? Would you make that deal? Again, probably not. Why is that?

Simple: we don't want to lose something we have, even if we're going to gain something of greater value later.

Psychologists refer to this as *loss aversion*, and it's a trap many would-be dieters in particular fall into.[12] When we're hovering over a doughnut, it sure seems a lot more desirable in the moment than a little extra weight loss at some indistinct point in the future.

We can turn this psychological quirk to our advantage, however, by reframing willpower challenges. Research shows that by thinking about the future reward at stake first and how giving in now will sacrifice progress toward it or some part of it, we can lower our chances of acting against our best long-term interests.[13]

For instance, when you face the prospect of putting down a few slices of piping hot pizza with all your favorite toppings—for the third time that week—you could take a moment to imagine having achieved your ideal body composition.

The more vividly you can experience this, the better. Really *feel* your rippling stomach, tighter thighs, and perky butt. Envision how your new clothes fit you, and how proud you are whenever you catch a glimpse of your new body in a reflection.

Then think about how digging into the pizza will mean giving all that up and watching your body bulge and bloat. Chances are the big grease wheel will suddenly look a lot less appetizing.

You can also institute the mandatory 10-minute wait we spoke about before indulging in an undesirable activity. If 10 minutes of waiting (and visualizing the long-term rewards at stake) isn't enough to squash the desire to indulge, then allow yourself to, but not before the 10-minute mark.

Another highly effective way to change your time preference is a strategy called *precommitment*, which entails taking action now to strengthen your dedication to a behavior and ward off any underhanded attempts at self-sabotage.[14]

Much like how Ulysses instructed his men to lash him to the mast of their ship to ensure he didn't fall prey to the beautiful songs of the sea Sirens, you too can create systems to protect you from your lower self.

With the right precommitment strategies, you can put safeguards in place that make it much harder to fail. These safeguards consist of anything you can do today that makes it difficult and uncomfortable to change your mind tomorrow.

By being proactive like this, you'll find it easier to keep your impulses and feelings under control and stay on course.

For instance, if you have trouble with procrastinating on the internet instead of working, you can download a program called Cold Turkey (www.getcoldturkey.com) that allows you to block specific websites and applications or turn your internet off altogether for a set period of time.

If sticking to a diet is your struggle, you can precommit by throwing out all tempting junk foods in the house and not rebuying them, preparing healthy lunches to bring to work every day, or putting money on the line on a website like www.dietbet.com.

If you want to precommit to exercising regularly, you can pay for an annual membership at your gym instead of going month-to-month, sign up for an online coaching service, or recruit a friend to join you in your journey.

Another tool that has helped many thousands of people precommit successfully to all kinds of goals is the website www.stickk.com.

Stickk allows you to set a goal and time frame, wager money, and decide what happens with it if you fail. (It could go to a charity, for example, or even an organization you don't like, which can be a stronger incentive.)

You can also designate a "referee" who will monitor your progress and confirm the truthfulness of your reports, and you can invite supporters to cheer you on.

LET'S ALL GET FAT AND JUMP OFF BRIDGES

According to several studies, just 10 percent of people eat enough fruit and vegetables to meet their bodies' most basic nutritional needs, and just 20 percent exercise enough to preserve their general health and well-being.[15]

What do they do instead?

32 percent eat fast food at least one to three times per week, 70 percent eat more sugar than they should, and 30 percent would rather do housework, file their tax returns, or clean out their garage than give time over to working out.[16]

Statistics like these are supposed to "scare us straight," but they can actually have the exact opposite effect because they remind us that "everyone else is doing it too." And when that's the case, how wrong can it really be?

Even if you're not inclined to think this way, don't assume you're immune to the underlying psychology. It's comforting to think that *we're* not like that, that *we* singularly chart our own courses in our lives, uninfluenced by how others think and act. This simply isn't true.

Extensive research shows that what others do—and even what we *think* they do—has a marked effect on our thoughts and behaviors whether we realize it or not, especially when the people we're observing are close to us.[17]

When we're not sure how to think or act, we tend to look at how other people think and act and follow along, even if subconsciously. We're all instinctively drawn to the idea that there's safety in numbers.

In the world of marketing, this effect is known as "social proof," and it's used in myriad ways to influence us. This is why customer reviews and testimonials are vital to every business ("if all these people say it's good, it must be good!"), why companies pay exorbitant sums to secure celebrity endorsements ("if David Beckham likes it, it must be good!"), and why media mentions are so powerful ("if *Forbes* has featured it, it must be good!").

This also occurs naturally in our everyday lives. Whenever we tell ourselves behaviors are acceptable because other people are doing them too, or because of how "normal" they are, we're using social proof.

According to research conducted by scientists at Dartmouth College, we can pick up anything from temporary solutions to long-term habits this way, and they can come from people we do and don't know, including even characters we see in movies.[18]

The reality is mindsets and habits are far more contagious than most of us realize. For example:

- Those with obese friends and family members are far more likely to become obese themselves.[19]

- The more a student believes that other students cheat on tests, the more likely they are to cheat (even if they're wrong).[20]

- The more people believe that others underreport income on their taxes, the more likely they are to cheat the IRS themselves.[21]

- The more teetotalers hang out with people who drink alcohol, the more likely they are to start drinking too.[22]

- The more nonsmokers hang out with smokers, the more likely they are to take up the habit.[23]

- The more time people spend with those who feel lonely, the more likely they are to feel lonely themselves.[24]

Even if overeating, drinking, or smoking isn't your thing, seeing others indulge in these vices can encourage you to give in to your impulses as well.[25]

Seeing someone overspend might subconsciously trigger you to overeat. Hearing about someone skipping class might help you justify skipping your workout. Reading about someone cheating on their partner might make it more acceptable for you to cheat on your diet.

We've all heard that we're the average of the five people we spend the most time with, and an abundance of scientific evidence says this is true to one degree or another for every single one of us.

Even if we don't directly adopt the negative attitudes, ideas, and behaviors of those we're around most, their mere presence will act on us in insidious ways, making it harder for us to do the things we want to do and become the people we want to be.

I've made the mistake of keeping a number of "toxic" people in my life for too long for one reason or another, and the blows and bruises I've suffered as a result have taught me that no matter how close you might have once been to someone or how interesting or "fun" they might be, there's a point where their fellowship is no longer worth the price.

Remember this when you begin your fitness journey, because such people are always the first to criticize and question it—and anything positive you might want to do, for that matter. I have a hardline policy for these types of folk—an abrupt and decisive parting of ways—but whatever you do, just don't let them stop you.

Fortunately, positive attitudes and behaviors are contagious as well. If we surround ourselves with people who are generally upbeat, uplifting, and possessed of higher than average willpower and self-control, we too can "catch" these traits.[26]

In fact, research shows that simply *thinking* about people with high levels of self-control can temporarily increase our willpower.[27]

So, whether you tend to struggle with diet and exercise compliance or not, you can make your life easier by doing three things:

1. Limit your exposure to instances of people failing willpower challenges.

    While this is generally good advice, watching others lose control can *increase* resolve in some people by prompting them to view such lapses as threats to long-term goals, not as tempting invitations to follow suit.[28] I happen to be one of these types of people. Other people's failures make me want to work harder to succeed, not waver and lose resolve.

    In fact, I view much of what most people consider "normal" as highly negative and undesirable. So much so that I believe that a reliable compass for decision-making is to first ask what "most" people would do in such a situation, and then considering the merits of doing the exact opposite.

2. Join forces with at least one person who's on the same path as you and making progress.

    You don't even have to physically make the journey together. Regular email check-ins can be enough to feed, and feed on, each other's success.

3. Read or listen to stories about how others have gotten fit. This is one of the reasons I interview men and women on my podcast who have used my programs, products, and services to transform their bodies and lives.

    I hear from listeners every week who write to tell me how motivating they find these interviews because they reinforce my promise that everyone listening—including you—can do it too.

THE TRAP OF BEING "GOOD" AND "BAD"

Have you ever told yourself that you were "good" when you did what you needed to do or stayed strong, but "bad" when you procrastinated or acted impulsively?

Have you ever used "good" behavior as permission to be "bad"?

Of course you have. Of course I have. Of course every human who has ever lived has.

Scientists call this *moral licensing*, and it can powerfully undermine our self-control. When we assign moral values to our actions, they become fodder for our desire to simply feel good (enough) about ourselves, even when we're sabotaging our long-term aims or harming others.

By being "good," we reckon, we "earn" the "right" to be a little (or a lot) "bad."

For example, if someone basks in the glow of having exercised and stuck to their meal plan for the day, they might find themselves oversleeping and overeating the next day while still feeling virtuous, guilt-free, and in control.

Interestingly, "good" behaviors that can justify the "bad" don't even have to be related. Studies show that shoppers who pass up a purchase are more likely to feel justified in splurging on indulgent foods; when reminded of their virtue, people tend to donate less to charity; and merely thinking about doing something good can increase the likelihood of immoral or excessive behavior.[29]

In an even stranger feat of mental contortion, when some people imagine what they could have done but didn't, they feel virtuous.[30] They could have eaten the entire cheesecake but only had a couple slices, or they could have skipped four workouts but only skipped three, or they could have bought the $2,000 suit but opted for the $700 one instead.

Just to illustrate how absurd moral licensing can get, can you figure out why, after adding healthier items to its menus, McDonald's began selling more Big Macs than ever?

According to research conducted by scientists at Baruch College, the mere opportunity to eat healthily gave people some of the satisfaction of actually doing it, which in turn permitted them to choose the cheeseburger.[31]

As you can see, the moment we feel an itch for moral permission to stray from our goals or standards, it's all too easy to find that emotional green light.

The irony, however, is that all these "licensed" harmful behaviors keep us from achieving what really matters—a fit body, a robust mind, a long life, a balanced budget, a completed project.

When we think this way, we're tricking ourselves into believing that squandering our health, money, time, effort, and opportunities is a "treat" to be "cherished," that self-subversion is okay so long as it *feels* okay. Who are we really kidding, though? Only ourselves.

To escape from this trap, we must first stop moralizing our behaviors. Instead of using fuzzy feelings of "right" and "wrong" and "good" and "bad" to guide our actions, we need to remember why we've committed to doing the hard things like exercising, following a meal plan, educating ourselves, sticking to a budget, and working overtime.

We need to view these actions as independent steps necessary for achieving the outcomes we desire, not as "good" behaviors that we can "cash in" for sins.

For our purposes here, remember that our goal isn't just good workouts or on-target eating. It's enjoying shopping for clothes again—especially for the breezy, summer, sleeveless stuff. It's throwing away the scale because you don't need it anymore. It's the surprise on people's faces when they haven't seen you in a while. It's the newfound intimacy in your love life.

In short, bingeing on chocolate and missing workouts aren't little "oopsies" that you can erase with the right thoughts. They're direct threats to your overarching objectives. Remember that when you come face to face with sticky willpower challenges.

THE CRYSTAL BALL OF DELUSION

Another favorite way for people to abandon their self-control is justifying their sins of the present with planned virtues of the future.

For example, research shows that simply planning to exercise later can increase the likelihood of cheating on a diet.[32] In another study, making a future commitment to volunteer three hours per week for a charity doubled people's likelihood of choosing to buy an extravagance like designer jeans over a practical item like an identically priced vacuum cleaner.[33] In yet another study, agreeing to tutor a fellow student decreased the amount of money that people donated to charity.[34]

This type of thinking not only smacks of moral licensing, but it also introduces another critical flaw into the mix: the assumption that we'll somehow make different decisions in the future than we do today.

"Today I'll eat more dessert," we might say, "but tomorrow I'll stick to my diet." Or "Today I'll skip my workout, but tomorrow I'll double up." Or "Today I'll binge on my favorite TV shows, but I won't watch any for the rest of the week."

Such optimism would be reasonable if we knew we could implicitly count on ourselves to follow through. But we both know that's not how it goes. When the future finally arrives, that noble, idealized version of ourselves is nowhere to be found, and the new burdens are more pressing than we imagined them to be.

What to do, then? Put it off again, of course, hoping that our savior will rescue us next time.

We simply give our future selves too much credit, counting on them to be able to do whatever we can't bring ourselves to do now. We're too quick to assume that we'll be more enthusiastic, energetic, willful, diligent, motivated, brave, morally strong—whatever—in a couple of days, weeks, or months, and often for no good reason in particular.

In this way, we burden Future Us with an impossible load of tasks and responsibilities.

Remember that Future You isn't some abstract entity whose emotions and desires will be radically different from Present You's. And when tomorrow comes, the chances of doing what you didn't do today are slim. More often than not, you're going to find yourself in the exact same state of mind, and you're going to respond in the exact same way.

This is why we can all benefit from improving our ability to connect our present actions with their future consequences.

Scientists call this *future self-continuity,* and research shows the better you can do it, the easier it'll be to get and stay in shape, and to do the many other creative, constructive things you want to do in your life.[35]

The following mental exercises found in research conducted by scientists at the University Medical Center Hamburg-Eppendorf, McMaster University, and Erasmus University are simple ways to improve your future self-continuity:[36]

You can think about how you will behave in the future.

Just thinking about the future—not even the rewards per se—can strengthen your willpower. Specifically, by imagining yourself in the future, doing what you should be doing or refraining from what you shouldn't be doing, you can increase your chances of success.

This has unlimited application. For example, if you're struggling to stick to a meal plan, you can imagine yourself shopping and eating differently, or if you're dreading the next day's workout, you can envision yourself getting it done despite how you feel, or if you're anxious about an upcoming holiday party where you're going to be surrounded by your favorite foods, you can picture yourself having a good time without being excessive.

You can write a letter to Future You.

In this letter, you should write about what you think Future You will be like, what your hopes for her are, what you're doing for her now that will pay off later, what she might say about Present You, and even what the consequences of failing now will mean for her down the line

If you want to make this more fun, use the website www.futureme.org, which allows you to write an email to yourself and choose a future date on which it will be delivered.

You can imagine Future You in vivid detail.

To do this, explore the future consequences of your current behaviors, both good and bad.

What will your Future Self look like if you don't commit to stopping the things you know you shouldn't be doing and starting the ones you know you should? What are the likely physical, mental, and emotional outcomes? Disease, regret, shame, ugliness, depression, and loneliness? Don't hold back.

And what if you do succeed in changing your ways in addition to continuing your current good behaviors? How will you look and feel? Will you be proud and thankful? What might your life be like? Again, explore the possibilities.

If you want a comprehensive, evidence-based, and guided method for doing this, check out the Self Authoring Program (www.selfauthoring.com) from Dr. Jordan Peterson.

Like physical exercise, the more you do these three drills, the stronger your future self-continuity will become, and the better you'll be able to deal with will-power challenges of all kinds, fitness-related and otherwise.

"OH, WHY NOT? I'M A LAZY IDIOT ANYWAY!"

What do people tend to do after a relatively minor misstep, like missing a workout or eating too many sweets?

Do they shrug it off and move on, or do they berate themselves, catastrophize the affair, and go whole hog?

Unfortunately, the latter is far more common. For many, the vicious cycle of slip up, regret, and splurge—called the *what-the-hell effect* by psychologists—seems inevitable and inescapable.[37]

This is how the extra handful of chips can become the whole bag, the nibbles of chocolate can continue until the entire bar is gone, and the glass of wine can be a prelude to the bottle … or two.

Whenever people confronted with a setback say to themselves, "I've already messed up, so what the hell," they're exhibiting this type of behavior. They give in, and then, to feel better, they indulge in earnest, which often triggers even worse feelings of shame and regret, which can lead to even bigger failures.

Well, I have good news for you: you're going to make mistakes in your fitness journey. You're going to eat too much at parties, skip workouts for no good reason, and give less than 100 percent sometimes.

Why is that good news? Because you have nothing to worry about.

Like most everything in life, you don't need to be anywhere near perfect to win in the fitness game. You just have to be good enough most of the time. Perfectionism isn't required, nor is it even desirable because it often makes the whole process more stressful than it needs to be.

So don't get down on yourself when you mess up. The "damage" is never as bad as you might think, and an abusive tirade of self-criticism will only make things worse.

For example, many people worry that they've "blown" their diets after a single instance of overeating, not realizing that the absolute amount of fat that they can gain from a single meal or day—no matter how much they've eaten—ranges from negligible in the case of a single "cheat meal" (a few ounces) to mildly irritating in the case of a day of feasting (0.5 to 1 pound).

Therefore, when you stumble (and you will), show yourself the same compassion and forgiveness that you would show a friend.

Research conducted by scientists at Carleton University and Duke University shows that this type of response in times of frustration and failure is associated with better willpower and self-control because it helps us accept responsibility for our actions and steam ahead, unfazed.[38]

NOTHING FAILS LIKE SUCCESS

Once we've set our sights on a goal, what do we crave most?

Progress, of course. We want to see positive change and forward movement, which, we hope, will give us the energy we need to keep going.

But that's not how it necessarily goes. Progress can cut both ways because the satisfaction it produces can become complacency, a powerful catalyst for weakening willpower.

Instead of reinvigorating us for another charge into the breach, progress can convince us that one step forward has earned us the privilege of taking two steps back.

This paradox has been demonstrated in a number of studies. For example, research conducted by scientists at the University of Chicago found that when people were led to believe they were closing in on their weight loss goals, they were 32 percent more likely to choose a chocolate bar for a snack over an apple.[39]

I've seen this many times over the years. All too often, people use weight loss progress as a license to loosen the dietary reins and hinder further progress.

How can we guard against the slackening effects of success?

According to another study conducted by the same team of scientists at the University of Chicago, we should avoid getting into the habit of patting ourselves on the back for all the work we've done.[40] Instead, we should view our wins as evidence of how important our goals are to us and how committed we are to seeing them through.

That is, we should look for reasons to keep going, not to slow down and take in the scenery.

This has been one of my personal "secrets" to success inside and outside the gym. I've always remained more focused on how much road I still have to travel to realize the future I want for myself and my family than on how far I've already come. I've always allowed myself to be contented, but never satisfied.

This has certainly increased the stress quotient in my life, but the payoff has been well worth it, and I don't just mean that in a financial sense. In fact, the nonfinancial rewards, which can be summed up in one word—self-actualization—mean a lot more to me than the money.

. . .

Human nature is full of paradoxes, and willpower and self-control are no exceptions.

We're drawn to both delayed and immediate gratification in the forms of long-term satisfaction and short-lived spurts of delight. We're inherently susceptible to temptation but also have the power to resist it. We're often juggling contradictory emotions like frustration, anxiety, and doubt intermingled with happiness, calm, and certainty.

We may or may not be able to fundamentally change ourselves through strengthening our willpower, but we certainly can improve our ability to conquer the demands of daily living with more mindfulness, effectiveness, and confidence.

In many ways, fitness is the ideal training ground for these virtues because its challenges and difficulties are fundamentally analogous to the obstacles and barriers we face everywhere else in our lives.

If you can develop the will to push through a punishing workout when every ounce of you wants to quit, to tackle dietary temptations large and small, and to successfully follow regimented diet and exercise plans, then chances are you'll also have what it takes to meet important deadlines, resist seductive invitations to overspend, and realize your greater ambitions for self-development and growth.

KEY TAKEAWAYS

- Regardless of the types of tasks performed, people's self-control is at its highest in the morning and steadily declines as the day wears on.

- We can increase our willpower by "training" it with regular, small acts of self-control.

- What we're really training when we exercise self-control is what psychologists call the "pause-and-plan response," which involves pausing before we act, noticing what we're about to do, and choosing wisely.

• A willingness to think thoughts and feel feelings without having to act on them is an effective method of dealing with a wide variety of challenges, such as mood disorders, food cravings, and addiction.

• Trying to suppress negative thoughts and feelings, like self-criticism, worries, sadness, or cravings, can lead to greater feelings of inadequacy, anxiety, depression, and even overeating.

• A successful strategy that's helped people cut back on smoking and other external coping mechanisms for stress and desire involves three steps: notice and accept the undesirable feelings, remind yourself that while you may not always be able to control where your mind wanders, you can always control how you respond, and remember the goal that's at stake and why you committed to abstaining in the first place.

• A simple way to implement this coping strategy in your life is to put a mandatory 10-minute wait time in place before you allow yourself to act on a craving or other impulsive urge to do something you know you shouldn't.

• If you're dreading something you know you need to do, commit to doing it for 10 minutes and then deciding whether to continue.

• People with a high time preference heavily discount the value of future rewards and care far more about immediate gratification than long-term consequences.

• People with a low time preference exhibit the opposite behaviors, caring more about future pleasure and foregoing immediate prizes to maximize it.

• Thinking about the future reward at stake first and how giving in now will sacrifice progress toward it or some part of it can lower your chances of acting against your best long-term interests.

• Another highly effective way to change your time preference is a strategy called precommitment, which entails taking action now to strengthen your position and commitment to a behavior and ward off any underhanded attempts at self-sabotage.

• Anything you can do today that makes it difficult and uncomfortable to change your mind tomorrow is going to help you keep your impulses and feelings under control so you can stay on course.

• What others do—and even what we think they do—has a marked effect on our thoughts and behaviors whether we realize it or not, especially when the people we're observing are close to us.

• Even if we don't directly adopt the negative attitudes, ideas, and behaviors of those we're around most, their mere presence will act on us in insidious ways, making it harder for us to do the things we want to do and become the people we want to be.

• If we surround ourselves with people who are generally upbeat, uplifting, and possessed of higher than average willpower and self-control, we too can "catch" these traits.

• You can make your life easier by limiting your exposure to instances of people failing willpower challenges, by joining forces with at least one person who's on the same path as you and making progress, and by reading or listening to stories about how others have gotten fit.

• Moral licensing refers to telling ourselves that by being "good," we reckon, we "earn" the "right" to be a little (or a lot) "bad."

• "Good" behaviors that can justify the "bad" don't even have to be related.

• Instead of using fuzzy feelings of "right" and "wrong" and "good" and "bad" to guide our actions, we need to remember why we've committed to doing the hard things like exercising, following a meal plan, educating ourselves, sticking to a budget, and working overtime.

• A favorite way for people to abandon their self-control is justifying their sins of the present with planned virtues of the future.

• We give our future selves too much credit, counting on them to be able to do whatever we can't bring ourselves to do now.

• Future self-continuity refers to our ability to connect our present actions with their future consequences.

• You can improve your future self-continuity by thinking about how you'll behave in the future, writing a letter to Future You, and imagining Future You in vivid detail.

• Whenever people confronted with a setback say to themselves, "I've already messed up, so what the hell," they're acting out the vicious cycle of slip up, regret, and splurge, or what psychologists call the what-the-hell effect.

• Like most everything in life, you don't need to be anywhere near perfect to win in the fitness game—you just have to be good enough most of the time.

• Many people worry that they've "blown" their diets after a single instance of overeating, not realizing that the absolute amount of fat that they can gain from a single meal or day—no matter how much they've eaten—ranges from negligible in the case of a single "cheat meal" (a few ounces) to mildly irritating in the case of a day of feasting (0.5 to 1 pound).

- When you stumble (and you will), show yourself the same compassion and forgiveness that you would show a friend.

- Progress can cut both ways because the satisfaction it produces can become complacency, a powerful catalyst for weakening willpower.

- We should view our wins as evidence of how important our goals are to us and how committed we are to seeing them through.

- In many ways, fitness is the ideal training ground for many of our most important virtues because its challenges and difficulties are fundamentally analogous to the obstacles and barriers we face everywhere else in our lives.

15

FINDING YOUR BIGGEST
FITNESS WHYS

"Be first and be lonely."
—GINNI ROMETTY

People with vague, unrealistic, or uninspiring fitness goals (or none at all) are always the first to quit.

These people are easy to spot too. They show up to the gym sporadically to sleepwalk through workouts, barely breaking a sweat. They constantly complain about how situations and circumstances "made" them fall off the wagon (pesky office potlucks!). They're always on the lookout for the newest fads and magic bullet fixes.

If you're going to succeed where the masses fail, if you're going to get into the best shape of your life and become a paragon of health and fitness, you need to inoculate yourself against these attitudes and behaviors, and that's why we're going to do a little soul-searching in this chapter.

Different people have different reasons for eating well and working out. Some like to push their bodies to the limit. Others just want to impress the opposite (or same) sex. Many want to boost their confidence and self-esteem. Most want to improve their general health and well-being.

These are all perfectly valid reasons to get fit—looking great, feeling great, having high energy levels, being more resistant to sickness and disease, living longer, and so forth—but it's important that you isolate and articulate *your* reasons.

In the last chapter, you learned about the power of visualizing your future, and how doing so can greatly enhance your ability to navigate your life more skillfully.

Let's put this into practice right now, starting with the dimension of fitness that most people find most alluring: the visual.

WHAT DOES YOUR IDEAL BODY LOOK LIKE?

Let's face it: a major reason why you're reading this book is you want to look a certain way. And there's nothing wrong with that.

Every single fit person I know—including myself—is motivated just as much by the mirror as anything else, if not more so. I value my health, but I'd be lying if I said I didn't care about how I look nearly as much as the many other benefits of regular exercise.

Don't mistake that for narcissism, either. There are plenty of self-absorbed fitness twits out there, but I don't see anything wrong with playing a bit to our vanity if looking great also helps us feel great (and it does).

So, let's talk about you. What does *your* ideal body look like?

I want us to go beyond trite words and hazy daydreams, too. I want us to establish this visually and precisely by finding a picture or two (or three or four!) of exactly what you want to look like. Then, I want you to save these pictures somewhere that's easily accessible, like your phone or Google Drive or Dropbox.

In other words, when you're on my *Thinner Leaner Stronger* program, I want you to feel that you're working toward a very real, very sexy body that's as concrete as the page you're reading, not an imaginary physique that could be described as "toned" or "defined."

If you already know where to go to find pictures of the type of body you really want, go collect them now. If you don't, head over to my "Great Female Physiques" board on my Pinterest (www.pinterest.com/mikebls/great-female-physiques), and you'll find a large gallery of fit women of all types to choose from.

WHAT DOES YOUR IDEAL BODY FEEL LIKE?

This question asks you to explore one of the many "hidden" benefits of fitness.

Few people are aware of it when they begin their transformations, but a fit, healthy body is far more pleasurable to inhabit than an unfit, unhealthy one.

The more in shape you are, the more you get to enjoy higher energy levels, better moods, more alertness, clearer thinking, fewer aches and pains, and higher-quality sleep, to name just a few of the advantages.

And then there's the deeper stuff like more self-confidence and self-esteem, more productivity and self-fulfillment, and more intimate and satisfying relationships.

I want you to take a few minutes now to imagine what this will be like for you, and then write it all down in the form of individual affirmations.

In case you're not familiar with affirmations, they're positive statements that describe how you want to be, like, "I'm full of energy all day" and "My mind is always quick, clear, and focused."

This might seem a bit woo-woo, but research shows that writing and reading affirmations can benefit you in several ways. For example, a study conducted by scientists at the University of Pennsylvania found that people who practiced affirmations exercised more than people who didn't, and research conducted by scientists at the University of Sussex found that performing self-affirmations improved working memory and cognitive performance.[1]

For the sake of completeness, you can organize your health and fitness affirmations into four broad categories:

- Physical
- Mental
- Emotional
- Spiritual

Physical affirmations are all about bodily function and physical energy levels, and they can include statements like, "I wake up rested every day," "My joints are pain-free," and "I rarely get sick."

Mental affirmations concern your mind's ability to remember and compute and your ability to focus on the present and tune out the "noise." They can include statements like, "I can focus deeply on the task at hand," "My memory is sharp," and "I can control my thoughts."

Emotional affirmations relate to your feeling of positive or negative sensations, and they can include statements like, "I find joy everywhere I go," "I bounce back quickly from bad news," and "I give and receive love openly."

Spiritual affirmations involve your sense of purpose and motivation, and they can include statements like, "I'm driven to build the body of my dreams," "I feel I'm on the right path," and "I know I will succeed."

Here are a few pointers for writing more effective affirmations:

- Keep your affirmations short so they're easier to process and remember.

Even four or five carefully chosen words can be powerful.

- Start your statements with "I" or "My."

Affirmations are all about you, so it's best to start with you. "I have no aches or pains in my joints" is much better than "The aches and pains in my joints have disappeared."

- Write your affirmations as though you're experiencing them right now, not in the future.

For example, "I fall asleep quickly and wake up feeling rejuvenated" is superior to "I will fall asleep quickly and wake up feeling rejuvenated" or "Within three months, I'm falling asleep quickly and waking up feeling rejuvenated."

- Don't begin your statements with "I want" or "I need."

You don't want to affirm needing or wanting, but *being*.

- Make sure your affirmations are positive statements.

In many cases, realizing your affirmations will require discarding negative behaviors and thoughts, but you don't want your statements to reflect this.

Think, "I'm calm, confident, and contented" and not "I'm no longer anxious and insecure," and "I wake up on time every day feeling refreshed" instead of "I don't sleep in anymore."

- Inject emotion into your affirmations by including, "I'm [emotion] about . . ." or "I feel [emotion]."

For example, you could say, "I'm excited to do my daily workouts."

- Create affirmations that are believable.

If you don't think your statement is possible, it won't have much of an effect on you, so make sure you can fully buy into it.

If you find a certain affirmation particularly incredible, you can start with a qualifier like, "I'm open to . . ." or "I'm willing to believe I could . . ."

So, are you ready to write your affirmations? Take as long as you need! I'll be here when you're done!

WHAT ARE YOUR WHYS?

One of my favorite things about being fit are the moments where you just stop for a second and think, "Wow, it's awesome I did that with my body."

These are the things that put a smile on your face and a spring in your step, and sometimes even make your day.

I'm not talking about stuff like "turning heads in the coffee shop" but rather "having my doctor ask me for fitness advice", "feeling way more productive," and "keeping up with my kids without getting tired." The small but meaningful things that confirm you're on the right track.

I've worked with thousands of women over the years, and here are a few examples of the fitness wins they've shared with me:

- Getting asked for advice in the gym

- Enjoying clothing shopping more
- Feeling sexier naked
- Surprising friends, family members, and colleagues with a hot new body
- Eating desserts guilt-free
- Looking fantastic in yoga pants
- Setting a good example for their kids
- Enjoying outdoor activities again
- Staying fit while pregnant
- Losing their postpregnancy baby weight

I love these. They're real, specific, and meaningful, and they're great examples of the more sincere and personal reasons to get into great shape.

How about you? Why do you want to achieve everything you just laid out in your affirmations?

Maybe you want to boost your confidence? Play sports better? Be more attractive? Enjoy the overcoming of physical barriers? Be more active with your kids? Avoid disease? Stay active well into your retirement years? Slow down the processes of aging and retain a youthful vitality? Just have a body that works the way it's supposed to? Heck, beat your male friends in arm-wrestling matches?

Brainstorm your reasons for getting in shape and write them down until you feel pumped up and ready to get into action, because in the next part of this book, you're going to learn how to use my *Thinner Leaner Stronger* program to make all your reasons a reality.

. . .

Remember the work you've done here whenever you need a pick-me-up, and it'll help you find the power to persevere.

Recall it when you're feeling too tired to train, when you're out with friends watching them stuff and drink themselves silly, when sugary treats are cooing your name, and when you roll out of bed in the morning like a log off a truck.

Regularly look at the pictures you've saved, read the affirmations you've written, and review the whys you've formulated, and you'll always feel a wind in your sails, propelling you ever closer to your best body ever.

And then, once you've achieved everything you've created here, repeat the process anew, charting another more exciting course for the next phase of your fitness and life.

To help get you there as quickly as possible, we must now return to the "outer game" and learn once and for all how to use food, exercise, and supplementation to transform your body and mind.

KEY TAKEAWAYS

- People with vague, unrealistic, or uninspiring fitness goals (or none at all) are always the first to quit.

- Different people have different reasons for eating well and working out—but it's important that you isolate and articulate your reasons.

- Establish what your ideal body looks like visually and precisely by finding a picture or two (or three or four!) of exactly what you want to look like and saving these pictures somewhere that's easily accessible, like your phone or Google Drive or Dropbox.

- Take a few minutes to imagine what it'll be like to be in the best shape of your life, and then write it all down in the form of individual affirmations.

- Affirmations are positive statements that describe how you want to be, like, "I'm full of energy all day" and "My mind is always quick, clear, and focused."

- You can organize your health and fitness affirmations into four broad categories: physical, mental, emotional, and spiritual.

- Physical affirmations are all about bodily function and physical energy levels, and they can include statements like, "I wake up rested every day," "My joints are pain-free," and "I rarely get sick."

- Mental affirmations concern your mind's ability to remember and compute and your ability to focus on the present and tune out the "noise." They can include statements like, "I can focus deeply on the task at hand," "My memory is sharp," and "I can control my thoughts."

- Emotional affirmations relate to your feeling of positive or negative sensations, and they can include statements like, "I find joy everywhere I go," "I bounce back quickly from bad news," and "I give and receive love openly."

- Spiritual affirmations involve your sense of purpose and motivation, and they can include statements like, "I'm driven to build the body of my dreams," "I feel I'm on the right path," and "I know I will succeed."

- Brainstorm your reasons for getting in shape and write them down until you feel pumped up and ready to get into action.

- Remember the work you've done here whenever you need a pick-me-up, and it'll help you find the power to persevere.

PART 4

THE LAST DIET ADVICE YOU'LL EVER NEED

16

WELCOME TO THE WONDERFUL WORLD OF FLEXIBLE DIETING

If you dread the idea of "dieting," I understand. Most diets feel more like self-denial than self-improvement.

Instead of educating you on how your metabolism works and giving you the tools you need to manage it effectively, most diets resort to browbeating, fear-mongering, and food restriction instead.

If you want to lose fat or build lean muscle, they say, you can kiss just about everything you like to eat goodbye. Grains, gluten, sugar, high-glycemic carbs, red meat, processed foods, dairy, caloric beverages—it's all gotta go. All your toys. Throw them all into the fire.

Maybe I'm not up to this, you might think as you contemplate starting such a program. *Maybe I'm not tough or dedicated enough. Maybe that beach body isn't really worth it ...*

Thinner Leaner Stronger isn't one of those kinds of programs, and I'm here to tell you that yes, you *are* up to it, you absolutely have what it takes, and looking better than you ever have before is worth far more than you probably realize.

To prove it, I'm going to teach you how to follow the easiest and most effective approach to dieting in the world: *flexible dieting*.

With flexible dieting, you can dramatically transform your body eating foods you want to eat, every day, seven days per week. All you have to do is follow a handful of simple guidelines, not starve or deprive yourself.

Even better, once you experience the power of flexible dieting firsthand, you'll thrill at the realization that you're now immune to the diet frustrations and anxieties plaguing most people, and that you're finally free to develop a positive, healthy relationship with food.

A big promise, I know, but I'm going to deliver on it in spades. Let's begin, shall we?

PUTTING DIET INTO PERSPECTIVE

How important is your diet to achieving your health and fitness goals?

Some people say it's everything. Others say it's not as important as exercise, genetics, or some other factor. Still others say it's 70, 80, or 90 percent of the game.

Well, I say it's 100 percent. And progressively overloading your muscles? That's also 100 percent. Having the right attitude is 100 percent too. And let's not forget getting adequate rest and sleep, because that's also 100 percent. (I know, we're at 400 percent so far . . .)

My point is this: the building blocks of a great body are more like pillars than puzzle pieces. If you weaken one enough, the whole structure collapses.

Your body won't positively adapt to your training if you don't support it with proper nutrition. You can't gain much muscle or strength if you don't train correctly. Your progress will be lackluster if you don't have the right attitude. Your workout performance will suffer if you don't maintain good sleep hygiene.

That's why I want you to go all-in on achieving your fitness goals. I want you to give 100 percent in each part of my program and achieve 100 percent of the potential results. Let other people train at just 60 percent, diet at just 30 percent, and give just 20 percent of their spirit. They're going to make you look that much better.

Arbitrarily assigned values aside, here's the practical answer to how important diet is in your fitness journey: your diet either works for or against you, multiplying or dividing the bottom-line results you get from your training.

No matter how much you get right in the gym, you'll never be fully satisfied with the results unless you also get things right in the kitchen. This is why so many people spend so much time exercising yet look like they've never even seen a barbell or bicycle, let alone touched one.

You can think of diet as a series of tollbooths along the highway of fat loss and muscle gain. Training moves you forward, but if you don't stop and pay your dues, you don't get to go any further.

Another helpful perspective on the relationship between diet, training, and body composition is this: diet is primarily how you lose fat, maintain a desirable body fat level, and boost muscle growth, and training is primarily how you gain and maintain muscle mass.

Many people get this mixed up and think that working out is mostly for calorie and fat burning, and thus fall into a frustrating and ultimately fruitless cycle of doing a lot of grueling exercise just to keep pace with all their eating.

If you've been there before or are there now, then I have very good news for you: it all ends here.

Soon, you're going to experience a whole new approach to diet and exercise that will make losing fat, building muscle, and staying healthy easier than ever before.

Soon, you're going to realize that you've finally found the answers you've been looking for.

THE FOUR PRINCIPLES OF FLEXIBLE DIETING

What kind of "diet" worth a damn has you be less strict about the foods you eat?

How can you possibly lose fat eating bucketfuls of carbs every day?

Which self-respecting "dieter" would dare eat candy or fast food with a clean conscience?

Such questions represent some of the common criticisms of flexible dieting. Much of the controversy stems from the fact that it means different things to different people.

So, for the sake of thoroughness, let's start with an outline for flexible dieting the *Thinner Leaner Stronger* way:

1. How much you eat is more important than what you eat.

2. You should eat foods that you like.

3. The majority of your calories should be nutritious.

4. You should eat on a schedule that works for you.

Basically, my approach to flexible dieting is a way to take your body's basic energy and nutritional needs and turn them into an eating regimen that you actually enjoy. It's about turning your diet into a lifestyle rather than a quick fix.

Let's take a closer look at each of these principles.

1. HOW MUCH YOU EAT IS MORE IMPORTANT THAN WHAT YOU EAT.

This refers to the prominence of energy balance (calories) and macronutrient balance (protein, carbohydrate, and fat).

Food choices do matter (more on that in a minute), but not for the reasons most people are told.

In short, this principle comes down to just two things:

1. Manipulating your calorie intake to lose, maintain, or gain weight as desired

2. Manipulating your protein, carbohydrate, and fat intake to optimize your body composition

Once you can do those two things well, you can gain complete control of your physique.

2. YOU SHOULD EAT FOODS THAT YOU LIKE.

No matter how perfect a diet might look on paper, if you can't stick to it, it's not going to work for you. Period.

That's why flexible dieting is a blessing for so many people. When you can eat foods you actually like, including indulgences, you never quite feel like you're "on a diet."

Instead of depriving yourself for months and then flaming out in a spell of gluttonous bingeing, you get to enjoy yourself along the way, heading hunger and cravings off before they can cause problems.

From time to time, you might be eating fewer or more calories than you'd like (depending on your goals), but on the whole, most people find that flexible dieting is a smooth, painless experience. Eventually, "diet" even loses its four-letter-word status.

That said, if you've spent any time in fitness circles on social media, you might think flexible dieting is all about eating copious amounts of junk food while still having abs.

This is foolish. Just because you can get ripped eating like a 12-year-old doesn't mean you should, and just because someone has low body fat levels or big biceps doesn't mean they're healthy.

There's far more to food than just calories and macros—it also provides our bodies with dozens of vital micronutrients that are needed to keep us healthy, happy, and performing our best.

That's why ...

3. THE MAJORITY OF YOUR CALORIES SHOULD BE NUTRITIOUS.

Will hitting the drive-thru or pizza joint every now and then or eating a bit of sugar or "empty calories" here and there hurt you in the long run? Decidedly not.

But will allotting a large portion of your daily calories to nutritionally bankrupt fodder? Absolutely.

Slowly but surely, you'll develop nutritional deficiencies that can lead to all kinds of health problems, impair mental and physical performance, and even blunt muscle gain by interfering with your body's ability to recover from your workouts.

In that sense, "clean eaters" get a lot right. They may not understand why it seems so hard to lose fat and gain muscle, but they do understand the importance of nourishment.

Hence, this third flexible dieting rule of thumb: You should get at least 80 percent of your daily calories from nutritious, relatively unprocessed foods.

In other words, most of what you eat should consist of whole foods that you clean, cut, and cook yourself, like lean protein, fruits, vegetables, whole grains, legumes, nuts, seeds, and oils. Then, if you feel so inclined, you can fill your remaining calories with your favorite treats.

A major reason why eating like this is so healthy is it provides your body with enough fiber, which is an indigestible type of carbohydrate found in many types of plant foods.

Fiber comes in two forms:

1. Soluble fiber
2. Insoluble fiber

Soluble fiber dissolves in water and tends to slow the movement of food through the digestive system.

Research shows that soluble fiber is metabolized by bacteria in the colon, and can increase fecal output by stimulating the growth of healthy intestinal bacteria and fatty acids.[1] Because of this, soluble fiber is an important source of fuel for the colon.[2]

Good sources of soluble fiber include beans; peas; oats; certain fruits like plums, bananas, and apples; and certain vegetables like broccoli, sweet potatoes, and carrots.

Insoluble fiber doesn't dissolve in water and bangs against the walls of the intestines, causing damage that must be repaired. Research shows this process stimulates cellular regeneration and helps maintain intestinal health and function.[3]

Good sources of insoluble fiber include whole-grain foods like brown rice, barley, and wheat bran; beans; certain vegetables like peas, green beans, and cauliflower; and the skins of some fruits like plums, grapes, kiwis, and tomatoes.

The importance of fiber in the diet has been known for a long time. For instance, the ancient Greek physician Hippocrates, who famously said, "Let food be thy medicine, and medicine be thy food," recommended whole-grain breads to patients to improve bowel movements.

Modern science has found that fiber is good for a lot more than that. In fact, the evidence is pretty clear at this point that eating enough fiber is vital to reducing the risk of many types of disease, including heart and respiratory disease, cancer, infection, and type 2 diabetes, and to generally living a longer, healthier life.[4]

This is why the Academy of Nutrition and Dietetics recommends that children and adults consume 14 grams of fiber for every 1,000 calories of food eaten.[5]

This is easy to do if you follow my flexible dieting guidelines. In fact, it'll happen naturally because, as you've just learned, the best sources of fiber are the nutritious plant-based foods that you should be eating plenty of every day.

4. YOU SHOULD EAT ON A SCHEDULE THAT WORKS FOR YOU.

When you eat doesn't matter nearly as much as many people believe. On the whole, so long as you're sticking to your daily numbers, meal timing isn't going to make much of a difference one way or the other.

There are some unique benefits to preworkout, postworkout, and prebed nutrition that you'll learn about soon, but the bottom line is you can get the body you want eating three or eight meals a day, eating a large breakfast or skipping it, and eating as much or little at night as you'd like.

. . .

Every so often, a new spate of headlines hits the shelves and airwaves proclaiming that "diets don't work."

According to one "expert" or study or another, we're told that no matter what people do, if it qualifies as "dieting," chances are it won't result in significant and long-term weight loss.

Heck, you may have even concluded this yourself based on your own experiences.

Well, the real problem isn't that "dieting" doesn't work, but that most diets suck.

Most have you eat too few calories, which leaves you feeling miserable; most have you eat far too little protein, which accelerates muscle loss; most severely restrict the foods you can eat, which is impractical and irritating; and most provide no off-ramp to help you successfully return to normal eating, which makes it easy to regain any fat you lost.

That's why a new approach to dieting is needed. One that sets you up for a guaranteed win, both physically and psychologically.

That new approach is *Thinner Leaner Stronger's* flexible style of dieting, and once you've gotten a taste (figuratively and literally), I think you'll never look back.

KEY TAKEAWAYS

- With flexible dieting, you can dramatically transform your body eating foods you want to eat, every day, seven days per week. All you have to do is follow a handful of simple guidelines, not starve or deprive yourself.

- Diet is primarily how you lose fat, maintain a desirable body fat level, and boost muscle growth, and training is primarily how you gain and maintain muscle mass.

- Once you can manipulate your calorie intake to lose, maintain, or gain weight as desired and manipulate your protein, carbohydrate, and fat intake to optimize your body composition, you can gain complete control of your physique.

- No matter how perfect a diet might look on paper, if you can't stick to it, it's not going to work for you.

- There's far more to food than just calories and macros—it also provides our bodies with dozens of vital micronutrients that are needed to keep us healthy, happy, and performing our best.

- You should get at least 80 percent of your daily calories from nutritious, relatively unprocessed foods.

- Most of what you eat should consist of whole foods that you clean, cut, and cook yourself, like lean protein, fruits, vegetables, whole grains, legumes, nuts, seeds, and oils.

- A major reason why eating like this is so healthy is it provides your body with enough fiber, which is an indigestible type of carbohydrate found in many types of plant foods.

- Good sources of soluble fiber include beans; peas; oats; certain fruits like plums, bananas, and apples; and certain vegetables like broccoli, sweet potatoes, and carrots.

- Good sources of insoluble fiber include whole-grain foods like brown rice, barley, and wheat bran; beans; certain vegetables like peas, green beans, and cauliflower; and the skins of some fruits like plums, grapes, kiwis, and tomatoes.

- Children and adults should consume 14 grams of fiber for every 1,000 calories of food eaten, which is easy to do if you follow my flexible dieting guidelines.

- On the whole, so long as you're sticking to your daily numbers, meal timing isn't going to make much of a difference one way or the other.

17

THE EASIEST WAY TO CALCULATE YOUR CALORIES AND MACROS

"You are right to be wary. There is much bullshit. Be wary of me too, because I may be wrong. Make up your own mind after you evaluate all the evidence and the logic."

—MARK RIPPETOE

Imagine someone tells you that she wants to drive across the country without paying attention to her gas tank.

She plans on stopping for gas whenever and wherever she feels like stopping, and pumping as much or as little gas as she feels like pumping.

How would you respond? You'd probably think she's nuttier than squirrel crap, right?

What if she picked up on that and snapped back with something like, "I hate feeling like a slave to the oppressive fuel meter. I should be able to drive as far as I want before refueling!"

Or "There has to be a better way. Who wants to constantly keep an eye on how much gas is left in their tank?"

Or "I read this book that said you don't have to watch how much gas you have left if you use organic, gluten-free, low-carb, non-GMO gasoline."

What would you do then? Gather up your toys and go play with someone else, right?

My point? When someone says they want to lose (or gain) weight without paying attention to their calories, or says that energy intake and expenditure have nothing to do with their weight, they're being just as silly.

Is it possible to lose weight without watching your calories? Sure. Is it likely to work well over the long term for most people? Absolutely not.

It takes a high intuitive awareness of how many calories you're eating and burning to make it work, and even then, it gets difficult as you get leaner and your body's natural desire for more food rises.

This is why you need to learn how to calculate how many calories you should be eating every day. From there, you can easily create meal plans that all but guarantee fat loss and muscle gain.

There are just three simple steps to figuring out how many calories you should eat every day:

1. Calculate your basal metabolic rate.

2. Calculate your total daily energy expenditure.

3. Calculate your target daily calorie intake.

Let's start with step one.

1. CALCULATE YOUR BASAL METABOLIC RATE.

Your basal metabolic rate (BMR) is the amount of energy your body would burn if you were to lie motionless for a day, without food. In other words, it's the minimum amount of energy it costs to stay alive for 24 hours.

It's called this because *basal* means "forming a base, fundamental."

Unless you're extremely active, your BMR constitutes the majority of your energy expenditure. Your brain alone burns about 10 calories per hour, for instance. This is why keeping your metabolism functioning optimally is a big part of successful weight loss and maintenance.

For example, I'm 34 years old and weigh 195 pounds, and my BMR is about 2,100 calories. I say "about" because you can never truly know how many calories you're burning every day without doing fancy lab tests.

Fortunately, you don't need to do that to achieve your goals. You just need to do some simple arithmetic to get a good enough guesstimate.

There are a number of mathematical formulas you can use to calculate your BMR.

The one I like most for our purposes here is known as the Mifflin-St. Jeor equation, which was introduced in 1990 by scientists from the University of Nevada to address some of the shortcomings of an older formula, the Harris-Benedict equation.[1]

Here's the Mifflin-St. Jeor equation for women:

BMR = 10 x weight (in kilograms) + 6.25 x height (in centimeters) – 5 x age (in years) – 161

If that looks like Greek to you, don't worry—all you have to do is solve from left to right, like this:

1. Multiply your weight in kilograms by 10.

2. Multiply your height in centimeters by 6.25.

3. Add these two numbers together.

4. Multiply your age in years by 5.

5. Subtract the result from the sum of steps 1 and 2.

6. Subtract 161 from the result.

Let's see how this plays out for a 160-pound woman who's 5 feet and 7 inches tall and 41 years old.

First, she needs to convert her weight into kilograms, which is accomplished by dividing the number of pounds by 2.2. So, 160 / 2.2 = 72.7, which we'll round up to 73 kilograms.

Then, she needs to multiply this by 10: 73 x 10 = 730.

Next, she needs to convert her height into centimeters, which is accomplished by multiplying the number of inches by 2.54. So, 67 x 2.54 = 170 centimeters.

Then, she needs to multiply this by 6.25: 170 x 6.25 = 1,062.

Next, she needs to add these two numbers together: 730 + 1,062 = 1,792.

After that is multiplying her age in years by 5 (41 x 5) and subtracting the result from the sum above: 1,792 - 205 = 1,587.

And last is subtracting 161 from that number: 1,587 - 161 = 1,426.

Thus, this woman's BMR is approximately 1,400 calories.

Want to know yours? Take a break and calculate it now! You'll need to know it soon anyway.

If math really isn't your forte, you can find a handy-dandy
BMR calculator on my website.
Go to www.thinnerleanerstronger.com/calculator.

2. CALCULATE YOUR TOTAL DAILY ENERGY EXPENDITURE.

Your total daily energy expenditure (TDEE) is exactly what it sounds like: the total number of calories you burn every 24 hours.

Your TDEE consists of your BMR plus all additional energy burned during physical activity and digesting and processing the food you eat.

"Eating food burns energy?" you might be wondering.

Yes ma'am, food costs energy to digest, process, and absorb, and different types of foods cost more energy than others.

Technically speaking, this is known as the *thermic effect of food*, or TEF, as well as *thermogenesis*, and research shows that it accounts for approximately 10 percent of TDEE.[2]

In this way, your metabolism does "speed up" when you eat, and the size of the boost depends on several factors:

- The types of foods eaten

  For example, protein costs the most energy to use and store, followed by carbohydrate and then dietary fat.[3]

  Studies also show that the thermic effect of highly processed foods is substantially less than their whole-food counterparts.[4]

  This is one of the contributing factors to the obesity epidemic because a diet of mostly processed foods results in less energy expenditure than one rich in whole foods, which makes it easier to accidentally overeat.[5]

- How much food you eat in one sitting

  Smaller meals result in smaller increases in energy expenditure and larger meals result in larger increases.

- Genetics

  Some people just have naturally faster metabolisms than others (bastards).[6]

This helps explain why a number of studies have shown that high-protein, high-carb diets are best for maximizing fat loss.[7] There are other factors, of course, but the significant boost in TEF is certainly one of them.

So, how do you calculate your TDEE?

First you need to know your BMR, which you just learned how to calculate, and then you need to account for the additional energy you're burning, which requires a little more work.

There are a number of ways to calculate how many calories you're burning through exercise and physical activity, including activity trackers, exercise machines, and mathematical methods. Let's take a look at each.

HOW ACCURATE ARE ACTIVITY TRACKERS?

Activity trackers are more popular than ever because the sales pitch sounds great. Wear a stylish band, do your thing, and know how many calories you're burning every day!

Unfortunately, studies show they're not nearly as precise as we're being told.

These devices contain an *accelerometer*, an instrument that registers the velocity of movements. Every time you take a step, the accelerometer wiggles, and raw data is run through an algorithm to estimate how many calories that movement burned.

The problem here is obvious: this primitive mechanism can't differentiate well between different types of activities. This is why most activity trackers can only be calibrated for one specific kind of activity, and doing anything else produces inaccurate data.

For instance, most pedometers are only good at measuring the calories you burn from walking at a certain pace.[8] If you walk faster or slower, they become less accurate.

They're even less precise for running and completely useless for something like weightlifting (heavy squatting burns a lot of energy but doesn't involve a lot of motion).[9]

Fancier fitness trackers aren't much better. According to a study conducted by scientists at the University of North Carolina, both Fitbit and Jawbone trackers underestimated steps, under- and overestimated calories burned during different kinds of exercise, and overestimated total sleep time.[10]

What about smartphone apps? Many are advertised as more accurate and convenient than dedicated fitness trackers, but the data says otherwise. Research shows that the measurements produced by many of these apps are off by 30 to 50 percent.[11]

It also doesn't help that the most accurate of tracking gizmos requires that you wear an unwieldy strap around your chest. Ones that measure heart rate via the wrist generally produce inferior results.

So, if you want to use an activity tracker to pay attention to steps or get a rough estimate of how many calories you're burning in your workouts and other physical activities, go for it.

But don't use any of that data to inform your calorie intake because it's probably going to lead you astray.

HOW ACCURATE ARE EXERCISE MACHINES?

Many people go into their cardio workouts with a target for calorie burning and rely on machine readouts to guide them there.

Little do they know that most of these machines overestimate the number of calories burned. By a lot.

For instance, an analysis conducted by scientists at the University of California-San Francisco found that, on average:

- Stationary bicycles overestimated calories burned by 7 percent.

- Stair-climbers overestimated by 12 percent.

- Treadmills overestimated by 13 percent.

- Elliptical machines overestimated by 42 percent (ouch).[12]

There are several reasons for these errors.

First, the algorithms used to estimate calorie expenditure differ from manufacturer to manufacturer, and some are better than others.

Then there's the fact that weight, age, gender, and fitness level affect how much energy is burned during exercise. Heavier people generally burn more energy than lighter people, and fitter people generally burn less than unfit.[13]

Few machines ask for any of that information, let alone all of it, and work off fixed data instead.

Wear and tear on the machines also matters. For example, the belts on treadmills and other machines tend to slip with age, which reduces the amount of resistance they provide. This makes them easier to use, which results in less energy expenditure.

User error also factors in, with the most common mistake being leaning heavily on the handrails on the stair-stepper, elliptical machine, and treadmill (especially when walking on an incline). This lessens the amount of weight that muscles have to move, thereby lessening the amount of energy burned.

Another example of user error is being passive with your upper body on the elliptical machine. The calorie calculations assume vigorous pumping with the arms, so if yours are just along for the ride, the readout is going to be wrong.

HOW ACCURATE ARE MATHEMATICAL METHODS?

You probably know the answer to this question as this is our last option, and yes, you're correct. Mathematical models are the ticket for calculating your total daily energy expenditure.

They can produce highly accurate estimates of how many calories you're burning every day, which allows you to move ahead in your meal planning with a fair amount of confidence that your body will respond positively.

There are a number of systems out there that you can use, and some are fairly complex.

For instance, you might have heard of methods that revolve around the *Metabolic Equivalent of Task,* or MET. Think of an MET like a calorie, but instead of representing the amount of energy required to heat one kilogram of water one degree Celsius, an MET equals the amount of energy an average-size person will burn while sitting still for one minute.

Different activities, then, have different MET scores. Walking at a slow pace for a minute burns about double the amount of energy as sitting still, and thus has an MET score of 2. Vacuuming is more vigorous, so it's listed at 3.5 METs, and so forth.

With these various scores, you can use formulas to calculate the total number of calories you burn throughout the day by first working out the calories burned for each type of physical activity you engage in, and then factoring in your basal metabolic rate and general activity levels.

Does this method work? Absolutely. Is it tedious? Indeed. So much so that you need a spreadsheet just to get through it.

Some people enjoy geeking out on numbers and details, but most prefer a workable back-of-the-napkin approach instead. Thankfully, this exists too, and it's called the *Katch-McArdle formula.*

This formula has an equation for calculating your BMR, but also contains BMR multipliers for estimating your TDEE based on your general activity levels.

This means that all you have to do to compute your approximate TDEE is multiply your BMR by a single number.

There's a problem with this formula, though. Its multipliers will probably overshoot the actual amount of energy you're burning. I don't have any research to directly back that statement up, but I've worked with thousands of people and consistently found it to be the case. It's also common knowledge among experienced bodybuilders.

This is why I recommend the following slightly modified activity multipliers when calculating your TDEE:

BMR x 1.15 = Sedentary (little or no exercise)

BMR x 1.2 to 1.35 = Light activity (1 to 3 hours of exercise or sports per week)

BMR x 1.4 to 1.55 = Moderate activity (4 to 6 hours of exercise or sports per week)

BMR x 1.6 to 1.75 = Very active (7 to 9 hours of exercise or sports per week)

BMR x 1.8 to 1.95 = Extra active (10+ hours of exercise or sports per week)

These calculations won't tell you how much energy you're burning on any given day, of course. To do that, you'd have to go the MET route we just discussed.

Instead, these equations estimate the average amount of energy you burn every day based on how active you are.

Fortunately, this snapshot of your average daily energy expenditure is all you need for reliable fat loss and muscle gain. It also makes creating meal plans a breeze, which works wonders for long-term compliance.

Let's see how this math works for me.

We already know that my BMR is about 2,100 calories, and I do four to six hours of moderate exercise per week.

Per the calculations above, my TDEE should be around 2,800 calories (2,100 x 1.4), give or take a hundred calories or so.

And that's empirically correct as my meal plan currently provides around 2,800 calories per day, which perfectly maintains my current body composition. What's more, when I intentionally eat less than this, I lose fat, and when I intentionally eat more, I gain fat.

You're up next! Take a few minutes to calculate your average TDEE, and then let's move on!

If math really isn't your forte, you can find a handy-dandy BMR
and TDEE calculator on my website.
Go to www.thinnerleanerstronger.com/calculator.

3. CALCULATE YOUR TARGET DAILY CALORIE INTAKE.

Once you've calculated your average TDEE, you're ready to figure out how many calories you should eat every day.

The first step in working this out is determining what you want to do with your body composition.

- If you want to lose fat, you need to eat fewer calories than you're burning.

  This is known as *cutting*.

- If you want to maintain your current weight and body composition, you need to eat more or less how many calories you're burning.

  This is known as *maintaining*.

- If you want to gain muscle as quickly as possible, you need to eat slightly more calories than you're burning.

  This is known as *lean bulking*.

Let's break down each.

HOW MANY CALORIES YOU SHOULD EAT TO LOSE FAT

As you know, you must be in a calorie deficit to lose fat, but how large should that deficit be? Ten percent? Twenty percent? Larger?

In other words, should you eat 90 percent of the calories you burn every day? Eighty percent? Less?

Some fitness folk advocate a "slow-cutting" approach where you use a mild calorie deficit and lax workout schedule to whittle down fat stores over the course of many months.

The advantages of this are claimed to be less muscle loss, more enjoyable workouts, and fewer issues related to hunger and cravings. And there's some truth here.

Slow cutting is at least slightly easier and forgiving in some ways than a more aggressive approach, but the upsides aren't all that significant in most people, and they come at a steep price: duration.

Namely, slow cutting is, well, *slow*, and for many dieters, this is more troubling than eating a bit less food every day.

For instance, all things being equal, by reducing your calorie deficit from 20 to 10 percent, you're halving the amount of fat you'll lose each week and doubling the amount of time it'll take to finish your cut.

This is a problem for most people, because the longer they remain in a calorie deficit of any size, the more likely they are to fall off the wagon due to life commotion, dietary slipups, scheduling snafus, and so on.

Furthermore, when you know what you're doing, you can maintain a significant calorie deficit that results in rapid fat loss without losing muscle, suffering in the gym, or wrestling with metabolic hobgoblins.

This allows you to enjoy faster results without having to sacrifice anything but calories, and this in turn allows you to spend more time doing the more enjoyable stuff (maintaining and lean bulking).

Therefore, my recommendation is an aggressive but not reckless calorie deficit of about 25 percent when cutting.

In other words, when you're cutting I recommend that you eat about 75 percent of your average TDEE. For most women, this comes out to 10 to 12 calories per pound of body weight per day.

For example, we established that my average TDEE is 2,800 calories, so when I cut, I should drop my calories to about 2,100 (2,800 x 0.75). And this is exactly what I do whenever I need to lose fat, and it has allowed me to get very lean without any muscle loss to speak of.

I didn't pick this 25 percent number out of thin air, either. Studies show that it works tremendously well for both fat loss and muscle preservation when combined with resistance training and high protein intake.

For instance, a study conducted by scientists at the University of Jyväskylä (Finland) split national- and international-level track and field jumpers and sprinters with low levels of body fat (at or below 10 percent) into two groups:[14]

1. Group one maintained a 300-calorie deficit (about 12 percent below TDEE).

2. Group two maintained a 750-calorie deficit (about 25 percent below TDEE).

After four weeks, the first group lost very little fat and muscle, and the second group lost, on average, about four pounds of fat and very little muscle. Neither group experienced any negative side effects to speak of.

More evidence of the effectiveness of my recommended approach can be found in a study conducted by scientists at Brigham and Women's Hospital with 38 overweight men.

After 12 weeks of maintaining a calorie deficit of about 20 percent, lifting weights about two hours per week, and eating a high-protein diet, the men lost, on average, 13 pounds of fat and gained 7 pounds of muscle.[15]

And just to take it to the extreme, a 90-day study conducted by scientists at the University of Nebraska with 21 obese, middle-aged women found that subjects eating just 800 calories per day and lifting weights just 90 minutes per week lost an average of 22 pounds and gained a significant amount of muscle mass.[16]

These findings are also in line with what I've experienced working with thousands of people.

When combined with a high-protein diet and rigorous workout schedule, a calorie deficit of about 25 percent allows for speedy fat loss and considerable muscle gain without any serious side effects.

HOW TO CALCULATE YOUR CUTTING MACROS

Once you have your cutting calories worked out, turning them into daily macronutrient targets is easy. Here's how:

- Forty percent of your calories should come from protein.
- Forty percent of your calories should come from carbohydrate.
- Twenty percent of your calories should come from dietary fat.

Protein and carbohydrate contain about four calories per gram, and dietary fat contains about nine calories per gram. Therefore, all you have do to figure out your macros is the following:

1. Multiply your target daily calorie intake by 0.4 and divide the result by 4 to figure out your target daily protein intake (in grams).

2. Multiply your target daily calorie intake by 0.4 and divide the result by 4 to figure out your target daily carbohydrate intake.

3. Multiply your target daily calorie intake by 0.2 and divide the result by 9 to figure out your target daily fat intake.

For most people, this comes out to around 1.1 grams of protein and carbohydrate per pound of body weight per day, and 0.25 grams of dietary fat per pound of body weight per day.

In fact, if you want to skip most of the math, you can just use those macro guidelines when starting a cutting phase and move on to the next step in the process (meal planning).

If you're very overweight, however, I don't recommend this "macro shortcut" because it'll have you eating far more protein than is necessary. In this case, use the 40/40/20 method instead.

Let's see how this works out for me. If I were cutting, my target daily calorie intake would be 2,100 calories, so:

1. 2,100 x 0.4 = 840 and 840 / 4 = 210 (grams of protein per day)

2. 2,100 x 0.4 = 840 and 840 / 4 = 210 (grams of carbohydrate per day)

3. 2,100 x 0.2 = 420 and 420 / 9 = 47 (grams of dietary fat per day)

Or with the macro shortcut:

1. 195 (pounds) x 1.1 = 215 (grams of protein per day)

2. 195 x 1.1 = 215 (grams of carbohydrate per day)

3. 195 x 0.25 = 49 (grams of dietary fat per day)

HOW MANY CALORIES YOU SHOULD EAT TO GAIN MUSCLE

You learned back in chapter 10 that a calorie surplus is conducive to muscle gain, and that the easiest way to accomplish this is to intentionally eat a bit more calories than you're burning every day.

This has been confirmed in a number of studies that show a calorie surplus boosts muscle protein synthesis, increases anabolic and decreases catabolic hormone levels, and improves workout performance.[17]

All of that adds up to significantly better muscle and strength gains over time.

You don't want to eat too many more calories than you're burning, however, because after a point, increasing food intake no longer boosts muscle growth but just fat gain instead.

This extra fat gain does more than hurt your ego, too. It even further accelerates fat storage and slows down muscle building, because as body fat levels rise, insulin sensitivity drops.[18]

The better your body responds to insulin's signals, the better it can do many things, including build muscle and resist fat gain. As the body's sensitivity to insulin falls, fat burning drops, the likelihood of weight gain rises, and protein synthesis rates decline.[19]

So, how large should your calorie surplus be to maximize muscle growth while minimizing fat gain?

Unfortunately, I've been unable to find any research that gives a tidy answer, but I've spent enough time in the natural bodybuilding scene and worked with enough people to know that the point of diminishing returns is somewhere around 110 percent of your average TDEE.

That is, you'll likely gain just as much muscle eating about 110 percent of your average TDEE as you would eating 120 or 130 percent but a lot less fat.

And so that's my recommendation for lean bulking: eat about 110 percent of your average TDEE. For most women, this comes out to 16 to 18 calories per pound of body weight per day.

For me, this would mean eating about 3,100 calories per day (2,800 x 1.1). And again, this is exactly what I do when I want to start a lean bulking phase, and it results in slow and steady muscle gain with minimal fat gain.

HOW TO CALCULATE YOUR LEAN BULKING MACROS

Here's how to turn your lean bulking calories into macros:

- Twenty-five percent of your calories should come from protein.
- Fifty-five percent of your calories should come from carbohydrate.
- Twenty percent of your calories should come from dietary fat.

To figure this out, do the following:

1. Multiply your target daily calorie intake by 0.25 and divide the result by 4 to figure out your target daily protein intake.

2. Multiply your target daily calorie intake by 0.55 and divide the result by 4 to figure out your target daily carbohydrate intake.

3. Multiply your target daily calorie intake by 0.2 and divide the result by 9 to figure out your target daily fat intake.

For most people, this comes out to around 1 gram of protein, 2.2 grams of carbohydrate, and 0.35 grams of dietary fat per pound of body weight per day.

Again, if you want to skip most of the math, you can just use those macro guidelines when starting a lean bulking phase and move on to the next step in the process (meal planning).

Let's see how this works out for me. If I were lean bulking, my target daily calorie intake would be 3,100 calories, so:

1. 3,100 x 0.25 = 775 and 775 / 4 = 194 (grams of protein per day)

2. 3,100 x 0.55 = 1,705 and 1,705 / 4 = 425 (grams of carbohydrate per day)

3. 3,100 x 0.2 = 620 and 620 / 9 = 70 (grams of dietary fat per day)

Or with the shortcut:

1. 195 (pounds) x 1 = 195 (grams of protein per day)

2. 195 x 2.2 = 429 (grams of carbohydrate per day)

3. 195 x 0.35 = 68 (grams of dietary fat per day)

HOW MANY CALORIES YOU SHOULD EAT TO MAINTAIN YOUR WEIGHT

This shouldn't really come into play until you've completed several cycles of cutting and lean bulking and more or less have the body you want.

You use your lean bulking phases to add muscle and your cutting phases to strip away fat, and along the way, assess your physique to see how far you still have to go to look the way you want to look.

Eventually, you'll cut down to a lean body fat percentage and absolutely love what you see in the mirror. This will be one of the most rewarding experiences you'll have in your fitness journey.

It'll continue to pay dividends, too, because from that point forward, you'll get to focus more on enjoying the fruits of your labor than the labor itself.

In other words, it takes a lot more work to build your best body ever than it does to maintain it.

Once you have your "maintenance body," you don't have to work out as much if you don't want to, you can do less weightlifting if you want to try other forms of resistance training, you have a lot more wiggle room in your diet, and the occasional dietary flubs don't even register in any meaningful way.

Keep all that in mind as you progress on my *Thinner Leaner Stronger* program because if you stick to it, you *will* get there. It's only a matter of when.

Calculating your maintenance calories is straightforward. There are two ways to do it:

1. Eat the same amount every day.

This would be your average TDEE, and for most women, it comes out to around 14 to 16 calories per pound of body weight per day.

Practical speaking, this will mean that some days you'll be in a slight calorie deficit and other days a slight surplus. That's fine. They will balance out to neither weight loss nor gain over the course of weeks, months, and even years if you so desire.

2. Eat more on the days that you're more active and less on the days that you're less active.

This requires that you estimate your energy expenditure each day and eat accordingly.

I prefer the first option because it's the simplest, but the second can be better for people who are very active on certain days and very inactive on others. If you're one of those people (or just want to give the second method a try), here's the easiest way to set it up:

BMR X 1.15 = SEDENTARY DAY

On days where you're not exercising or otherwise physically active, eat 115 percent of your BMR.

This should be around 12 calories per pound of body weight.

BMR X 1.2 TO 1.35 = LIGHTLY ACTIVE DAY

On days where you do 30 to 45 minutes of vigorous exercise or other physical activity (or about 60 to 90 minutes of light activity), eat 120 to 135 percent of your BMR.

This should be around 13 calories per pound of body weight.

BMR X 1.4 TO 1.55 = MODERATELY ACTIVE DAY

On days where you do 45 to 60 minutes of vigorous exercise (or about 90 to 120 minutes of light activity), eat 140 to 155 percent of your BMR.

This should be around 15 calories per pound of body weight.

BMR X 1.6 TO 1.75 = VERY ACTIVE DAY

On days where you do 60 to 90 minutes of vigorous exercise (or about 120 to 180 minutes of light activity), eat 160 to 175 percent of your BMR.

This should be around 17 calories per pound of body weight.

BMR X 1.8 TO 1.95 = EXTRA ACTIVE DAY

On days where you do 90-plus minutes of vigorous exercise (or 180-plus minutes of light activity), eat 180 to 195 percent of your BMR.

This should start around 19 calories per pound of body weight and go as high as 24-plus depending on how active you are.

HOW TO CALCULATE YOUR MAINTENANCE MACROS

Here's how to turn your maintenance calories into macros:

- Thirty percent of your calories should come from protein.
- Forty-five percent of your calories should come from carbohydrate.
- Twenty-five percent of your calories should come from dietary fat.

Which means all you have to do to figure out your macros is the following:

1. Multiply your target daily calorie intake by 0.3 and divide the result by 4 to figure out your target daily protein intake.

2. Multiply your target daily calorie intake by 0.45 and divide the result by 4 to figure out your target daily carbohydrate intake.

3. Multiply your target daily calorie intake by 0.25 and divide the result by 9 to figure out your target daily fat intake.

For most people, this comes out to around 1 gram of protein, 1.6 grams of carbohydrate, and 0.4 grams of dietary fat per pound of body weight per day.

And again, if you want to skip most of the math, you can just use those macro guidelines when starting a maintenance phase and move on to the next step in the process (meal planning).

Let's see how this works out for me. If I were maintaining, my target daily calorie intake would be 2,800 calories, so:

1. $2,800 \times 0.3 = 840$ and $840 / 4 = 210$ (grams of protein per day)

2. $2,800 \times 0.45 = 1,260$ and $1,260 / 4 = 315$ (grams of carbohydrate per day)

3. $2,800 \times 0.25 = 700$ and $700 / 9 = 78$ (grams of dietary fat per day)

Or with the shortcut:

1. 195 (pounds) $\times 1 = 195$ (grams of protein per day)

2. $195 \times 1.6 = 312$ (grams of carbohydrate per day)

3. $195 \times 0.4 = 78$ (grams of dietary fat per day)

"DO I REALLY NEED TO EAT THAT MUCH PROTEIN?"

If you're like most women, you're not used to eating anywhere near the amount of protein I've just recommended, regardless of whether you're looking to cut, lean bulk, or maintain.

You're probably also wondering if it's really necessary, or even healthy, to eat that much protein every day.

The short answer is yes, it's necessary if you want to enjoy maximum muscle gain and fat loss, as well as less mood disturbance, stress, fatigue, and diet dissatisfaction.[20] And yes, it's perfectly healthy too.

A significant amount of research has been done on the protein needs of people who are physically active, and a fantastic summary of the literature was coauthored by my friend Dr. Eric Helms.[21] Here's an excerpt from the paper:

> The collective agreement among reviewers is that a protein intake of 1.2-2.2 g/kg is sufficient to allow adaptation to training for athletes whom are at or above their energy needs.

In other words, when you're maintaining or lean bulking, a protein intake of 1.2 to 2.2 grams per kilogram of body weight per day—0.55 to 1 gram of protein per pound of body weight per day—is adequate.

As you've just learned, I prefer the upper end of this range because the downsides of not eating enough protein (less muscle growth, less satiety, and less bone density, to name a few) are far greater than the downsides of eating a little more protein than you need (fewer calories for carbs and fat, mostly).

And what about protein intake when you're cutting? Also from that paper:

> In a review by Phillips and Van Loon, it is suggested that a protein intake of 1.8-2.7 g/kg for athletes training in hypocaloric conditions may be optimal.

That is, when athletes are restricting their calories for fat loss, they should eat more protein than when they're not in a calorie deficit—in the range of 1.8 to 2.7 grams of protein per kilogram of body weight per day, or 0.8 to 1.2 grams of protein per pound of body weight per day.

"CAN I REALLY EAT THAT MANY CARBS AND LOSE FAT?"

If you're having trouble shaking this out of your mind despite everything we've covered so far, I understand.

According to most people, including so-called diet experts, carbs and fat loss go together like Chinese food and chocolate pudding or cocaine and waffles (Talladega Nights, anyone?).

I could cite even more weight loss research showing that carbohydrate intake has no impact on fat loss, like a study conducted by scientists from Harvard University that found the following:

> Reduced-calorie diets result in clinically meaningful weight loss regardless of which macronutrients they emphasize.[22]

Or maybe an extensive review of 19 weight loss trials conducted by scientists from several universities, including Stellenbosch University, the University of Cape Town, and the Liverpool School of Tropical Medicine, which concluded:

> Trials show weight loss in the short-term irrespective of whether the diet is low CHO [carbohydrate] or balanced. There is probably little or no difference in weight loss and changes in cardiovascular risk factors up to two years of follow-up when overweight and obese adults, with or without type 2 diabetes, are randomised to low CHO diets and isoenergetic balanced [calorically equal] weight loss diets.[23]

But I don't think reviewing another litany of studies is really necessary.

Instead, I'm just going to ask you to suspend your disbelief for the next four weeks, because that's all it's going to take for you to see noticeable changes on my Thinner Leaner Stronger program.

You will lose fat on a high-carb diet, easily and rapidly. Full stop.

"SHOULDN'T I BE EATING MORE DIETARY FAT?"

Dietary fat is the macronutrient du jour.

No matter what you want to fix with your body or do in the gym, eating more fat can purportedly help. Fat loss, vitality, libido, muscle and strength gain—it can all be yours if you follow this "one weird diet trick."

This makes for a powerful marketing message because it's simple, counterintuitive, and provides logical cover for what many people want to do anyway (eat deliciously fatty foods).

Hence the thriving industry of high-fat diets, cookbooks, food products, and supplements.

As you now know, the biggest hook used to sell people on high-fat dieting—faster fat loss—is scientifically bankrupt. And when it does work, it's only due to a significant reduction in calorie intake resulting in a larger calorie deficit, not metabolic voodoo.

Another hook is hormones. Specifically, some people claim that a high-fat diet optimizes your hormone profile, which in turn enhances every aspect of your health and well-being.

For men, the focus is usually on testosterone and its effects on body composition, and for women, reproductive hormones and their effects on fertility and menstruation.

While it's true that eating too little fat impairs hormone production and increasing intake can improve it, the effects are far less dramatic than you might think.

Furthermore, the physiological differences between a moderate-fat diet, such as one that provides 20 percent of daily calories from fat, and a high-fat diet, such as one that provides twice that, are downright negligible.

This was clearly demonstrated in a study organized by the National Institute of Child Health and Human Development, which included scientists from a number of universities including Harvard University, George Mason University, University at Buffalo, and Portland State University.[24]

After analyzing the hormone levels of 259 women 16 times throughout two menstrual cycles, researchers found those who ate the most fat (36 to 49 percent of daily calories) had just 4 percent higher testosterone levels than those who ate the least (18 to 32 percent of daily calories).

The differences in estrogen, progesterone, follicle-stimulating hormone, and luteinizing hormone—all involved in fertility and menstruation—were also so small as to be insignificant.

So, while some people might consider my dietary recommendations "low-fat," and too low at that, just know that they only appear low in the context of the current high-fat craze.

What's more, science clearly shows that my macronutrient guidelines not only provide adequate fat for general health and performance but also leave enough room for adequate amounts of protein and carbohydrate.

. . .

Are you getting excited yet?

I am because you've just taken a major stride toward a thinner, leaner, and stronger you and cleared one of the largest hurdles—one that trips up millions of people every year and prevents them from ever achieving the results they really desire.

Soon, after a few more leaps and bounds, you'll be officially off to the races, so let's keep going! Pre- and postworkout nutrition is next!

KEY TAKEAWAYS

- It's possible to lose weight without watching your calories, but it's unlikely to work well over the long term for most people.

- There are just three simple steps to figuring out how many calories you should eat every day: calculate your basal metabolic rate, calculate your total daily energy expenditure, and calculate your target daily calorie intake.

- Your basal metabolic rate (BMR) is the amount of energy your body would burn if you were to lie motionless for a day, without food. It's the minimum amount of energy it costs to stay alive for 24 hours.

- The Mifflin-St. Jeor equation for women is BMR = 10 x weight (in kilograms) + 6.25 x height (in centimeters) – 5 x age (in years) – 161

- Your total daily energy expenditure (TDEE) is the total number of calories you burn every 24 hours.

- Food costs energy to digest, process, and absorb, and different types of foods cost more energy than others.

• Protein costs the most energy to use and store, followed by carbohydrate and then dietary fat.

• Don't use any of the data from activity trackers and exercise machines to inform your calorie intake because it's probably going to lead you astray.

• Mathematical models are the ticket for calculating your total daily energy expenditure.

• Use my slightly modified activity multipliers when calculating your TDEE.

• The first step in working out how many calories you should eat is determining what you want to do with your body composition.

If you want to lose fat, you need to eat fewer calories than you're burning.

If you want to maintain your current weight and body composition, you need to eat more or less how many calories you're burning.

If you want to gain muscle as quickly as possible, you need to eat slightly more calories than you're burning.

• When cutting, eat about 75 percent of your average TDEE. For most women, this comes out to 10 to 12 calories per pound of body weight per day.

• When cutting, forty percent of your calories should come from protein, forty percent should come from carbohydrate, and twenty percent should come from dietary fat.

For most people, this comes out to around 1.1 grams of protein and carbohydrate per pound of body weight per day, and 0.25 grams of dietary fat per pound of body weight per day.

• When lean bulking, eat about 110 percent of your average TDEE. For most women, this comes out to 16 to 18 calories per pound of body weight per day.

• When lean bulking, 25 percent of your calories should come from protein, 55 percent should come from carbohydrate, and 20 percent should come from dietary fat.

For most people, this comes out to around 1 gram of protein, 2.2 grams of carbohydrate, and 0.35 grams of dietary fat per pound of body weight per day.

• Use your lean bulking phases to add muscle and your cutting phases to strip away fat, and along the way, assess your physique to see how far you still have to go to look the way you want to look.

• When maintaining, either eat the same amount of calories every day (for most women, this comes out to around 14 to 16 calories per pound of body weight per day) or eat more on the days that you're more active and less on the days that you're less active.

• When maintaining, 30 percent of your calories should come from protein, 45 percent should come from carbohydrate, and 25 percent should come from dietary fat.

For most people, this comes out to around 1 gram of protein, 1.6 grams of carbohydrate, and 0.4 grams

• The physiological differences between a moderate-fat diet, such as one that provides 20 percent of daily calories from fat, and a high-fat diet, such as one that provides twice that, are downright negligible.

18

THE TRUTH ABOUT PREWORKOUT AND POSTWORKOUT NUTRITION

*"I am building a fire, and every day I train, I add more fuel.
At just the right moment, I light the match."*

—MIA HAMM

Years ago, my pre- and postworkout meals were sacred, inviolable rituals to be observed without deviation.

A protein shake before and after every workout was crucial, I believed, and especially after, when your body's "anabolic window" was rapidly closing and with it your opportunity for maximum muscle and strength gain.

Chances are you've heard something similar.

Bodybuilders and gymbros alike have been singing pre- and postworkout nutrition's praises for decades. How important are these meals, though? Does eating before or after workouts actually matter?

The long story short is this: Eating before and after workouts isn't vital, but it's not entirely without merit, either.

And in this chapter, you're going to get the whole story, including why pre- and postworkout nutrition are even a "thing," the ideal type of pre- and postworkout meals, the truth about the "anabolic window," and more.

Let's start with preworkout nutrition.

SHOULD YOU EAT PROTEIN BEFORE YOU WORK OUT?

If you haven't eaten protein in the three to four hours preceding your workout, then it's a good idea to eat 30 to 40 grams before you train.

If you have eaten protein in the last few hours, though, then you don't need to eat more. You can just eat after your workout.

Let's take a few minutes to unpack this advice, because it not only helps you understand preworkout nutrition better, but nutrition and muscle building on the whole.

We recall that as far as muscle building goes, eating protein does two vital things:

1. It bumps up muscle protein synthesis rates and suppresses muscle protein breakdown rates.

2. It provides your body with the raw materials needed to build muscle tissue (amino acids).

That's why you need to make sure that you eat enough protein every day if you want to maximize muscle growth.

While there's evidence that eating protein before a resistance training workout can magnify its effects on muscle protein synthesis rates, the effects don't appear to be strong enough to support the claim that having protein before a workout is clearly superior to not having it beforehand.[1]

Instead, preworkout protein should be viewed in the context of your entire diet.

If you haven't eaten protein three to four hours preceding your workout, your body's muscle protein synthesis rates are going to be at a low baseline level. This means that your body's muscle-building machinery will be idle, waiting for the next feeding of protein to kickstart it into action.

Think of any time where this apparatus is dormant as lost production time. Your body could have been building muscle if only it were given the right stimulus and supplies.

Ideally, then, you'd eat another serving of protein more or less immediately after muscle protein synthesis rates bottom out. By doing this, you'd effectively keep muscle protein synthesis elevated throughout the entirety of your waking hours. (And you'd also ideally eat protein before going to bed to boost them while you sleep.)

If you go into a workout several hours after eating, you're letting that muscle-building equipment remain inactive even longer. And if you wait too long to eat after the workout, muscle protein breakdown rates will rise to exceed synthesis rates, which can ultimately result in muscle loss.[2]

This is why you should eat protein before you train if it has been a few hours since you last ate some. It'll get your body building muscle again, and as I mentioned, it may even prime it to receive a larger anabolic boost from the training.[3]

If you have eaten protein an hour or two before a workout, however, amino acids will still be in your bloodstream, insulin levels will still be elevated, and muscle protein synthesis rates will still be humming. Thus, eating protein again won't accomplish much.

This is why a study conducted by scientists at the University of Tartu found that weightlifters who simply added two protein shakes before and after their workouts on top of their regular diet didn't gain more muscle or strength than weightlifters who consumed protein shakes five-plus hours before and after their workouts.[4]

SHOULD YOU EAT CARBS BEFORE YOU WORK OUT?

Yes. The research on eating carbs before a workout is clear: it improves performance.

Specifically, eating carbs 15 to 60 minutes before working out will help you push harder in your training and may also aid in postworkout recovery and muscle growth.

Eating carbs before training provides your body with an abundance of glucose to burn for immediate energy. This helps you in three ways:

1. The more glucose that's available for your muscles to burn, the better you're going to perform in your workouts (especially if they're longer).[5]

2. Elevating blood glucose levels helps preserve the glycogen stored in your muscles, because your body doesn't need to draw from these glycogen stores as heavily to fuel your training.[6]

This, in turn, improves performance.

3. Research suggests that maintaining higher levels of muscle glycogen improves cellular signaling related to muscle building.[7]

So, by eating carbs before you train, you'll have more energy in your workouts, which will help you put up better numbers and thus progress faster, and it may also enhance your body's ability to build muscle.

What eating carbs before a workout won't do, however, is directly cause more muscle growth. Unfortunately, carbs don't have the same anabolic properties of protein.

How much carbohydrate should you eat before working out and what types are best?

Studies show that for our purposes, 30 to 40 grams of any type of carbohydrate eaten about 30 minutes before a workout will get the job done.[8]

And by "any," I mean any: fruit, starch, simple sugars, etc. Choose whatever you enjoy most and is easiest on your stomach.

You don't need to buy fancy, overpriced preworkout carbohydrate supplements. They're usually little more than tubs of simple sugars like maltodextrin or dextrose, which aren't bad sources of preworkout carbs per se, but don't offer any special benefits, either.

My favorite preworkout carbs are nutritious whole foods like oatmeal, bananas, dates, figs, melons, white potatoes, white rice, raisins, and sweet potatoes.

SHOULD YOU EAT FAT BEFORE YOU WORK OUT?

You can, but you don't need to.

There are several theories about how eating fat before a workout can improve performance, but the scientific literature disagrees.

A good summary of the existing research on the matter can be found in a study conducted by scientists at Deakin University.[9] Here's their conclusion:

> Thus, it would appear that while such a strategy can have a marked effect on exercise metabolism (i.e., reduced carbohydrate utilization), there is no beneficial effect on exercise performance.

Chalk up yet another strike against high-fat, low-carb dieting

SHOULD YOU EAT PROTEIN AFTER YOU WORK OUT?

Yes, it's a good idea to eat 30 to 40 grams of protein within an hour or two of finishing a workout.

We recall that after we finish training, muscle protein breakdown rates go on the rise, quickly surpassing synthesis rates.

Muscle gain can't occur until this reverses (synthesis rates outstrip breakdown rates), and eating protein causes exactly that by:

1. Providing the amino acid *leucine*, which directly stimulates muscle protein synthesis.[10]

2. Stimulating the release of insulin, which suppresses muscle protein breakdown rates.[11]

Studies also show that protein eaten after a workout causes more muscle protein synthesis than when eaten otherwise.[12]

SHOULD YOU EAT CARBS AFTER YOU WORK OUT?

Maybe.

We're often told to eat carbs after working out to spike insulin levels, which is supposed to supercharge muscle growth in various ways.

Unfortunately, studies suggest this doesn't work, and adding carbs to your postworkout meals doesn't accelerate muscle gain.[13]

Only moderate elevations of insulin are needed to minimize muscle protein breakdown rates, and you can easily achieve this with a sufficient dose of protein.[14]

That said, adding carbs to your postworkout meal will keep insulin levels elevated for longer, which is desirable from a muscle-building standpoint because, as you know, insulin suppresses muscle protein breakdown.

This is one of the reasons why high-carb diets are better for gaining muscle than low-carb ones. Research shows that high-carb diets result in generally higher insulin levels, which results in generally lower muscle protein breakdown rates, which in turn produces more muscle gain.[15]

One other benefit to eating carbs after a workout is refilling your muscles with glycogen. This whole-body glycogen replenishment can give you a nice postworkout pump and mood boost, but it doesn't appear to improve overall workout performance unless you'll be training again later in the same day.[16]

It's also worth noting that the body won't store carbs as fat until glycogen stores have been refilled, which is why people often recommend eating your most carb-rich meals immediately after you work out.[17]

How much this can actually benefit your body composition over time is debatable, but it certainly won't hurt.

SHOULD YOU EAT FAT AFTER YOU WORK OUT?

Sure, if you want to.

Some people claim that you shouldn't because it slows down the process of digesting and absorbing the postworkout protein and carbs that your body so desperately needs.

While it's true that adding fat to a protein- or carb-rich meal slows down the rate at which food is cleared from the stomach, it's not true that this makes for less effective postworkout nutrition.[18]

For example, several studies have shown that the fat content of a meal has no effect on glycogen replenishment rates, and that whole milk may be more anabolic than nonfat milk.[19]

WHAT ABOUT THE "ANABOLIC WINDOW"?

No discussion of postworkout nutrition is complete without mentioning the anabolic window.

The idea here is that once you've finished a workout, you need to eat within a certain amount of time (30 to 60 minutes, generally) to maximize muscle gain. If you don't, the story goes, you'll gain less muscle from the workout.

How true is this, though? It depends on when you last ate protein.

If you haven't eaten protein in the three to four-plus hours preceding your workout, it's likely that muscle protein synthesis is going to be at a low baseline level. It would make sense, then, to eat protein soon after you finish in the gym. If you don't, you're not missing a special opportunity to gain muscle faster, but your body can't start building muscle until you eat.

If you have eaten protein within a few hours of starting your workout, however, then the timing of your postworkout meal is less important. Your body will still be processing the food you ate, so you can eat immediately after your workout if you want, but you can also wait until it has been up to three to four hours since your last meal.

. . .

It's long been said that your pre- and postworkout meals are the most important meals of the day.

This simply isn't true.

So long as your diet is set up properly on the whole, no individual meal ranks high above another. In other words, so long as your daily calories and macros are on point, when you eat isn't going to greatly influence your results one way or another.

That said, getting your pre- and postworkout nutrition right can give you a slight edge over the long term, so why not take every advantage you can get?

KEY TAKEAWAYS

- If you haven't eaten protein in the three to four hours preceding your workout, then it's a good idea to eat 30 to 40 grams before you train.

- If you've eaten protein an hour or two before a workout, eating protein again won't accomplish much.

- Eating carbs 15 to 60 minutes before working out will help you push harder in your training and may also aid in postworkout recovery and muscle growth.

- Eat 30 to 40 grams of any type of carbohydrate about 30 minutes before a workout.

• Choose whatever kind of carbohydrate you enjoy most and is easiest on your stomach.

• There are several theories about how eating fat before a workout can improve performance, but the scientific literature disagrees.

• It's a good idea to eat 30 to 40 grams of protein within an hour or two of finishing a workout.

• Protein eaten after a workout causes more muscle protein synthesis than when eaten otherwise.

• Adding carbs to your postworkout meal will keep insulin levels elevated for longer, which is desirable from a muscle-building standpoint because insulin suppresses muscle protein breakdown.

• High-carb diets result in generally higher insulin levels, which results in generally lower muscle protein breakdown rates, which in turn produces more muscle gain.

• One other benefit to eating carbs after a workout is refilling your muscles with glycogen.

This whole-body glycogen replenishment can give you a nice postworkout pump and mood boost, but it doesn't appear to improve overall workout performance unless you'll be training again later in the same day.

• The body won't store carbs as fat until glycogen stores have been refilled, which is why people often recommend eating your most carb-rich meals immediately after you work out.

How much this can actually benefit your body composition over time is debatable.

• While it's true that adding fat to a protein- or carb-rich meal slows down the rate at which food is cleared from the stomach, it's not true that this makes for less effective postworkout nutrition.

• The idea behind the anabolic window is that once you've finished a workout, you need to eat within a certain amount of time (30 to 60 minutes, generally) to maximize muscle gain.

• If you haven't eaten protein in the three to four-plus hours preceding your workout, it makes sense to eat protein soon after you finish in the gym.

• If you've eaten protein within a few hours of starting your workout, you can eat immediately after if you want, but you can also wait until it has been up to three to four hours since your last meal.

• So long as your daily calories and macros are on point, when you eat isn't going to greatly influence your results one way or another.

19

HOW TO MAKE MEAL PLANS THAT REALLY WORK

"Don't measure yourself by what you have accomplished, but by what you should have accomplished with your ability."

—JOHN WOODEN

You now know how your metabolism really works and how to use food to help you build muscle, lose fat, and optimize your health and performance.

You have in your possession everything you need to forever escape the diet roller coaster that keeps millions of people overweight, unhappy, and unhealthy.

You might be a little intimidated, though, and I understand.

Few people venture this far down the rabbit hole, and those who do are often expert trainers, dietitians, and nutritionists who work with celebrities and top-tier athletes. Soon, you're going to be able to give yourself this same world-class service for the rest of your life.

In this chapter, you're going to learn how to make meal plans that really work. That is, you're going to learn how to take your calorie and macronutrient targets and turn them into precise, meal-by-meal eating plans that help you lose fat and gain muscle like clockwork.

You don't *need* to plan all your meals the way I'm going to teach you to get results, but I don't recommend "on-the-fly" tracking with an app like MyFitnessPal or "eating by feel" until you've successfully cut, lean bulked, and maintained with meal planning.

There are two reasons for this:

Meal planning is the simplest and most effective way to put everything you've learned so far into practice. So long as you've done your math right and stick to the plan, your body composition *will* change.

Meal planning familiarizes you with the calorie and macronutrient profiles of various foods you like to eat, what different levels of calorie intake feel like, and how your body responds to changes in energy balance.

One for one, the people I've worked with over the years who have done the best eating intuitively were master meal planners.

I should also mention that many people, including myself, follow meal plans even though we have the knowledge and "freedom" to eat more spontaneously.

For me, meal planning is actually liberating because I don't have to waste any time or energy wondering about food—what I'm going to eat and when, how many calories or macros I have left for the day, how many I want to "spend" on one meal versus others, etc.

This is significant because research shows that the average person makes over 200 food decisions per day, and this can contribute to what psychologists call *decision fatigue.*[1]

Remember, your willpower is similar to a muscle in that it can only do so much work before running out of steam. All the decisions you make every day, large and small, bring you closer to that failing point, and any effort expended on deliberating over food could be used on other, more productive or enjoyable tasks.

Meal planning is the easiest way to reclaim that mental and emotional energy.

So, now that you understand the value of meal planning, let's learn how to do it.

MEAL PLANNING MADE EASY

When many people find out about flexible dieting, they're excited because it sounds so easy.

You have protein, carb, and fat targets for the day, and all you have to do is throw together a collection of meals that comes close to those numbers.

When people sit down to do this, though, the questions—and headaches—often begin.

How do you figure out the calories and macros of various foods? What's the best way to deal with recipes? What about eating out? Is alcohol a problem? Which meals in your plan should you create first? What if you want more variety?

All are good questions, and all have simple answers. Let's dig in.

HOW TO CALCULATE WHAT'S IN FOOD

The first thing you'll need to know to make great meal plans is how to look up the nutritional facts of various foods.

If the food came in a package, you can use the numbers provided on the label.

Most of your meals shouldn't come in packages, though. They should consist of relatively unprocessed foods that you prepare and cook yourself, and for those, the following websites are good resources:

- CalorieKing (www.calorieking.com)
- SELF Nutrition Data (nutritiondata.self.com)
- The USDA Food Composition Databases (ndb.nal.usda.gov)

One of the things I really like about these tools is that they contain many individual brands of foods (Quaker Oats oatmeal, for example), and in the case of CalorieKing, the average calories and macros for all brands as well.

Finding information on foods on these sites is straightforward:

1. Search for the food, and if the exact brand or product is listed, use that.

2. If the exact brand or product isn't listed but an "average for all brands" is, use that.

3. If neither the exact brand or product nor an average for all brands is listed, check multiple entries for the type of item to get an idea of the range. Choose numbers that are in the middle.

For example, if you want to add a cup of Uncle Ben's rice to your meal plan, you can find this exact food listed on CalorieKing. If it's a cup of bulk rice, though, you can search for the type of rice it is and choose the average for all brands.

It's critical that your food calculations are accurate, and that's why you want to weigh everything you eat before cooking to determine its calories and macros, and when preparing multiple servings, weigh again after cooking to determine portion sizes.

For instance, if you need to cook a pound of chicken for four meals, you would first weigh out 454 grams of raw chicken, cook it all together, and then divide it into four portions of more or less equal weight (which isn't going to be 454 divided by 4, because cooked chicken weighs less than raw due to moisture loss).

For meals that don't require cooking, you simply weigh them before you eat.

Remember that when you measure by volume as opposed to weight (cups and spoons versus ounces and grams), small measurement inaccuracies can significantly skew your numbers.

For example, a heaping tablespoon of peanut butter doesn't look much different from a properly measured tablespoon, but it could add 50 to 100 calories to the meal.

You also must include in your meal plan absolutely everything you're going to eat. *Everything* counts—vegetables, fruits, condiments, dabs of oil and butter, and every other bit of food that will go into your mouth every day.

One thing many readers of previous editions of this book have asked for is a quick reference guide of the calories and macros of some of the most commonly eaten foods. I thought this was a good idea, so here it is:

PROTEIN					
FOOD	AMOUNT	CALORIES	PROTEIN	CARBS	FAT
Skinless boneless chicken breast	100 grams	120	23	0	3
Skinless boneless chicken thigh	100 grams	121	20	0	4
93/7 ground beef	100 grams	152	21	0	7
93/7 ground turkey	100 grams	150	19	0	8
Plain nonfat Greek yogurt	100 grams	59	10	4	0
Sirloin, trimmed of visible fat	100 grams	127	22	0	4
1% cottage cheese	100 grams	72	12	3	1
Skim milk	100 grams	34	3	5	0
Whey protein isolate	100 grams	345	76	10	0
Whole egg	100 grams	143	13	1	10

CARBS					
FOOD	AMOUNT	CALORIES	PROTEIN	CARBS	FAT
Sweet potato	100 grams	86	2	20	0
Potato	100 grams	69	2	16	0
White pasta	100 grams	371	13	75	2
White rice	100 grams	365	7	80	1
Brown rice	100 grams	367	8	76	3
White bread	100 grams	266	9	49	3
Pearled barley	100 grams	352	10	78	1
Oatmeal	100 grams	379	13	68	7
Quinoa	100 grams	368	14	64	6
Lentil	100 grams	352	25	63	1

FAT					
FOOD	AMOUNT	CALORIES	PROTEIN	CARBS	FAT
Avocado	100 grams	160	2	9	15
Almond	100 grams	579	21	22	50
Walnut	100 grams	619	24	10	59
70 to 85% dark chocolate	100 grams	598	8	46	43
Creamy peanut butter	100 grams	598	22	22	51
Olive oil	100 grams	884	0	0	100
Canola oil	100 grams	884	0	0	100
Butter	100 grams	717	1	0	81
Half-and-half	100 grams	131	3	4	12
Cheddar cheese	100 grams	403	23	3	33

FRUITS					
FOOD	AMOUNT	CALORIES	PROTEIN	CARBS	FAT
Banana	100 grams	89	1	23	0
Grape	100 grams	69	1	18	0
Strawberry	100 grams	32	1	8	0
Watermelon	100 grams	30	1	8	0
Orange	100 grams	47	1	12	0
Pear	100 grams	57	0	15	0
Blueberry	100 grams	57	1	15	0
Apple	100 grams	52	0	14	0
Raspberry	100 grams	52	1	12	0
Cantaloupe	100 grams	34	1	8	0

VEGGIES					
FOOD	AMOUNT	CALORIES	PROTEIN	CARBS	FAT
Broccoli	100 grams	34	3	7	0
Zucchini	100 grams	17	1	3	0
Carrot	100 grams	41	1	10	0
Brussels sprout	100 grams	43	3	9	0
Lettuce	100 grams	17	1	3	0
Tomato	100 grams	18	1	4	0
Green bean	100 grams	31	2	0	0
Onion	100 grams	40	1	9	0
Mushroom	100 grams	22	3	3	0
Asparagus	100 grams	20	2	4	0

CONDIMENTS					
FOOD	AMOUNT	CALORIES	PROTEIN	CARBS	FAT
Mayonnaise	100 grams	680	1	1	75
Ketchup	100 grams	101	1	27	0
BBQ sauce	100 grams	172	1	41	1
Pesto	100 grams	418	10	10	38
Mustard	100 grams	60	4	6	3
Horseradish	100 grams	48	1	11	1
Balsamic vinegar	100 grams	88	0	17	0
Soy sauce	100 grams	60	11	6	0
Tabasco sauce	100 grams	12	1	1	1
Sriracha sauce	100 grams	93	2	19	1

HOW TO CALCULATE WHAT'S IN RECIPES

The only way to "safely" include recipes in your meal plans is to total the calories and macros for each ingredient and divide the sums by the number of servings.

If this isn't possible due to exotic ingredients or some other reason, skip the recipe. Stick with ones that you can easily and accurately measure.

For this reason, the simpler a recipe is, the better it will generally be for meal planning. Stay away from gourmet recipes that take considerable time, skill, and money to make; that don't store and reheat well; or that are hard to measure and quantify.

Remember that when it comes to cooking, more—more ingredients, more steps, and more time—doesn't always mean better food. A well-made, simple recipe beats a poorly executed, fancy one every time.

This is why the best meal plan recipes are easy and fast to make, require relatively few ingredients, and allow you to prepare large amounts of food with minimal equipment and work.

You can find scores of recipes that fit this bill in my cookbook *The Shredded Chef* (www.shreddedchefbook.com), as well as on my websites Muscle for Life (www.muscleforlife.com/category/recipes) and Legion Athletics (www.legionathletics.com/category/recipes).

If a recipe you like contains too many calories, there are several ways you can lighten it:

1. If it's not a baked good, reduce (or remove, if possible) the butter or oil.

An easy way to do this is to use cooking spray or a nonstick pan instead.

2. Replace sugar with a zero-calorie sweetener of your choice.

I like Truvia because it bakes well. Pure stevia extract mixed with egg whites can also work well in the oven.

3. Swap whole-fat dairy with low- or nonfat dairy.

Try skim milk instead of whole, 0 or 2 percent Greek yogurt instead of plain whole-fat yogurt, half-and-half instead of cream, etc.

4. Swap fatty meats for leaner cuts (or poultry).

WHAT ABOUT EATING OUT?

Generally speaking, the less you eat out, the better the results you're going to see with your diet.

The reason for this is obvious: eating out makes it harder to control your calories.

For example, a palm-sized piece of meat usually has at least 120 to 150 more calories than you'd expect due to the oil and butter absorbed during cooking.

A cup of plain pasta or potato ranges from 180 to 200 calories, but when there's a sauce or other source of fat, that can easily double.

Even vegetable dishes can contain a lot of "hidden calories" in the form of high-fat additions like butter, oil, and cheese. (The better the veggies taste, the more likely they are to be soaked in one or more of these.)

As for desserts, a good rule of thumb is 25 to 50 calories per tablespoon.

This is why you have to watch what you order when you eat out, especially if you're like me and can eat a lot of food in one sitting. If I let my stomach do the thinking, I can easily put down 200 or more grams of fat and a few thousand calories in one go.

The first step to becoming a skilled eater-outer (that's a word, right?) is familiarizing yourself with the nutritional realities of the types of foods you like to eat when you dine out.

You can do this on a website like CalorieKing, which has an entry for just about any type of dish you could want to eat. If you're eating at a chain restaurant, the exact meal might be listed there as well. Olive Garden's fettuccine alfredo, for example, is listed at 1,219 calories with 75 grams of fat and 47 grams of saturated fat.

When you can find the exact dish you want to eat, I recommend that you add 20 percent to the calories listed, because many restaurants underreport the actual number of calories in their food.[2]

When the exact restaurant's take on the dish isn't listed, search for it on CalorieKing, look for "Average All Brands," and, again, add 20 percent to the calories.

If there's no average for all brands, look at a handful of the entries, choose one in the middle of the pack, and add 20 percent to it.

The more you do this, the better you'll get at estimating calories and macros when eating out, and eventually, you'll know at a glance what is and isn't workable on just about any menu.

Even then, though, the more you eat out, the harder it'll be to accurately estimate your daily calorie intake.

WHAT ABOUT ALCOHOL?

According to some people, if you drink even lightly and sporadically, you're going to struggle with your weight. End of story.

This is an odd statement considering that moderate alcohol consumption is associated with lower, not higher, body weights.[3]

Furthermore, research shows that calories from alcohol itself don't impact body fat levels in the same way as other calories do.

For example, scientists at the University of Sao Paulo analyzed the diets of 1,944 adults aged 18 to 74 and were surprised to find that an increase in calories from alcohol alone didn't result in the weight gain that would normally occur if those calories had been from food.[4]

In fact, thanks to regular alcohol consumption, drinkers took in an average of 16 percent more calories than nondrinkers and had more or less the same levels of physical activity but weren't any fatter than their alcohol-free counterparts.

It's almost as if the calories from the alcohol simply "didn't count."

A similar result was seen in a study conducted by scientists at the University of Hohenheim with obese women on a weight loss diet.[5] Researchers split the women into two groups:

1. Group one got about 10 percent of their daily calories from white wine.

2. Group two got about 10 percent of their daily calories from grape juice.

After three months, the white wine group had lost about two pounds more than the grape juice group.

There are two likely reasons for these findings.

First, it's known that alcohol can reduce your appetite, which is conducive to weight loss, and can improve insulin sensitivity, which can positively impact fat burning.[6]

More importantly, however, the body has no way to directly convert alcohol into body fat.[7] That is, calories provided by ethanol (alcohol) simply can't produce fat gain in the same way that calories from food can.

We recall from chapter 7, however, that alcohol blunts fat oxidation and increases the conversion of carbs into body fat. In these ways, alcohol absolutely can contribute to fat gain.

Therefore, if you want to drink alcohol without interfering with your fat loss or accelerating fat gain, follow these three tips:

1. Don't drink more than one day per week.

2. Lower your carb and fat intakes that day. (Eat more protein than you normally would.)

3. Try not to eat while drinking and stay away from carb-laden drinks like beer and fruity stuff. (Stick to dry wines and spirits.)

HOW TO CREATE YOUR FIRST MEAL PLAN

Now that you know the ropes, let's learn how to tie the knots.

The first step in creating a meal plan is creating a list of your preferred sources of protein, carbs, and fats; your favorite fruits, veggies, and whole-grain foods (if you haven't already listed them under your preferred carbs); any recipes that you might want to use; and any treats that you want to include.

For example, my list would look like this:

• Protein: chicken, pork, turkey, eggs, lean beef, dairy, and protein powder

• Carbs: strawberries, bananas, blueberries, potatoes, sweet potatoes, pasta, English muffins, rice, oatmeal, and beans

• Fat: olive oil, cheese, butter, avocado, nuts, meat, dairy, and fish oil (supplement)

• Vegetables: onion, garlic, broccoli, mushrooms, peppers, carrots, cauliflower, green beans, peas, and Brussel sprouts

• Recipes: Creamy Blueberry-Banana Smoothie, Curry Chicken, and Chicken and Broccoli Stir-Fry (all from *The Shredded Chef*, of course!)

• Treats: dark chocolate, bread (I'm weird), low-calorie ice cream (Enlightened Sea Salt Caramel, I love you), and cereal

The easiest way to create your list, and everything else in this chapter, is to use Google Sheets or Excel.

The free bonus material that comes with this book (www.thinnerleanerstronger.com/bonus) contains a simple meal-planning template I like to use. You may want to download it now and fiddle with it as you read.

As you'll see if you download the template, I have a worksheet for my favorite whole foods, which are grouped together by their primary macronutrient, along with the calories and macros for each, like this:

FOOD	AMOUNT	CALORIES	PROTEIN	CARBS	FAT
Oatmeal	40 grams	152	5	27	3

And I keep my favorite recipes (along with their numbers) on another worksheet formatted in the same way.

RECIPE	AMOUNT	CALORIES	PROTEIN	CARBS	FAT
Adobo Sirloin from *The Shredded Chef*	1 serving	237	39	2	7

Next, you should familiarize yourself with the nutritional facts of your chosen foods using CalorieKing, SELF Nutrition Data, or the USDA Food Composition Databases.

As you do this, you'll probably find that some foods and recipes are too high calorie or macronutritionally imbalanced to fit your needs. Remove these from your list.

Now you have a list of foods and dishes that seem like good candidates for your meal plan, which means you're ready to start building it. Here's how I like to do it:

1. Set up your pre- and postworkout meals first.

2. Add your primary sources of protein to the rest of your meals.

3. Add your fruits and vegetables.

4. Add any additional carbs and caloric beverages that aren't dessert or junk.

5. Tweak your protein intake as needed.

6. Add additional fat as needed.

7. Add treats if desired.

And in the end, you want to be within 50 calories of your target intake when cutting and within 100 calories when lean bulking and maintaining.

Let's look at each of these steps in more detail.

1. SET UP YOUR PRE- AND POSTWORKOUT MEALS FIRST.

I like to start here because these two meals are simple and straightforward, and they usually account for a fair chunk of your daily protein and carbohydrate intake.

2. ADD YOUR PRIMARY SOURCES OF PROTEIN TO THE REST OF YOUR MEALS.

The goal here is to meet most (80 percent or more) of your protein needs with your primary preferred sources of protein (meat, fish, eggs, high-protein dairy products, soy, powders, etc.).

You don't need to reach 100 percent of your protein needs just yet, however, because your carbs are going to add protein as well.

You should also keep an eye on your saturated fat intake while adding your protein. (Remember that it shouldn't be more than 10 percent of your total calories).

3. ADD YOUR FRUITS AND VEGETABLES.

If you're going to give your body adequate nutrition, including vitamins, minerals, and fiber, you're going to need to eat several servings of fruit and vegetables every day.

In this step, your goal is to work at least one to two servings (cups) of fruit and at least two to three servings of fibrous vegetables into your meal plan.

Fibrous vegetables include basically everything your mother said you had to eat before dessert:

- Arugula
- Asparagus
- Bok choy and other Asian greens
- Broccoli
- Brussels sprouts
- Cabbage
- Carrots
- Cauliflower
- Celery
- Cucumber
- Eggplant
- Garlic
- Green beans
- Kale
- Leeks
- Lettuce
- Mushrooms
- Onion
- Radish
- Spinach
- Swiss chard
- Zucchini

It's also smart to eat a variety of fruits and veggies—especially colorful ones—because some are richer in certain nutrients than others.

4. ADD ANY ADDITIONAL CARBS AND CALORIC BEVERAGES THAT AREN'T DESSERT OR JUNK.

The next foods to layer into your plan are additional nutritious carbs, like whole grains (bread, rice, oats, pasta, etc.), legumes (beans and peas), and tubers (potato and other root vegetables), as well as caloric beverages that have at least some nutritional value, like fruit juice, milk, sports drinks, and alcohol.

If you're cutting, I don't recommend that you include any caloric beverages in your meal plan because they don't trigger satiety like food.[8]

You can drink 1,000 calories and be hungry an hour later, whereas eating 1,000 calories of food, including a good portion of protein and fiber, will keep you full for a number of hours.

This is why studies show that people who drink calories are much more likely to overeat than those who don't, and that there is a clear association between a greater intake of sugar-sweetened beverages and weight gain in both adults and children.[9]

5. TWEAK YOUR PROTEIN INTAKE AS NEEDED.

If your protein is still short after adding your nutritious carbs, now's a good time to top it off.

The easiest way to do this is by increasing the serving size of one or more of your primary sources of protein.

6. ADD ADDITIONAL FAT AS NEEDED.

Next, you should bolster your fat intake with (healthy) fatty foods of your choice, such as butter, cheese, oils, nuts, seeds, and avocado (my go-tos).

Remember to ensure that your saturated fat intake doesn't end up too high.

By the end of this step, you should have met your protein and nutritional needs and accounted for most of your carbs and fats as well. And unless your TDEE is *very* high, you should have also allocated 80 to 90 percent of your total daily calories.

What, then, should you do with the calories and macros that remain?

You can play with the serving sizes of everything you've done so far, or you can ...

7. ADD TREATS IF DESIRED.

Any calories left at this point are "discretionary," meaning you can use them on whatever you'd like.

Again, you can find delicious and calorie-friendly options in my cookbook *The Shredded Chef* (www.shreddedchefbook.com), as well as on my websites Muscle for Life (www.muscleforlife.com/category/recipes) and Legion Athletics (www.legionathletics.com/category/recipes).

PUTTING IT ALL TOGETHER

Meal planning is much like putting together a jigsaw puzzle.

You can dump the pieces into a heap and try to muddle your way through it, or you can shortcut the process by being more systematic—start with the edges, sort the tabs and blanks, separate into color groups, and so forth.

Following are several examples of effective and well-made meal plans for cutting and lean bulking. They're also included in the free bonus material that comes with this book (www.thinnerleanerstronger.com/bonus).

CUTTING MEAL PLAN FOR A 140-POUND WOMAN						
MEAL	**FOOD**	**AMOUNT**	**CALORIES**	**PROTEIN**	**CARBS**	**FAT**
Preworkout Meal	Plain nonfat Greek yogurt	170 grams	100	17	6	0
	Banana	136 grams	121	2	31	1
Total			221	19	37	1
Workout						
Breakfast	Plain nonfat Greek yogurt	170 grams	100	17	6	0
	Unsweetened almond milk	262 grams	39	1	3	3
	Blueberry	74 grams	43	1	11	0
Total			182	19	20	4
Lunch	Skinless boneless chicken breast	198 grams	237	45	0	5
	Roasted Garlic Twice-Baked Potato from *The Shredded Chef*	1 serving	216	6	39	5
	Butter	14 grams	102	0	0	12
Total			555	51	39	22
Dinner	Skinless boneless chicken breast	198 grams	237	45	0	5
	Curried Potatoes and Cauliflower from *The Shredded Chef*	1 serving	230	12	47	1
Total			467	57	47	6
Daily Total			1,425	145	143	32
Daily Target			1,400	140	140	31

MEAL	FOOD	AMOUNT	CALORIES	PROTEIN	CARBS	FAT
	LEAN BULKING MEAL PLAN FOR A 100-POUND WOMAN					
Preworkout Meal	Egg white	100 grams	52	11	1	0
	Cooked bacon	13 grams	60	6	0	4
	Whole grain bread	28 grams	80	4	14	0
	Jam	20 grams	56	0	14	0
	Butter	5 grams	34	0	0	4
	Total		278	21	29	8
	Workout					
Postworkout Shake	Plain nonfat Greek yogurt	170 grams	100	17	6	0
	Unsweetened rice milk	240 grams	113	1	22	2
	Banana	136 grams	121	2	31	1
	Blueberry	148 grams	84	1	21	1
	Total		418	21	81	3
Lunch	Chicken Pesto Pasta from *The Shredded Chef*	1 Serving	412	31	38	17
	Total		412	31	38	17
Snack	Apple	182 grams	95	0	25	0
	Total		95	0	25	0
Dinner	Sirloin, trimmed of visible fat	100 grams	126	22	0	4
	Brown rice	70 grams	218	5	39	2
	70 to 85% dark chocolate	14 grams	85	1	7	6
	Total		464	28	60	12
	Daily Total		1,704	101	232	40
	Daily Target		1,700	106	234	38

MAINTENANCE MEAL PLAN FOR A 130-POUND WOMAN						
MEAL	**FOOD**	**AMOUNT**	**CALORIES**	**PROTEIN**	**CARBS**	**FAT**
Preworkout Meal	Whole egg	100 grams	143	13	1	10
	Egg white	130 grams	68	14	1	0
	Oatmeal	40 grams	152	5	27	3
	Unsweetened almond milk	240 grams	36	1	3	2
	Strawberry	140 grams	45	1	11	0
	Total		444	34	43	15
Workout						
Postworkout Meal	Plain nonfat Greek yogurt	340 grams	201	35	12	1
	Banana	136 grams	121	2	31	1
	White bread	28 grams	74	3	14	1
	Avocado	60 grams	96	1	5	9
	Total		492	40	62	12
Lunch	Chunky Chicken Quesadillas from *The Shredded Chef*	1 serving	315	30	28	9
	Total		315	30	28	9
Snack	Grape	120 grams	83	1	22	0
	Total		83	1	22	0
Dinner	Farmed Atlantic salmon	112 grams	233	23	0	15
	Brown rice	70 grams	253	5	53	2
	Broccoli	300 grams	102	9	20	1
	Total		588	37	73	18
Daily Total			1,922	141	228	54
Daily Target			1,950	146	219	54

If you haven't already, make your first meal plan now.

Take as much time as you need—most people need thirty to sixty minutes to create their first meal plans and considerably less time going forward. Come back when you're done, and we'll continue.

If you'd like one-on-one help with creating meal plans (and everything else discussed in this book), check out my personal coaching service at www.muscleforlife.com/coaching.

HOW TO ADD VARIETY TO YOUR MEAL PLAN

If you're new to the *Thinner Leaner Stronger* method of meal planning, back-burner this bit. Eat the same foods every meal, every day, and you'll be much less likely to accidentally overeat or undereat.

If the thought of that routine sends a shiver through your taste buds, you might be surprised at how easy it is when you're eating foods that you actually like. You don't get sick of them as quickly as you might think.

Furthermore, if you look at your diet now, you'll probably find that you're already eating a lot of the same foods regularly. Most people tend to rotate through a number of staple meals for breakfast, lunch, dinner, and snacks. Creating a meal plan simply organizes this habit around a goal.

If you really want variety in your plan, however, or just feel up to the challenge, you can create alternative options for individual meals in your plan (breakfast, lunch, dinner, etc.).

The best way to do this is to work within the calorie and macronutritional restraints of the meals you're replacing.

For example, if your breakfast currently contains 30 grams of protein, 50 grams of carbs, and 15 grams of fat, work with those numbers when creating alternative breakfasts. That way, you don't have to adjust the rest of your plan for each meal option.

. . .

You now know how to create a "miracle meal plan"—one that meets your calorie and micro- and macronutritional needs, that allows you to eat the foods you like, and that fits your lifestyle.

If we ended this part of the book here, you'd be well equipped to succeed with your diet. We have one more topic to talk about, however, and it's an important one: "cheating."

Specifically, how to "cheat" on your diet without ruining it. Let's find out.

KEY TAKEAWAYS

- I don't recommend "on-the-fly" tracking with an app like MyFitnessPal or "eating by feel" until you've successfully cut, lean bulked, and maintained with meal planning.

- Meal planning is the simplest and most effective way to put everything you've learned so far into practice. So long as you've done your math right and stick to the plan, your body composition will change.

- If a food came in a package, you can use the numbers provided on the label.

- Most of your meals shouldn't come in packages. They should consist of relatively unprocessed foods that you prepare and cook yourself.

- The following websites are good resources for meal planning: CalorieKing (www.calorieking.com), SELF Nutrition Data (nutritiondata.self.com), and the USDA Food Composition Databases (ndb.nal.usda.gov).

- Weigh everything you eat before cooking to determine its calories and macros, and when preparing multiple servings, weigh again after cooking to determine portion sizes.

- When you measure by volume as opposed to weight (cups and spoons versus ounces and grams), small measurement inaccuracies can significantly skew your numbers.

- Include in your meal plan absolutely everything you're going to eat. Everything counts—vegetables, fruits, condiments, dabs of oil and butter, and every other bit of food that'll go into your mouth every day.

- The only way to "safely" include recipes in your meal plans is to total the calories and macros for each ingredient and divide the sums by the number of servings.

- The best meal plan recipes are easy and fast to make, require relatively few ingredients, and allow you to prepare large amounts of food with minimal equipment and work.

- If a recipe you like contains too many calories, there are several ways you can lighten it: if it's not a baked good, reduce (or remove, if possible) the butter or oil, replace sugar with a zero-calorie sweetener of your choice, swap whole-fat dairy with low- or nonfat dairy, and swap fatty meats for leaner cuts (or poultry).

- Generally speaking, the less you eat out, the better your results are going to be with your diet.

- The body has no way to directly convert alcohol into body fat, which means that calories provided by ethanol (alcohol) simply can't produce fat gain in the same way that calories from food can.

- Alcohol blunts fat oxidation and increases the conversion of carbs into body fat.

• If you want to drink alcohol without interfering with your fat loss or accelerating fat gain, follow these three tips: don't drink more than one day per week, lower your carb and fat intakes that day (eat more protein than you normally would), and try not to eat while drinking and stay away from carb-laden drinks like beer and fruity stuff (stick to dry wines and spirits).

• When creating a meal plan, you want to be within 50 calories of your target intake when cutting and within 100 calories when lean bulking and maintaining.

• If you're new to the *Thinner Leaner Stronger* method of meal planning, eat the same foods every meal, every day, and you'll be much less likely to accidentally overeat or undereat.

• If you really want variety in your plan, however, or just feel up to the challenge, you can create alternative options for individual meals in your plan (breakfast, lunch, dinner, etc.).

20

HOW TO "CHEAT" ON YOUR DIET WITHOUT RUINING IT

> *"Most champions are built by punch-the-clock workouts rather than extraordinary efforts."*
> —DAN JOHN

Sometimes it feels great to just let go. To stop striving and trying to control everything and just give in to our impulses.

You know . . . to just "be human" now and then.

When it comes to dieting, that means ignoring the plan and "cheating." No counting calories. No guesstimating macros. And no worrying about what we are and aren't "supposed" to eat.

There are quite a few opinions on cheating.

Some people believe that even mild deviations from your diet plan can prevent you from reaching your goals. Others are of the mind that you can stray so long as you don't turn to certain forbidden foods. Still others say it's okay to throw caution to the wind every week and gorge on anything and everything you can fit into your belly.

All these opinions are incorrect.

You certainly can have "cheat meals" without ruining your progress and you don't have to stick to a short list of "approved" foods, but you can't eat yourself unconscious every week without paying a price.

When done correctly, cheating can make it easier to stick to your diet and see results. When done incorrectly, however, it can cause considerable trouble.

In this chapter, you're going to learn how to have your cake and eat it too—how to get maximum enjoyment out of cheating while minimizing the potential downsides.

WHAT IS "CHEATING," ANYWAY?

When I talk about cheating on your diet, I'm not talking about eating sugar or dairy or some other food deemed "unclean" by one of the many pied pipers of the diet industry.

All you and I care about are the calories, macronutrients, and micronutrients of what you're eating.

When you eat more calories than you planned on eating, regardless of what foods you eat, that's cheating. And when you replace a large portion of your nutritious calories with nonnutritious ones, that's cheating too.

In other words, cheating consists of eating a lot more calories or a lot less nutritious food than you normally would eat.

The drawbacks of cheating are obvious. Eat too many calories too frequently, and you'll fail to lose weight as desired (or will gain weight too quickly), and disregard nutrition too frequently, and you'll increase the risk of developing nutritional deficiencies.

That doesn't mean you shouldn't stray from your meal plan from time to time, however. You absolutely should if you want to, but you need to know how to do it productively.

This begins with avoiding the five most common mistakes people make when cheating on their diets.

THE FIVE BIGGEST CHEATING MISTAKES YOU CAN MAKE

Cheating itself isn't a mistake or something to feel guilty about.

Occasionally allowing yourself to loosen up can make your diet as a whole more enjoyable and improve dietary compliance and long-term results.

That said, *how* you cheat matters. If you make any of the following mistakes, it becomes detrimental:

1. Cheating too frequently
2. Eating too much in a cheat meal
3. Indulging in cheat *days*, not meals
4. Eating too much fat
5. Drinking alcohol

Let's take a closer look at each.

1. CHEATING TOO FREQUENTLY

This one is pretty self-explanatory.

Overeat too often, and you'll erase either most or all of your calorie deficit and hamstring (or even halt) your fat loss. And if you're lean bulking, you'll balloon your calorie surplus and gain too much fat too quickly.

And on the nutritional side, neglect food quality often enough and you can erode your health and face a number of problems, including bone loss, anxiety and brain fog, fatigue and muscle weakness, and cardiovascular disease.[1]

2. EATING TOO MUCH IN A CHEAT MEAL

Many people don't realize how many calories are in the foods they eat in their cheat meals.

This is particularly true when eating at restaurants, because a professional chef's job is to produce delicious—not calorie-conscious—food. And when that's the goal, butter, oil, and sugar are a cook's best friends.

A good example of this is a study conducted by scientists at Tufts University that involved the analysis of 360 dinner entrees at 123 nonchain restaurants in San Francisco, Boston, and Little Rock between 2011 and 2014.[2]

They found that the restaurant dishes contained, on average, about 1,200 calories. American, Italian, and Chinese restaurants were the worst offenders, with an average of nearly 1,500 calories per meal.

Even more flagrant offenders can be found in an analysis of restaurant foods conducted by scientists at the Center for Science in the Public Interest.[3]

The Cheesecake Factory, for instance, makes a bruléed French toast with a side of bacon that weighs in at 2,780 calories, 93 grams of saturated fat, and 24 teaspoons of sugar. It also offers a creamy farfalle pasta with chicken and roasted garlic, which is a bit lighter at just 2,410 calories and 63 grams of saturated fat.

Let's also not forget that those are just individual entrees, which, for many people, aren't the entirety of their cheat meals. Add in some bread, an appetizer, and dessert, and the numbers can swell to horrific highs.

It should come as no surprise, then, that research conducted by scientists at the University of Illinois at Urbana-Champaign concluded that calorically speaking, there's not much of a difference between fast food and full-service dining.[4]

So, my point is this: if you don't pay attention to your calorie intake when having a cheat meal, you can seriously set yourself back.

3. INDULGING IN CHEAT DAYS, NOT MEALS

You just saw how easy it is to rack up a few thousand calories in just one trip to your favorite restaurant, so you can only imagine just how deep you can dig in an entire day of off-plan eating.

For example, here are the approximate calorie counts for a number of popular cheat-meal foods:

- Deep-dish pizza: 480 calories per slice
- Ice cream: 270 calories per half cup
- Bacon cheeseburger: 595 calories per burger
- Traditional cheesecake: 400 calories per slice
- French fries: 498 calories per large serving
- Chocolate chip cookies: 220 calories per large cookie
- Creamy pasta: 593 calories per cup
- Loaded nachos: 1,590 calories per plate
- Pecan pie: 541 calories per slice

As you can see, just a few hearty portions of any of those is all it takes to push your calorie intake into the stratosphere.

4. EATING TOO MUCH FAT

Many people think that eating a lot of carbs is the surest way to gain fat, but they're wrong. And that's true even when you're cheating.

What *is* the surest way to gain fat, though, is eating a large amount of dietary fat.[5] To understand why this is, we have to review the physiology of what happens in the body when you eat carbs and fat.

Chemically speaking, glucose is very different from the molecules that compose body fat (lipids). This is why glucose must be heavily processed in the body before it can be stored as fat. This process of carb-to-fat conversion is known as *de novo lipogenesis* (DNL).

Surprisingly, research shows that DNL rarely occurs under normal dietary conditions.[6] Furthermore, research shows that carbohydrate intake has to be absolutely sky high (700 to 900 grams per day for several days) for DNL to result in significant fat gain.[7]

There are exceptions, such as very large infusions of pure glucose and people with hyperinsulinemia (a condition where the amount of insulin in the blood is higher than normal), but in healthy individuals following a normal diet, carbs are rarely converted into body fat.[8]

How does this square with energy balance, you're wondering?

Well, just because it's hard to gain fat through DNL doesn't mean that eating carbs can't contribute to fat gain. We know it can, of course.

Here's how this works: when you eat carbs, fat oxidation decreases, which means that most of the dietary fat you eat with the carbs will be stored as body fat.[9]

Now, what about dietary fat? How is it metabolized compared to carbohydrate?

We recall that dietary fat is metabolized very differently and stored very easily as body fat, which explains why research shows that a high-fat meal causes more immediate fat gain than a high-carb meal.[10]

All this also helps explain why research conducted by scientists at the National Institutes of Health found that calorie for calorie, low-fat dieting is more effective for fat loss than low-carb (at least in the short term), and why studies show that it's easier to overeat on a high-fat diet, and that obesity rates are higher among high-fat dieters than low-fat.[11]

Oh, and in case you're wondering if you can "hack" your metabolism by eating a diet very high in carbs and very, very low in fat, I applaud your creative thinking, but don't bother.

Not only would doing so be bad for your health, but research shows that when fat intake is too low, DNL ramps up, increasing fat storage.[12]

5. DRINKING ALCOHOL

In chapter 7, you learned that alcohol blunts fat oxidation and triggers DNL, and when you mix this double whammy with overeating—especially the greasy, fatty foods that most people like to eat when drinking—you get maximum fat gain.

Just one or two large alcohol-infused cheat meals per week can be enough to wipe out all fat loss and stick you in a rut.

HOW TO CHEAT WITHOUT RUINING YOUR DIET

Now that you know what you're *not* supposed to do, let's look at how to cheat correctly.

1. Cheat once per week.

2. When cutting, try not to exceed your average TDEE for the day.

3. When lean bulking, try not to exceed 130 percent of your average TDEE for the day.

4. Try to keep your fat intake under 100 grams for the day.

5. Drink alcohol intelligently.

Let's review each of these points separately.

1. CHEAT ONCE PER WEEK.

Whether you're cutting, lean bulking, or maintaining, cheat just once per week, whether in a single meal or spread throughout an entire day, and you'll be able to loosen up and enjoy yourself without anything to worry about.

2. WIIEN CUTTING, TRY NOT TO EXCEED YOUR AVERAGE TDEE FOR THE DAY.

This gives you plenty of room to eat foods you normally wouldn't eat when cutting, especially if you're putting all those extra calories into just one or two meals.

You can also "save up" calories if you want to eat a lot in one meal by eating more or less nothing but protein leading up to (and after) it. This tip is great for people like me who like to eat one large cheat meal.

For example, my cheat meals are almost always dinners, so throughout the day, I'll eat a serving of protein every few hours but skip the carbs and fats that I would normally eat. This way, when I get to dinner, I have a large buffer of carbs and fat (and thus calories) before I even come close to my average TDEE for the day.

When I cheat at breakfast, the strategy is the same: I eat most of my carbs and fat for the day in that one meal and then have mostly protein from there on out.

In case you're wondering, here are some of my favorite cheat meals in no particular order:

1. Margarita pizza from a local restaurant that imports ingredients from Italy

2. Homemade pancakes covered in syrup (I love Kodiak Cakes' Whole Wheat Oat & Honey mix)

3. Jeni's Brambleberry Crisp ice cream

4. Fleming's steak and chocolate lava cake

5. Delicious bread rolls and pastries from a local baker

6. Plain ol' Five Guys cheeseburger with fries

And great, now I'm drooling. Time to practice some of those inner-game techniques we learned earlier ...

3. WHEN LEAN BULKING, TRY NOT TO EXCEED 130 PERCENT OF YOUR AVERAGE TDEE FOR THE DAY.

When you're in a calorie surplus, your body is primed for both muscle and fat gain.

This is why cheating can catch up with you very quickly when lean bulking. Give yourself too much dietary latitude, and you'll watch your waistline expand rather rapidly.

Thus, when cheating on a lean bulk phase, you can bump your calorie intake up a bit, but don't go to town.

Truth be told, when I'm lean bulking, I try not to exceed my normal daily calorie intake by using the "saving up" tip I just shared.

4. TRY TO KEEP YOUR DIETARY FAT INTAKE UNDER 100 GRAMS FOR THE DAY.

This not only helps you keep your calories under control (remember that a gram of fat contains about 9 calories), but it also helps you minimize fat gain.

So instead of doubling down on your favorite fatty foods when you cheat, go high carb instead. This will result in less immediate fat storage, and it also has other benefits when you're cutting.

One of the downsides of keeping your body in a calorie deficit is that it reduces the levels of a hormone called *leptin*, which is produced by body fat.[13]

In simple terms, leptin tells your brain that there's plenty of energy available, and that your body can expend energy freely, eat normal amounts of food, and engage in normal amounts of physical activity.

When you restrict your calories to lose fat, however, the drop in leptin tells your body that it's in an energy-deficient state and must expend less energy and consume more.

It accomplishes this through several mechanisms, including lowering the basal metabolic rate, reducing general activity levels, and stimulating the appetite.[14]

Raising leptin levels reverses these effects, which is one of the reasons you feel better when you stop restricting your calories and return to normal eating.

To fully reverse the dip in leptin that comes with cutting, you have to come out of a calorie deficit. You can temporarily boost leptin production, however, by acutely increasing your calorie intake for a day or two, giving your metabolism a shot in the arm.[15]

Research shows that eating a large amount of carbohydrate (two grams or more per pound of body weight per day) is particularly effective for this.[16]

This is known as "refeeding," and it's a win-win. It lets you load up on your favorite carbs and enjoy a physical and psychological boost.

5. DRINK ALCOHOL INTELLIGENTLY.

As you learned in the last chapter, the smart way to drink alcohol is to:

1. Not drink more than one day per week.

2. Lower your carb and fat intakes that day. (Eat more protein than you normally would.)

3. Try not to eat while drinking and stay away from carb-laden drinks like beer and fruity stuff. (Stick to dry wines and spirits.)

In other words, don't drink too often and don't combine it with cheat meals.

. . .

Cheating incorrectly is one of the major reasons why so many people "mysteriously" can't lose weight "no matter what they do," and why so many people have "mysterious" health problems despite "eating pretty healthily."

They don't realize that you can borderline starve yourself all week and, in one weekend, regain all the fat you lost, and that a smattering of fruits and vegetables here and there can't make up for general nutritional negligence.

Cheat correctly, though, and you can have the best of all worlds.

You can enjoy the satisfaction of indulging regularly without the penalties of excessive fat gain and impaired health, as well as the pleasure that comes from having a strong, vital body that looks and feels exceptional.

KEY TAKEAWAYS

- When done correctly, cheating can make it easier to stick to your diet and see results. When done incorrectly, however, it can cause considerable trouble.

- Cheating consists of eating a lot more calories or a lot less nutritious food than you normally would eat.

- Eat too many calories too frequently, and you'll fail to lose weight as desired (or will gain weight too quickly), and disregard nutrition too frequently, and you'll increase the risk of developing nutritional deficiencies.

- If you don't pay attention to your calorie intake when having a cheat meal, you can seriously set yourself back.

- The surest way to gain fat is eating a large amount of dietary fat.

- When you eat carbs, fat oxidation decreases, which means that most of the dietary fat you eat with the carbs will be stored as body fat.

- Dietary fat is chemically similar to the lipids in body fat and thus can be converted and stored very easily as body fat. This explains why a high-fat meal causes more immediate fat gain than a high-carb meal.

- Alcohol blunts fat oxidation and triggers DNL, and when you mix this double whammy with overeating—especially the greasy, fatty foods that most people like to eat when drinking—you get maximum fat gain.

- Just one or two large alcohol-infused cheat meals per week can be enough to wipe out all fat loss and stick you in a rut.

- Whether you're cutting, lean bulking, or maintaining, cheat just once per week, whether in a single meal or spread throughout an entire day.

- When cutting, try not to exceed your average TDEE for the day.

- You can "save up" calories if you want to eat a lot in one meal by eating more or less nothing but protein leading up to (and after) it.

- When lean bulking, try not to exceed 130 percent of your average TDEE for the day.

- When I'm lean bulking, I try not to exceed my normal daily calorie intake by using the "saving up" tip.

- Try to keep your dietary fat intake under 100 grams for the day.

- One of the downsides of keeping your body in a calorie deficit is that it reduces the levels of a hormone called leptin, which tells your brain that there's plenty of energy available, and that your body can expend energy freely, eat normal amounts of food, and engage in normal amounts of physical activity.

- You can temporarily boost leptin production by acutely increasing your calorie intake for a day or two, giving your metabolism a shot in the arm.

- Eating a large amount of carbohydrate (two grams or more per pound of body weight per day) is particularly effective for this.

- Don't drink too often and don't combine it with cheat meals.

PART 5

THE LAST EXERCISE ADVICE YOU'LL EVER NEED

21

THE ULTIMATE WORKOUT PLAN FOR WOMEN — STRENGTH TRAINING

"I love to see a young girl go out and grab the world by the lapels. Life's a bitch. You've got to go out and kick ass."

—MAYA ANGELOU

If you're like most women, you want a very specific type of body.

You want to be lean but not too skinny (and most definitely not "skinny fat").

You want a toned upper body but don't want to look like a "bulky" weightlifter.

You want a flat, defined stomach. You want tight, shapely legs.

And last but most definitely not least, you want that perfect, gravity-defying butt.

Well, you—yes, lil' ol' you—can have all these things. You don't need top-shelf genetics or a lifetime of training to look like a million bucks.

You have to know what you're doing, though, because you don't become a "goddess" by starving yourself and doing endless cardio.

Instead, you need to take a completely different approach in the gym than most women, and believe it or not, a much healthier, more enjoyable, and sustainable one at that.

We're going to break it all down in this chapter, and it begins with a simple formula that looks like this:

$$2-3 \mid 8-10 \mid 9-15 \mid 2-4 \mid 3-5 \mid 1-2 \mid 8-10$$

No, that isn't a secret code that you have to break, but it does contain the "secrets" to building the body you've always wanted.

As you know, my *Thinner Leaner Stronger* program revolves mostly around smart and effective weightlifting, and this formula outlines the protocol you're going to follow.

There are many other types of weightlifting blueprints out there, and some are far better than others. But if you're like most women, this one is all you need to grab your brass ring because it's simple, straightforward, and delivers head-turning results, and fast.

Once you're rocking your best body ever, if you want to take your strength and fitness to the next level, there's a lot more you can learn about effective training, but we can save that for another time and another book.

For now, I want to keep things as practical as possible, and I want to guarantee you rapid and remarkable results. That's why I'm going to give you a very specific training prescription that follows the numeric recipe above.

Let's go through it one piece at a time, followed by several other essential training components, including progression, exercise tempo, and more.

2-3

TRAIN 2 TO 3 MAJOR MUSCLE GROUPS PER WORKOUT

There are many different ways to organize your workouts.

For instance, you can train your entire body several times per week ("full-body split"), your upper and lower body on different days ("upper/lower split"), or different major muscle groups on different days ("body-part split").

Thinner Leaner Stronger utilizes what's known as a "push-pull-legs" or "PPL" split, which has you train two to three major muscle groups per workout.

This type of routine has stood the test of time for several reasons:

- It trains all major muscle groups.

- It allows plenty of time for recovery.

- It can be easily tailored to fit different training goals, schedules, and histories.

It's easy to understand, too. At bottom, a push-pull-legs routine separates your major muscle groups into three different workouts:

1. Chest, shoulders, and triceps (push)

2. Back and biceps (pull)

3. Legs (including glutes, usually)

And this routine has you train anywhere from three to six times per week, depending on how much your body can take, what you're looking to achieve with your physique, and how much time you can spend in the gym.

8–10

DO 8 TO 10 REPS PER HARD SET

First, some clarification on the lingo.

"Rep" is short for "repetition," which is a single raising and lowering of a weight.

For example, if you're doing dumbbell biceps curls and curl the weights up from your sides and then lower them back to their starting positions, you've done one rep.

A "set" is a fixed number of repetitions of a particular exercise.

For instance, if you do six reps of biceps curls and stop, you've done one set (of six reps).

And a "hard set" is a heavy, muscle- and strength-building set that's taken close to technical failure (the point where you can no longer continue with proper form).

Thinner Leaner Stronger is going to have you work in the rep range of 8 to 10 reps, meaning that most hard sets for all exercises are going to entail doing at least 8 reps but not more than 10.

For most women, this means working with weights that are around 70 to 75 percent of their one-rep max.

Why this rep range? Two reasons:

1. Research shows that it's highly effective for gaining muscle and strength.[1]

2. It's heavy but not so heavy that you're going to struggle to control the weights properly.

Chances are *Thinner Leaner Stronger* will have you handling much heavier weights than you're used to, which is exactly what we want.

Many weightlifting programs for women involve lifting very light weights for a high number of reps. This can result in muscle growth, but as you learned in chapter 10, it's far less practical than lifting heavier weights for fewer reps.

Therefore, if you wanted to deviate from my recommended 8-to-10-rep range, you'd be better off going with heavier weights and fewer reps, not the other way around.

9–15

DO 9 TO 15 HARD SETS PER WORKOUT

Each *Thinner Leaner Stronger* workout will have you warm up and perform 9 to 15 hard sets.

This isn't as minimalist as some programs out there, but it's a lot less than many women are used to. For example, poke around magazines and websites and you'll find workout after workout for women that call for 25 to 30 sets.

I'm not going to ask you to do anywhere near that many sets in each workout because when you're lifting heavy weights and pushing close to technical failure in each set, you don't need to do as much to produce a powerful muscle-building stimulus, and you can only do so much before it becomes counterproductive.

2–4

REST 2 TO 4 MINUTES IN BETWEEN HARD SETS

Most people are in the gym to move and sweat, so sitting around in between sets seems like a waste of time.

This is why they tend to keep rest periods as short as possible or, in some cases, eliminate them altogether, preferring to always stay in motion.

Short or no rest periods is fine if you're looking to merely burn calories, but if you're there to build muscle and get stronger, it's a mistake.

Strength training involves pushing your muscles to their limits, and resting enough in between sets is a vital part of this process because it prepares your muscles to exert maximum effort in each set.

This has been clearly demonstrated in a number of studies.

For instance, scientists at the Federal University of Parana (Brazil) found that when people performed the bench press and squat with two-minute rest intervals, they were able to perform significantly more reps per workout than when rest intervals were shortened in 15-second increments (1:45, 1:30, 1:15, and so forth).[2]

This is significant because the total amount of reps performed over time is a major contributor to muscle growth.[3]

Additionally, an extensive review of weightlifting studies conducted by scientists at the State University of Rio de Janeiro found the following:

> In terms of acute responses, a key finding was that when training with loads between 50% and 90% of one repetition maximum, 3-5 minutes' rest between sets allowed for greater repetitions over multiple sets.

Furthermore, in terms of chronic adaptations, resting 3-5 minutes between sets produced greater increases in absolute strength, due to higher intensities and volumes of training. Similarly, higher levels of muscular power were demonstrated over multiple sets with 3 or 5 minutes versus 1 minute of rest between sets.[4]

Similar findings were demonstrated in a study conducted by scientists at Eastern Illinois University.[5] In this case, researchers concluded the following:

> The findings of the present study indicate that large squat strength gains can be achieved with a minimum of 2 minutes' rest between sets, and little additional gains are derived from resting 4 minutes between sets.

I could go on, but the evidence is clear: when you're lifting heavy weights to gain muscle and strength, you want to rest around three minutes in between each hard set.

The reason why this piece of the formula is "2–4" and not just "3" is you can rest slightly less (two minutes) in between hard sets for smaller muscle groups like the biceps, triceps, and shoulders, and slightly more (four minutes) in between hard sets for your larger muscle groups like your back and legs if your heart rate hasn't settled down, or if you simply feel you need a little more time before you can give maximum effort on your next hard set.

If you're used to mainstream weightlifting programs for women, this is going to feel very strange at first. You might even feel a bit guilty, like you're sitting around more than you're actually working out.

This is normal, and once you see how well your body responds to this type of training, you'll stop worrying and start enjoying your downtime. If I'm working out alone, I like to read on my phone (Kindle app) in between sets. I can get through an extra 15 to 25 pages per day this way!

3-5

TRAIN MOST MAJOR MUSCLE GROUPS ONCE EVERY 3 TO 5 DAYS

Many people think that training frequency is a major factor in muscle building.

To them, it's black and white: if you're not directly training every major muscle group in your body two to three times per week, you're not going to get very far.

This makes for good tweets and YouTube snippets, but it also misses the forest for the trees. How frequently you can and should train each major muscle group depends on several things:

- Your workout schedule
- Your physique goals

- Your workout intensity (how heavy the weights are)
- Your workout volume (how many hard sets you do)

For instance, if you can lift weights three days per week and are much more interested in developing your lower body than your upper body, it doesn't make sense to do three whole-body workouts per week.

Instead, you'll want to focus the majority of your time and effort on your lower body.

The relationship between intensity, volume, and frequency is fairly complicated, and there are many viable ways to design a workout routine, but here's an overarching, nonnegotiable rule that will govern the results:

The higher the intensity and volume of the individual workouts, the less frequently you can do them.[6]

So yes, you can squat or bench press three times per week, but you can't do 10 heavy sets of each per workout.

Furthermore, and more importantly, really, when it comes to gaining muscle and strength, research shows that training frequency isn't nearly as important as how heavy the weights generally are and how many hard sets you generally perform each week.[7]

In other words, so long as you're lifting heavy weights, frequency is mostly a tool you use to reach your target weekly volume for each major muscle group. Whether you reach that volume target in one workout or three has a far smaller effect on muscle growth than many people realize.

As you'll see, in *Thinner Leaner Stronger*, you're going to train your lower body more frequently than your upper body because if you're like, well, every woman I've ever known, it's going to take a lot more work to get the legs and glutes you want than the chest, shoulders, back, and arms you desire.

Don't worry, though—your upper body isn't going to fall behind or look underdeveloped. The weekly volume for your upper body will be more than enough to develop plenty of muscle definition in everything above the waist (not to mention the fact that many lower-body exercises benefit the upper body as well!).

1–2

TAKE 1 TO 2 DAYS OFF PER WEEK

Search the hashtag #nodaysoff, and you'll see a lot of very fit people bragging about their undying dedication and determination.

While I applaud the effort, for most of us, training seven days per week is a one-way street to physical and psychological burnout (especially when cutting).

Heavy weightlifting can feel pretty brutal at times. Hard sets are *hard*. Your muscles take a beating. Your joints and tendons ache. Your nervous system is regularly redlined.

All this is healthy and a necessary part of the adaptation process that makes your muscles stronger and more defined. It also accumulates nonmuscular fatigue in the body, however, that leads to reductions in speed, power, and the ability to perform technical movements and exercises.[8]

In layman's terms: intense training wears you out.

Some research indicates that this may be more of a sensation or emotion rather than a purely physical phenomenon, but it's real, and you need to know how to deal with it.[9]

If you ignore it and keep forging ahead, you can develop a number of symptoms related to overtraining, including:[10]

- Soreness, fatigue, and weakness that doesn't go away with rest
- Trouble sleeping
- Loss of appetite and unintended weight loss
- Irritability, anxiety, impatience, and restlessness
- Irregularly slow or fast heart rate
- Inability to focus
- Depression

This is why I recommend no more than six days of serious exercise per week (resistance training and higher-intensity cardio), with one day of no intense physical activity whatsoever (very low-intensity cardio or sports, however, like swimming, walking, or golf is fine).

I also recommend two days off resistance training per week when in a calorie deficit.

8–10

TAKE IT EASY EVERY 8 TO 10 WEEKS

Another effective way to avoid symptoms related to overtraining is dialing back your workouts every so often. There are two easy ways to do this:

1. Periodically reduce your workout intensity or volume (known as *deloading*).
2. Periodically take five to seven days off weightlifting.

In *Thinner Leaner Stronger*, I'm going to have you try both and see which works best for you. And don't worry—a week off the weights isn't going to cause fat gain or muscle loss.

Now that we've gone through the entire formula I introduced you to earlier, let's discuss several other vital aspects of *Thinner Leaner Stronger* training.

THE DOUBLE PROGRESSION MODEL

As you learned in chapter 10, one of the most important aspects of weightlifting is progression.

No matter how much thought you put into frequency, intensity, volume, or any other factor related to workout programming, if you don't get progression right, you won't make it very far.

It's the key to avoiding stagnation and breaking through the many training plateaus that will occur throughout your fitness journey.

There are a number of ways to progress in your weightlifting workouts, but one of my favorite models is known as *double progression*.

In double progression, you work with a given weight in a given rep range, and once you hit the top of that rep range for a certain number of hard sets (one, two, or three, usually), you increase the weight.

Then, if you can at least come to within a rep or two of the bottom of your rep range in your first hard set with the new, heavier weight, you work with that weight until you can hit the top of your rep range again.

If you can't get to within at least a rep or two of the bottom of your rep range with that new weight, however, you have a couple of options that we'll discuss later in this book.

With this model of progression, you work to increase your reps, and then "cash in" that progress to increase your weights. Hence, "double progression."

To see how this works in action, let's say you're squatting in the 8-to-10-rep range, and on your first (or second) hard set of your workout, you get 10 reps with 100 pounds.

In *Thinner Leaner Stronger*, you're going to progress after hitting 10 reps for one hard set, so that means it's time to increase the weight!

You then add 5 pounds to the bar, rest a few minutes, and get 8 reps on your next hard set.

Hooray! The progression succeeds and you now work with 105 pounds until you can squat it for one hard set of 10 reps, move up in weight, and so on.

Simple enough, but here's a key question: How difficult are these hard sets supposed to be?

If you want to get the most out of double progression, you want to end each of your hard sets one or two reps shy of technical failure, which again, is the point where you can't do another rep with proper form.

In other words, you want your hard sets to be pretty dang hard.

Why not go to absolute muscle failure? Mostly because it's not necessary for muscle and strength gain and often leads to a breakdown in form, which increases the risk of injury.[11]

As our muscles become fatigued, we lose the ability to accurately feel what we're doing with our bodies and can think we're maintaining good form when we're not.[12]

This is especially true in the case of compound exercises like the deadlift, squat, and bench press, which require more technical skill than simpler isolation exercises.

We'll talk about progression in more detail in chapter 29 and learn what to do if you don't get your eight reps after moving up in weight or run into other snags.

THE RIGHT REP TEMPO

"Rep tempo" refers to how quickly you lower and raise the weights, and there are two basic schools of thought on it:

1. You should perform reps fairly quickly.
2. You should perform reps fairly slowly.

People who advocate for a slow tempo often say that "muscles don't know weight, only tension," and the more tension they're subjected to, the more they'll grow in response.

Furthermore, by slowing your reps down, you increase the amount of time your muscles remain under tension, and this, they claim, produces more muscle gain than faster reps.

While it's true that slow reps do indeed increase time under tension, it turns out that this isn't important enough to warrant special attention.

The primary reason for this is that the slower you perform an exercise with a given weight, the fewer reps you can do with it.[13] Depending on how slow your tempo is, you might get half the reps or even fewer than you would at a faster tempo.

This is important because, as we've noted earlier in this book, the total reps performed with a given muscle group over time is a major factor in muscle gain.[14]

Some people would say that super-slow training compensates for the reduction in reps by increasing the difficulty of the reps you do perform.

While slow reps do feel more difficult than normal ones, research shows that they result in less work done, which reduces the muscle- and strength-building potential of the exercise.[15]

Slow-rep training has also been directly put to the test in a number of studies, which show that it produces inferior results compared to normal tempo training. For instance:

- A study conducted by scientists at the University of Sydney found that people following traditional "fast" training on the bench press gained more strength than with slow training.[16]

- A study conducted by scientists at the University of Wisconsin found that even in untrained people, a traditional training tempo resulted in greater strength gains in the squat.[17]

- A study conducted by scientists at the University of Oklahoma found that four weeks of traditional resistance training was more effective for increasing strength than slow-training.[18]

Therefore, I recommend that you follow the traditional "1–1–1" rep tempo for all weightlifting exercises.

This means the first part of each rep (either the *eccentric*, or lengthening phase, or in some cases, the *concentric*, or contraction phase) should take about one second, followed by a one-second (or shorter) pause, followed by the final part of the rep, which should also take about one second.

For example, if we apply this to the squat, it would mean sitting to the proper depth in about one second, pausing for a moment, and standing up quickly.

HOW TO WARM UP FOR YOUR WORKOUTS

What many people do to warm up for their resistance training workouts is rather pointless.

You know, 20 minutes on the treadmill, followed by stretching; rubber-banded twisting, hopping, and bending; and so forth.

There are much more productive ways to warm up, and that's what we're going to talk about here.

Most people think that you warm up to make sure your muscles don't tear when you work out. By raising the temperature of your muscle tissue, it should be less injury prone, right?

Animal studies have suggested this is true.[19] When rabbits' muscles and tendons are warmer, for example, they can handle more force before they tear.

We're not big rabbits, though, which is why animal research can't be applied directly to humans.

When you work out, your body isn't whistling Dixie while you load it with heavier and heavier weights until it breaks. It has a complex system to manage how its muscles contract, and it involves a lot more than muscle temperature.

In other words, we don't know if warming up our muscle tissue before loading it actually makes it more resistant to injury.[20]

Some studies indicate that it does, while others suggest otherwise. When viewed as a whole, there seems to be a slight trend toward the former findings, but it's insignificant in the bigger picture.

That doesn't mean that warming up can't decrease your risk of injury, though. While warming up properly may not help prevent an acute injury to muscle fibers, it absolutely can help prevent injury on the whole.

The reason for this is simple: it helps you improve your technique. If you've ever done any heavy compound weightlifting, you know how hard it can be to maintain proper form as you approach technical failure.

You've probably felt your knees cave in while squatting, your wrists go crooked while benching, and your lower back curve while deadlifting.

One of the best ways to avoid these mistakes is to do warm-up sets before your hard sets to troubleshoot your form and "groove in" proper movement patterns.

Think of your warm-up sets as practice, which is, of course, the best way to get better at anything. The more times you squat, bench, and deadlift perfectly, the more that will become your default way to squat, bench, and deadlift.[21]

This is especially important for beginners. When you first start weightlifting, you can get away with bad technique because you're not strong enough to cause major damage. It's hard to get hurt when you're squatting half your body weight for 10 reps.

As you get stronger, though, that all changes. Weights get heavier, and poor form becomes more dangerous.

Studies also show that a short warm-up routine can significantly boost performance levels, which can translate into more muscle and strength gain over time.[22]

Your muscle cells are powered by tiny chemical reactions that are affected by temperature, and a little warmer than normal appears to be better for contracting effectively.[23]

Warming up also increases blood flow to your muscles, which enables your body to deliver them more oxygen and nutrients that are needed for generating energy.

So, how should you warm up for your *Thinner Leaner Stronger* workouts, then?

To ensure that each of the major muscle groups you're going to train in a workout is warmed up and primed for optimum performance, you're going to do several warm-up sets with the first exercises for each of those muscle groups.

For instance, let's say you show up to do a lower-body workout that entails squatting, lunging, and hip thrusting, in that order.

You would first warm up for the squat, and then do your hard sets. Next is the lunges, but you won't need to warm up first because the major muscle groups involved are the same as the squat's. The same goes for the hip thrusting—your glutes will be more than ready to go after the squatting and lunging.

In this way, your warm-up sets for the squat serve as your warm-up sets for the entire workout.

Let's say you were going to do a whole-body workout, however, that entails squatting, bench pressing, and shoulder pressing, in that order.

In this case, you would warm up for the squat, do your hard sets, and then warm up on the bench press before doing your hard sets because squatting doesn't involve your "push" muscles. Then, you would move directly into your hard sets of shoulder pressing because the shoulders are a major player in the bench press.

One more example for the sake of clarity. Let's say you're going to do a "pull" workout that calls for deadlifting, barbell rowing, and biceps curling, in that order. Based on what you now know, how would you do this workout?

You've got it. Warm up on the deadlift first, followed by your hard sets, followed by the hard sets of the next two exercises without any further warm-up sets because they train the same muscles as the deadlift.

The last question to answer, then, is how to warm up on any given exercise.

Here's an easy and effective routine that will warm you up without doing so much that your performance on your hard sets is compromised:

1. Do 10 reps with about 50 percent of your hard set weight, and rest for a minute.

2. Do 10 reps with the same weight at a slightly faster pace, and rest for a minute.

3. Do 4 reps with about 70 percent of your hard set weight, and rest for a minute.

And that's it. You're now ready to do your hard sets.

INTENSITY AND FOCUS:
YOUR TWO SECRET WEAPONS

You probably know what a great workout feels like. You're full of energy, you're completely focused on the task at hand, the weights feel light, you're able to push yourself a bit harder than you expected, and you leave the gym feeling invigorated, not wiped out.

Most people assume that physical factors alone determine whether you have a great workout or not. They're wrong. While eating right, getting enough sleep, minimizing stress, and so forth are major ingredients, there are mental components as well.

Two of the bigger ones are training with intensity and focus.

I'm not talking about grunting and groaning your way through every hard set with death metal blaring in your headphones or putting on a show before stepping into the squat rack.

By intensity, I mean the level of physical and mental effort you give to your workout. It's how intent you are on pushing yourself to make progress.

A high-intensity workout is one where you feel like you didn't leave anything in the tank. You hit every set with determination and didn't miss reps that you could have gotten if you had really tried.

By focus, I mean the amount of concentration you apply to the task at hand.

A focused workout is one where you have your attention on the work in front of you, not on the TV show you watched last night, the party you're throwing later that night, or the argument you had with your partner.

I don't want to get too "woo-woo" on you and say you need to mentally visualize every set before you perform it—although research shows this actually can increase performance[24]—but there's definitely something to be said for just doing what you're doing while you're doing it.

I designed *Thinner Leaner Stronger* to help you maintain a high level of intensity and focus in your workouts, but the program can't supply them. You have to.

THE DELOAD WEEK

A deload week is a weeklong reduction in training intensity (weight lifted) or volume (number of hard sets).

For example, if your training routine consists of 80 hard sets per week, a deload week might cut the volume in half (40 sets, for instance) or dramatically reduce the intensity (50 percent of your normal hard set weight is common).

The primary purposes of deloading are fourfold:

1. Alleviating "accumulated" nervous system fatigue
2. Reducing joint and ligament strain
3. Reducing the risk of injury
4. Reducing psychological stress

A distant fifth would be reducing the demands placed on your muscles, but this isn't as important as the other points.

The basic theory of deloading is based on research on how the body deals with physical stress. Here's the basic outline:

1. You provide a stimulus (exercise).
2. You remove the stimulus (rest and recovery).
3. Your body adapts to deal with the next stimulus better.

This adaptation is what allows you to gain muscle and strength, increase speed and agility, and improve technique, and it's known as *supercompensation*. Here's how this process looks visually:

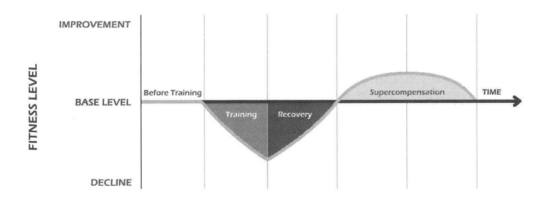

Like maintaining good sleep hygiene and managing energy balance properly, deloading is a tool that falls under #2 above (removing stimulus), and its purpose is to help with #3 (adapting).

There's no "one-size-fits-all" answer to how often you should plan deload weeks because some people's bodies can take more or less of a beating than others' before needing a break.

That said, a reasonable recommendation is to plan a deload week every 8 to 10 weeks of heavy, intense training. If you're in a calorie deficit, make this once every 6 to 8 weeks due to the added physical stress and impaired recovery.

Age and training history are factors too. One of the major (but not only) shifts that occurs with working out in your 40s and beyond is you need to give more attention to recovery.

You can probably train just as hard as the boys and girls in their 20s, but you probably can't recover as quickly.

I've also found that, rather counterintuitively, people new to weightlifting need to deload less frequently than veteran weightlifters. In fact, in some cases, people new to lifting haven't felt the need for a break in 6, 8, even 10 months. And that's fine.

As you progress in your training, your workouts get harder and harder, both in absolute weight moved and willingness and confidence to push yourself to your limits. This puts more and more stress on your body, which increases the need for deloading.

Regardless, if you're new to weightlifting, you should plan regular deload weeks. This will ensure you don't accidentally slip into a state of overtraining by being stubborn and refusing to cut back (guilty as charged).

As you learn more about how your body responds to training, though, you can get a bit looser with your deload timing.

You'll begin to recognize the need for a deload—the most common signs being that your progress is stalling, your body is extra achy, your sleep quality has declined, you have less motivation to train, and your workouts feel much harder than they should. And you can respond accordingly.

HOW TO AVOID WEIGHTLIFTING INJURIES

Many weightlifting injuries aren't caused by training too intensely in any individual workout, but by failing to fully recover from previous workouts.[25]

Sure, you can find videos of people who have ripped a pec while benching, collapsed while squatting a bending barbell, or jackhammered their lower back with a heavy deadlift, but these worst-case scenarios rarely happen.

The reality is most weightlifting injuries are insidious and give you plenty of time to change course before the bottom falls out.

For example, your knee feels a little stiff the day after heavy squats, but you shrug it off and keep going. A few weeks later, it's starting to hurt while you squat. "No pain, no gain," you say, and keep going. A few more weeks and, well, now it just hurts all the time.

These are called *repetitive stress injuries,* or RSIs, and they're the bane of every athlete. They're not painful enough to put you on the sidelines, but they cause just enough trouble to hinder your performance and progress.

Fortunately, a bit of rest is all it usually takes to eliminate RSIs. In fact, that's the only way to do it. Once an RSI has set in, you must avoid the activity that caused it (and will continue to aggravate it), along with any other activities that will prolong it.

This usually means avoiding a specific exercise but sometimes requires that you stop training a muscle group altogether until the injury has healed.

You learned in chapter eight that weightlifting isn't nearly as dangerous as many people think. As with any strenuous physical activity, however, if you do it enough, you're probably going to experience an RSI of one type and severity or another along the way.

In other words, while true injuries aren't necessarily inevitable, minor aches, stresses, and strains are. That doesn't mean we can't take preventive actions to stave them off for as long as possible, though.

Let's learn how to do that.

IF IT HURTS, DON'T DO IT

This might seem like common sense, but we all know that "common" sense isn't really all that common.

The rule here is simple: if something hurts, stop immediately.

I'm not talking about muscle soreness or the burning sensation that occurs as you approach technical failure, but *pain.* If a rep hurts enough to make you wince, that means you need to stop. Pain is a warning that something is wrong, and if you don't listen to it, you're asking for trouble.

So, when you hit pain, stop, rest for a couple of minutes, and try the exercise again.

If it still hurts, do something else and come back to it next workout and see how it goes. If it's still a problem, substitute it with a different exercise. Don't think that you "have" to do any specific exercise in any workout, even if it hurts.

If you aren't sure if what you're feeling qualifies as pain or the normal discomfort of training, ask yourself these two questions:

1. Is the pain on both sides of my body or just one?

When you perform exercises correctly, both sides of your body are fairly equally subjected to stress.

Thus, if one side starts to hurt more than the other, it's more likely a sign of trouble rather than merely muscle burn or fatigue.

2. Is the pain concentrated around a joint or other specific spot?

These are the types of pains that you're most likely to encounter because muscle strains and tears are uncommon.

Muscle and joint aches and stiffness generally go away if you warm up properly, but genuine pains won't (in fact, they'll often get worse).

Therefore, when localized pain strikes and lingers, back off and rest the affected area(s) until the pain is completely gone.

PROGRESS GRADUALLY

One of the easiest ways to get hurt in weightlifting is getting greedy.

Maybe you're feeling particularly strong one day, or you want to impress or one-up someone in the gym or just progress faster, so you load the bar with a weight that makes your spidey senses tingle.

This is almost always a bad idea. It increases the likelihood that your form will break down, it can place more stress on your joints and ligaments than they can safely handle, and it can make fully recovering from your training harder.

A much smarter, and ultimately more effective, approach to progression is one that's slow and steady.

If you're new to weightlifting and you can add five pounds to your big lifts every week or two for the first several months, you're doing great.

If you're an experienced weightlifter on a lean bulk, gaining just one rep per week on these exercises (and thus adding weight every few weeks) is good progress.

BE A STICKLER FOR GOOD FORM

Want to know one weird trick for immediately increasing your whole-body strength by at least 10 percent?

Use crappy form!

"Cheat reps" are an easy way to add weight to the bar, but they also reduce the quality of the training and increase the risk of injury.

Remember the goal in weightlifting isn't to haphazardly lift as much weight as possible, but to carefully control heavy loads through a full ranges of motion.

This not only protects you from injury but also makes every rep, exercise, and workout more conducive to muscle and strength gain.

This is especially important with compound exercises like the squat, deadlift, and bench press because while they're not inherently dangerous, they involve the heaviest weights and most technical skill.

There's a big difference between cheating on the last rep or two of isolation exercises like the dumbbell curl and lateral raise versus a barbell pull or press.

So, don't sacrifice form for the sake of progression. Instead, learn proper form for every exercise you do and stick to it.

. . .

You now have in your possession a powerful blueprint for long-term strength-training success.

A lean and toned torso. A tight and curvy behind. A strong and sculpted set of legs. All this can be yours if you follow this plan.

In fact, this might be the last weightlifting strategy you ever need, because it has enough horsepower to radically transform your body.

Perhaps more importantly, it will also help you enjoy the process. With this approach, you get to do relatively short, invigorating workouts that you actually look forward to because they produce consistent results and never leave you feeling exhausted or burned out.

If you've ever had a falling-out with weightlifting or resistance training, here's your chance to fall back in love with it. And if this is your first foray, you're in for a good time.

KEY TAKEAWAYS

- You don't need top-shelf genetics or a lifetime of training to look like a million bucks.

- *Thinner Leaner Stronger* utilizes what's known as a "push-pull-legs" or "PPL" split, which has you train two to three major muscle groups per workout.

- At bottom, a push-pull-legs routine separates your major muscle groups into three different workouts: chest, shoulders, and triceps (push); back and biceps (pull); and legs (including glutes, usually).

- "Rep" is short for "repetition," which is a single raising and lowering of a weight.

- A "set" is a fixed number of repetitions of a particular exercise.

- A "hard set" is a heavy, muscle- and strength-building set that's taken close to technical failure (the point where you can no longer continue with proper form).

- *Thinner Leaner Stronger* is going to have you work in the rep range of 8 to 10 reps, meaning that most hard sets for all exercises are going to entail doing at least 8 reps but not more than 10.

- For most women, this means working with weights that are around 70 to 75 percent of their one-rep max.

- If you wanted to deviate from my recommended 8-to-10-rep range, you'd be better off going with heavier weights and fewer reps, not the other way around.

- When you're lifting heavy weights to gain muscle and strength, you want to rest around three minutes in between each hard set.

- Training frequency isn't nearly as important as how heavy the weights are and how many hard sets you perform each week.

- I recommend no more than six days of serious exercise per week (resistance training and higher-intensity cardio), with one day of no intense physical activity whatsoever (very low-intensity cardio or sports, however, like swimming, walking, or golf is fine).

- I recommend two days off resistance training per week when in a calorie deficit.

- Another effective way to avoid symptoms related to overtraining is dialing back your workouts every so often.

There are two easy ways to do this: periodically reduce your workout intensity or volume (known as deloading) and periodically take five to seven days off weightlifting.

- In double progression, you work with a given weight in a given rep range, and once you hit the top of that rep range for a certain number of hard sets (one, two, or three, usually), you increase the weight.

- If you want to get the most out of double progression, you want to end each of your hard sets one or two reps shy of technical failure.

- Going to absolute muscle failure isn't necessary for muscle and strength gain and often leads to a breakdown in form, especially in higher-rep ranges, which increases the risk of injury.

- Slow-rep tempo training produces inferior results compared to normal tempo training.

- I recommend that you follow the traditional "1–1–1" rep tempo for all weightlifting exercises.

- To ensure that each of the major muscle groups you're going to train in a workout is warmed up and primed for optimum performance, do several warm-up sets with the first exercises for each of those muscle groups.

- A reasonable recommendation is to plan a deload week every 8 to 10 weeks of heavy, intense training.

If you're in a calorie deficit, make this once every 6 to 8 weeks due to the added physical stress and impaired recovery.

- One of the major (but not only) shifts that occurs with working out in your 40s and beyond is that while you can probably train just as hard as the boys and girls in their 20s, you probably can't recover as quickly.

- As you learn more about how your body responds to training, you'll begin to recognize the need for a deload—the most common signs being that your progress is stalling, your body is extra achy, your sleep quality has declined, you have less motivation to train, and your workouts feel much harder than they should.

- Once an RSI has set in, you must avoid the activity that caused it (and will continue to aggravate it), along with any other activities that will prolong it.

- When you hit pain, stop, rest for a couple of minutes, and try the exercise again.

- If you're new to weightlifting and you can add five pounds to your big lifts every week or two for the first several months, you're doing great.

- If you're an experienced weightlifter on a lean bulk, gaining just one rep per week on your key exercises (and thus adding weight every few weeks) is good progress.

- Don't sacrifice form for the sake of progression.

22

THE ULTIMATE WORKOUT PLAN FOR WOMEN — CARDIO

> *"If you obey all the rules, you miss all the fun."*
> —KATHARINE HEPBURN

When it comes to working out, most people assume more is always better.

If you want more muscle, you should spend more time lifting heavy things, right? And if you want more definition, you should spend more time on the Stairmaster, no?

Not quite.

That mentality has some relevance to resistance training because you do have to continue overloading your muscles to keep improving, but it can easily lead to overtraining if you don't know what you're doing.

Cardio is different, though. The only reason to do a lot of cardio is to improve your cardiovascular endurance. If you just want to build muscle, lose fat, and be healthy, however, cardio is far less important than you might realize.

You're going to learn why in this chapter and get answers to all your most pressing cardio questions, like:

- How much cardio should you do to lose weight?
- What about building muscle? Is cardio good or bad for this?
- How much cardio is too much? What happens when you do too much?
- What type of cardio is best and why?

And by the end of this chapter, you're going to know how to create the perfect cardio routine for you and your goals.

HOW MUCH CARDIO SHOULD YOU DO TO LOSE WEIGHT?

For decades, women have been taught that they should all be running, stepping, and dancing their way to being fit.

This, combined with a low-fat diet, was the mission statement and prevailing practice of the nineties. Fatty foods were sinful and anything less than an hour per day on the treadmill was just plain lazy.

It didn't work out so well. Obesity rates have continued to soar and people are more confused than ever about what it really takes to "shift" fat and get in shape.

Thanks mainly to the scientific advances and the efforts of the evidence-based fitness community to disseminate the research, we now know better.

We know, for example, that eating fat doesn't necessarily make us fat and that pounding the pavement doesn't necessarily make us lean.

And that's why my position on cardio is this:

If you don't particularly enjoy cardio, you should do as much as it takes to achieve your goals and no more.

And if you do enjoy it, then you do you, but not so much that it impairs your strength training, recovery, or health.

THE BEST TYPE OF CARDIO FOR LOSING FAT FASTER

What would you rather do: four to six 30-second sprints with 4-minute rest periods or 60 minutes of incline walking?

I don't know about you, but I'll take the sprints. Give me short and hard over long and boring any day. (Wait, that didn't sound right ...)

Now the more important question: Which of those workouts do you think would burn more fat? Most people would say the walking, and they're wrong.

Research conducted by scientists at the University of Western Ontario shows that the sprinting burns significantly more fat.[1] This wasn't a one-off occurrence, either. These results have been replicated in a number of other studies as well.[2]

If you do the math here, that's pretty impressive. A 17-to-27-minute session of high-intensity cardio, which mostly consists of low-intensity cooldown periods, burns more fat than 60 minutes of traditional "bodysculpting" cardio.

Research also shows that this style of cardio is particularly good for getting rid of abdominal fat, including visceral fat—fat covering your organs, which can be particularly dangerous to your health.[3]

This high-intensity style of cardio is known as *high-intensity interval training*, or HIIT, and the science is clear: it's significantly more time effective for losing fat than traditional *low-intensity steady-state* cardio (LISS).

HIIT involves alternating between periods of (almost) all-out-intensity sprinting and low-intensity recovery. The idea is simple: during your high-intensity bouts, you're pushing yourself almost as hard as you can, and during your low-intensity intervals, you're catching your breath to prepare for the next dash.

Although the exact mechanisms behind HIIT's fat-burning advantages aren't fully understood yet, scientists have isolated several factors, including the following:[4]

- Increased metabolic rate for up to 24 hours
- Increased insulin sensitivity in the muscles
- Increased fat burning in the muscles
- Increased growth hormone levels
- Increased catecholamine (fat-burning chemicals) levels
- Decreased postexercise appetite

These days, most people have heard about high-intensity interval training and its special fat-burning powers, but don't know how to do it correctly.

You yourself have probably wondered things like how "intense" the high-intensity intervals need to be, how "restful" the rest periods should be, how long the workouts should be, and how frequently you should do HIIT sessions.

Let's find out, starting with how hard your high-intensity intervals should be.

When you review the research on HIIT, you'll often find that exercise intensity is discussed in terms of percentage of "VO_2 max." This is the maximum rate of oxygen consumption during exercise and a major factor in determining your endurance.

In most studies on HIIT, people reached between 80 and 100 percent of their VO_2 max during their high-intensity intervals. This isn't a very practical insight, however, because VO_2 max is hard to approximate while exercising.

It's tough to know with any certainty whether you're at, let's say, 60 or 80 percent of VO_2 max without being hooked up to a fancy machine (metabolic cart).

A more useful way of prescribing intensity in your HIIT training is basing it on your *ventilatory threshold* (VT). This is the level of intensity where breathing becomes labored and you feel like you can't bring in as much air as your body wants. It's about 90 percent of your "all-out" effort.

Your goal during your high-intensity intervals is to reach your ventilatory threshold.

That is, you need to get moving fast enough that your breathing becomes labored and you can't quite suck in air as quickly as you feel you need to. And then you need to hold that speed for a period of time.

As you can imagine, this requires a significant amount of effort.

Repeatedly achieving and sustaining this level of exertion is the whole point of HIIT. If you don't do this—if you can chat away on the phone during your "high-intensity" periods—you're not doing HIIT.

You should also know that the total amount of time you exercise at your VT determines the overall effectiveness of your HIIT workouts.

If an individual workout racks up just a minute or two of VT-level exertion, it's not going to be as effective as one that involves double that amount.

HOW TO CREATE AN EFFECTIVE HIIT ROUTINE

Now that you know how HIIT works, let's talk about making it work for you. Specifically, how to create a HIIT routine that will amplify your fat loss in just an hour or two per week.

There are five things to consider when creating a HIIT routine:

1. The type of cardio performed
2. The duration and intensity of the high-intensity periods
3. The duration and intensity of the rest periods
4. The duration of the workouts
5. The frequency of the workouts

Let's look at each point individually.

1. THE TYPE OF CARDIO PERFORMED

While you can use HIIT principles with any type of cardio, if your goal is to preserve muscle and strength, your best choices are biking and rowing.

The reason I've chosen these exercises is studies show that the type of cardio you do has a significant effect on your ability to gain muscle and strength in your weightlifting.[5]

There are two likely reasons for this:

1. Cardio that mimics the movement patterns of muscle-building exercises can enhance weightlifting performance.

The reason why muscles fatigue during exercise is extremely complicated, but we know that both *aerobic* (with oxygen present) and *anaerobic* (without oxygen present) capacities are major factors.[6]

Even when you're doing a highly anaerobic activity like sprinting or weightlifting (which outstrip your body's ability to supply sufficient oxygen for energy), your body's aerobic system is still producing a significant amount of energy.

Thus, if you improve a muscle's aerobic capabilities through certain aerobic exercises, you'll see an improvement in your anaerobic capabilities as well.

2. Cardio that is low impact doesn't require much recovery.

Low-impact cardio causes very little soft tissue damage and adds little additional stress for the body to cope with.

Biking and rowing check both of these boxes. They imitate the movement patterns of the squat and deadlift, respectively, and involve no impact.

If you can't or don't want to bike or row, however, feel free to use other low-impact methods of cardio for your HIIT workouts. Swimming, jump roping, elliptical, and bodyweight circuits are popular choices.

I don't recommend sprinting, though, as it causes too much muscle and joint soreness, which will get in the way of progress in your lower-body workouts.

2. THE DURATION AND INTENSITY OF THE HIGH-INTENSITY PERIODS

As you now know, the intensity target of your high-intensity intervals is your ventilatory threshold, and the total number of minutes spent at this level of exertion dictates the effectiveness of your HIIT workouts.

Too little time at this near-peak effort level results in a "kinda-high-intensity" workout, and too much can lead to exhaustion and overtraining.

Don't slowly build up to this level of effort when you launch into a high-intensity interval. Give it everything you've got right out of the gate. You should be breathing hard within 10 to 15 seconds.

It's also worth noting that you want to adjust your speed in your training more than the resistance settings offered by various machines.

The goal of HIIT is to go fast and hard, not slow and hard. (And there I go again ...)

In terms of the duration of your high-intensity intervals, 50 to 60 percent of the total amount of time that you can maintain VT intensity is sufficient if your goal is losing fat and improving metabolic health.

This total amount of potential VT exertion is known as your "T_{MAX}."

So, for example, my T_{MAX} on the bike is about three minutes, so my high-intensity intervals are 90 to 120 seconds long (yeah, it's tough!).

To determine the proper length of your intervals, you can either test your T_{MAX} (all you need is your phone's clock app), or if you're new to HIIT and want to keep it simple, start with one-minute high-intensity periods.

If you also want to significantly improve your conditioning, you'll need to make your HIIT workouts progressively tougher. As you get fitter, your T_{MAX} is going to improve, and as it improves, the duration of your high-intensity intervals will need to increase if you want to continue increasing your cardiovascular capacity.

As you can imagine, this can get pretty dang intense for experienced athletes. In several HIIT studies conducted with highly trained cyclists, for instance, high-intensity intervals were *five minutes long* and resulted in improved performance.[7] In contrast, other research conducted with endurance athletes found that two- and one-minute intervals (hard!) weren't enough to improve performance.[8]

3. THE DURATION AND INTENSITY OF THE REST PERIODS

Your rest periods should consist of active recovery, which means you should keep moving, not come to a standstill.

Studies show that this helps you reach your ventilatory threshold easier during your high-intensity intervals, which makes your HIIT workouts more effective.[9]

As far as duration goes, start out with a 1:2 ratio between high- and low-intensity intervals. For example, one minute at high-intensity and two minutes at low.

As your conditioning improves, you can work toward a 1:1 ratio.

4. THE DURATION OF THE WORKOUTS

The great thing about HIIT is how much you can get out of relatively small amounts of it. It can be quite stressful on the body, though, which means you don't want to do too much (especially when you're lifting weights as well, and especially if you're also cutting).

So, start your HIIT workouts with 2 to 3 minutes of low-intensity warm-up, and then do 20 to 25 minutes of intervals, followed by 2 to 3 minutes of warm-down, and you're done.

5. THE FREQUENCY OF THE WORKOUTS

How often you should do HIIT workouts depends on your goals and what other types of exercise you're doing.

I've found that four to seven hours of exercise per week is plenty for losing fat quickly and efficiently, and of course, you want to spend most of that time on resistance training, not cardio.

Thus, when I'm cutting, I like to do four to five hours of weightlifting and one and a half to two hours of HIIT per week. This allows me to get as lean as I want without risking overtraining or burnout.

THE SECOND-BEST TYPE OF CARDIO FOR LOSING FAT FASTER

If your goal is maximum fat loss and you have the energy and will to endure an hour or two of HIIT per week, that's your best bet.

If you can't or don't want to do that much HIIT, however, or any at all, you have another option.

You're not going to need any special equipment, gadgets, or skills. You're not going to need to track your heart rate, time your intervals, or log your miles. All you're going to do is something that you've been doing every day since you were a toddler, and that you'll do for the rest of your life.

It's walking, of course, and while it's not the best way to lose fat rapidly, it's definitely the easiest way to burn additional calories and lose fat faster.

That's why many people don't think walking qualifies as a bonafide "cardio workout." When it comes to exercise, "easy" is usually equated with "worthless." That's true in certain contexts, but not this one.

For instance, a study conducted by scientists at California State University found that people who ran a 10-minute mile burned about 190 calories.[10] People who walked a 19-minute mile burned fewer calories, of course, but not as few as you might think—about 111.

This isn't going to impact your fat loss like HIIT will, but if you go for several walks per week, it can make a significant difference over time.

Walking has other benefits too.

WALKING IS VERY EASY ON THE BODY

Managing stress levels is an important part of minimizing muscle loss while restricting calories to lose fat.

Walking is great in this regard because, unlike more intense forms of exercise, it places very little stress on the body. In fact, research shows that walking can counteract the effects of stress and reduce cortisol levels.[11]

Thus, if walking were your only form of exercise while dieting, you probably couldn't do enough to risk overtraining. Moreover, you can also safely add several hours of walking per week on top of an already rigorous exercise schedule.

WALKING MINIMALLY IMPACTS MUSCLE GAIN

As you know, cardio workouts can directly impair strength and muscle gain.

This is why strength athletes dramatically reduce or eliminate cardio altogether leading up to a competition, and why many bodybuilders generally keep cardio to a minimum while lean bulking.

We also recall that not all forms of cardio are equally detrimental to weightlifters. For example, running clearly impairs muscle and strength building but cycling and rowing don't seem to.[12]

In the case of walking, it doesn't mimic a muscle-building movement and so won't likely improve your performance in the gym, but it's as low impact as you can get.[13] And that means you can use it to burn calories without getting in the way of your progress in your weightlifting.

WALKING PREFERENTIALLY BURNS FAT

Walking may not burn many calories, but the calories it does burn come primarily from fat stores.

You burn both fat and carbohydrate when you exercise, and the proportions vary with the intensity.[14] As intensity increases, so does the reliance on muscle glycogen (carbohydrate) for energy over fat stores.[15]

This is why a very low-intensity activity like walking taps mainly into fat stores, whereas high-intensity exercise pulls much more heavily from glycogen stores.

This is also why some people think low-intensity steady-state cardio is best for fat loss. You now know it's not (HIIT is), but it's certainly the easiest and least stressful way to augment weight loss.

HOW MUCH WALKING SHOULD YOU DO?

The biggest downside to walking is it doesn't burn all that much energy (about 300 to 350 calories per hour).

That means you'd need to do quite a bit of walking (several hours per week) to see noticeable changes in your body composition. Every calorie burned matters, however, so even relatively small amounts of walking will help you reach your fat loss goals faster.

This is especially true if you do other exercise as well. For example, if you add weightlifting to the mix, you can dramatically increase fat loss. Just four heavy sets of deadlifts can burn over 100 calories, and that's not taking into account the additional energy expenditure that occurs after (the "afterburn effect").[16]

I've worked with many people who've used a combination of weightlifting, high-intensity interval training, and walking to lose fat rapidly. The most successful approach looks like this:

- Three to five one-hour weightlifting sessions per week
- One to three 25-to-30 minute HIIT sessions per week
- Two to three 30-to-45-minute walks per week

. . .

Medicine has known the value of regular exercise for thousands of years, but only recently have we gained a better understanding of how much is enough and how much is too much.

If you do at least a few hours of resistance training per week, you should view cardio as supportive, not essential, and you should do enough to reach your goals (and enjoy yourself, if you like endurance exercise) but not more.

For most people, that means doing no more than one to two hours of HIIT or three to four hours of walking per week, or some combination thereof.

Not only will this regimen help you get into the best shape of your life, it'll also leave you with plenty of free time to invest in other activities and pursuits, including relationships, family, and hobbies.

Remember that your health and fitness routines should enhance you and your life, not consume them!

KEY TAKEAWAYS

- If you just want to build muscle, lose fat, and be healthy, cardio is far less important than you might realize.

- If you don't particularly enjoy cardio, you should do as much as it takes to achieve your goals and no more.

- A 17-to-27-minute session of high-intensity cardio, which mostly consists of low-intensity cooldown periods, burns more fat than 60 minutes of traditional "bodysculpting" cardio.

- This high-intensity style of cardio is known as *high-intensity interval training*, or HIIT, and the science is clear: it's significantly more time effective for losing fat than traditional *low-intensity steady-state* cardio (LISS).

- HIIT involves alternating between periods of (almost) all-out-intensity sprinting and low-intensity recovery.

- Your goal during your high-intensity intervals is to reach your ventilatory threshold.

- The total amount of time you exercise at your VT determines the overall effectiveness of your HIIT workouts.

- While you can use HIIT principles with any type of cardio, if your goal is to preserve muscle and strength, your best choices are biking and rowing.

- If you can't or don't want to bike or row, however, feel free to use other low-impact methods of cardio for your HIIT workouts like swimming, jump roping, elliptical, and bodyweight circuits.

- In terms of the duration of your high-intensity intervals, 50 to 60 percent of the total amount of time that you can maintain VT intensity is sufficient if your goal is losing fat and improving metabolic health.

- Your rest periods should consist of active recovery, which means you should keep moving, not come to a standstill.

- Start out with a 1:2 ratio between high- and low-intensity intervals.

- Start your HIIT workouts with 2 to 3 minutes of low-intensity warm-up, and then do 20 to 25 minutes of intervals, followed by 2 to 3 minutes of warm-down, and you're done.

- Four to seven hours of exercise per week is plenty for losing fat quickly and efficiently, and of course, you want to spend most of that time on resistance training, not cardio.

- If you can't or don't want to do that much HIIT or any at all, you can walk instead.

This isn't going to impact your fat loss like HIIT will, but if you go for several walks per week, it can make a significant difference over time.

- I've worked with many people who've used a combination of weight-lifting, high-intensity interval training, and walking to lose fat rapidly, and the most successful approach looks like this:

Three to five one-hour weightlifting sessions per week

One to three 25-to-30 minute HIIT sessions per week

Two to three 30-to-45-minute walks per week

23

THE BEST EXERCISES FOR BUILDING YOUR BEST BODY EVER

"There is no reason to be alive if you can't do the deadlift!"
—JÓN PÀLL SIGMARSSON

Of the hundreds of resistance training exercises that you can do, a minority stand head and shoulders above the rest.

And of those, a handful are the absolute breadwinners.

This is great news for us because it means we can disregard most of what we see people doing in magazines, YouTube videos, and the gym, and focus on a relatively short list of exercises instead.

In this chapter, I'm going to share those superior exercises with you, and in the next chapter, we're going to have an in-depth discussion about three of them in particular—the "Big Three," as they're often called.

As you'll see, most of the exercises I recommend are compound exercises, which are those that involve multiple joints and muscles.

Isolation exercises—those that involve just one joint and a limited number of muscles—are included to help develop smaller, stubborn muscle groups like the shoulders and arms and to support the growth of larger muscle groups.

Let's begin our discussion with how we're going to categorize these exercises. I like to group exercises by the major muscle group they train, because it helps us better organize and prioritize our workouts based on our physique goals.

Here are the seven major muscle groups that you'll be focusing on in my *Thinner Leaner Stronger* program:

1. Legs
2. Glutes

3. Core

4. Arms

5. Shoulders

6. Chest

7. Back

Let's go over each one by one, learning the anatomy first, followed by the best exercises for developing each.

And just to show how deeply sensitive I am to female interests and needs (just ask my wife! Well, on second thought …), I'm going to start with the muscle group you probably care the most about …

LEGS

Your legs consist of three major muscle groups:

   1. Quadriceps (quads)

   2. Hamstrings

   3. Calves

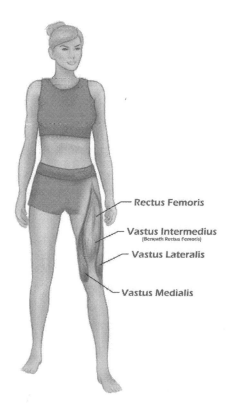

Rectus Femoris

Vastus Intermedius
[Beneath Rectus Femoris]

Vastus Lateralis

Vastus Medialis

Each one is best trained by different exercises and has "special needs" if you're going to achieve maximum development and definition.

The quadriceps are a set of four large muscles on the front of your legs:

1.   Vastus lateralis

2.   Vastus medialis

3.   Vastus intermedius

4.   Rectus femoris

(Interestingly, research indicates there's a fifth muscle involved, so maybe we should be talking about the quintraceps instead![1])

Here's how they look:

Together these muscles work to extend the knees and flex the hips. Thus, quads exercises bring the hips from an extended (straight) to a flexed (bent) position, and the knees from a flexed to an extended position.

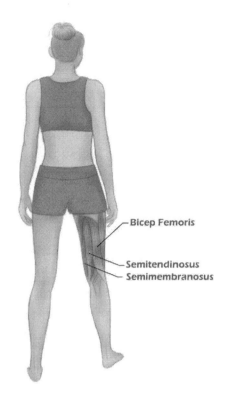

Bicep Femoris

Semitendinosus
Semimembranosus

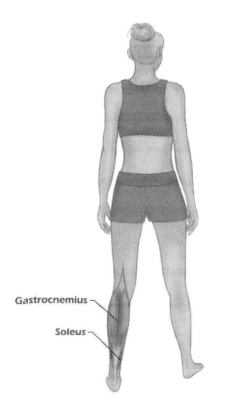

Gastrocnemius

Soleus

The hamstrings are a group of three muscles on the back of your legs:

1.   Semitendinosus

2.   Semimembranosus

3.   Biceps femoris

The hamstrings work in the opposite fashion of the quadriceps, flexing the knees and extending the hips.

The biceps femoris is split into two "heads" or sections, just like the biceps in your arms. Unlike those biceps, however, the hamstrings tend to be one of the more neglected muscles among weight-lifters.

The quads get most of the attention for the lower body because they're larger and more visible, and this can create a muscular imbalance between the front and back of the thighs that looks strange and may increase the risk of injury.[2]

The calves are made up of two powerful muscles:

1.   Gastrocnemius

2.   Soleus

The gastrocnemius is the large (or not so much in my case—thanks, genetics) muscle you see when you look at your calf. The soleus is a deep muscle that lies underneath the gastrocnemius.

These two muscles work together to manipulate the foot and ankle joint and are involved in knee flexion as well.

THE BEST LEG EXERCISES YOU CAN DO

Barbell Squat

Barbell Front Squat

Hack Squat (Sled, Not Barbell)

Single-Leg Split Squat (Barbell or Dumbbell)

Leg Press

Lunge (Dumbbell or Barbell, Walking or In-Place,
Forward or Reverse)

Romanian Deadlift

Leg Curl (Lying or Seated)

Standing Calf Raise

Seated Calf Raise

Leg Press Calf Raise

You've probably heard there's just one rule to properly training your legs: always do squats. While I agree that the squat is the single best leg exercise you can do, I also think it's smart to include other exercises in your lower-body workouts.

For instance, while the squat does involve the hamstrings, the quads do the lion's share of the work.[3] A good rule of thumb, then, is to always include exercises in your routine that target your hamstrings in addition to your squatting (and other quads-dominant exercises).

GLUTES

The gluteus muscles, or *glutes*, are composed of three muscles that form your butt:

1. Gluteus maximus

2. Gluteus minimus

3. Gluteus medius

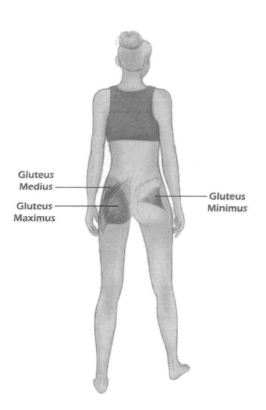

Gluteus Medius

Gluteus Maximus

Gluteus Minimus

They're for more than just show, too. Together, they play a key role in stabilizing your body during all kinds of movements, and generating force in exercises like the deadlift and squat.

If you're training your lower body correctly, you don't necessarily have to do additional training for your glutes. That said, if you feel your glute development is particularly weak, or if you just want a great butt as quickly as possible, you'll want to include exercises that specifically target it.

As you'll see, I include glute-specific training in *Thinner Leaner Stronger* because most women I've spoken to and worked with have wanted to give their booties as much of a boost as possible.

THE BEST GLUTE EXERCISES YOU CAN DO

Barbell Squat

Barbell Front Squat

Barbell Deadlift

Romanian Deadlift

Lunge (Dumbbell or Barbell, Walking or In-Place, Forward or Reverse)

Single-Leg Split Squat (Barbell or Dumbbell)

Hip Thrust (Barbell or Dumbbell)

Glute Blaster

Step-Up (Barbell or Dumbbell)

Weighted Back Hyperextension

Forget the endless lunge and leg lift variations and everything else you see in those flashy Pinterest infographics. Get strong on the exercises listed here, and you'll get the kind of butt that can "melt the internet."

As you can see, there's quite a bit of overlap here with the list of best leg exercises because the glutes are heavily involved in most of them.

That said, there are four glute-specific exercises that you're going to do in *Thinner Leaner Stronger*: the hip thrust, glute blaster, step-up, and weighted back hyperextension.

CORE

Your *core* is the following group of muscles around your midsection:

1. Rectus abdominis

2. Transverse abdominis

3. Internal and external obliques

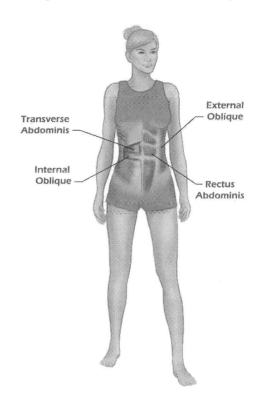

Transverse Abdominis

Internal Oblique

External Oblique

Rectus Abdominis

These muscles work to stabilize and flex the spine (bring your chest closer to your hips).

When people talk about "abs," they're usually referring to the pair of muscles that make up the rectus abdominis. Most ab exercises target these muscles. To have the whole package, however, you want to develop the other muscles that frame them.

If you're properly training the other six major muscle groups discussed here, your core muscles will do plenty of work. This is why many people think they don't need to do core exercises because they squat and deadlift.

Why, then, do so many of these people have unimpressive midriffs?

Research shows that compound exercises, even when performed with heavy loads, don't involve the "show" muscles of the rectus abdominis, transverse abdominis, and external obliques as much as people think.[4]

This is probably why I've found that most gals have to do quite a bit of targeted core work to achieve the look they really want.

Remember too that body fat percentage is crucial here. No matter how much you work on your core or how developed it is, it's not going to look "ripped" until you're around 20 percent body fat or lower.

THE BEST CORE EXERCISES YOU CAN DO

Captain's Chair Leg Raise

Hanging Leg Raise

Lying Leg Raise

Crunch

Cable Crunch

Weighted Sit-Up

Plank

Abdominal Rollout

There aren't hundreds of ab exercises out there because you need the variety. It's simply a matter of supply and demand.

People are obsessed with getting abs—"ab exercises" and related searches get over 50,000 Google searches per month. That's why you have thousands of websites, magazines, and trainers creating list after list of the "best ab exercises ever" in hopes of nabbing new readers and followers.

I've kept my list of core exercises short and simple because this is all we really need to get killer abs and accompaniments.

ARMS

There are two major muscle groups in your arms that we're most interested in developing:

1. Biceps

2. Triceps

The biceps is made up of two muscles, the *biceps brachii* and *biceps brachialis*, which look like this:

The biceps' job is to flex the arm (bring your forearm closer to your upper arm), and to supinate your elbow (turn your hand palm up).

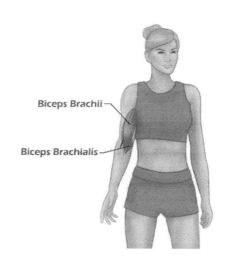

Biceps Brachii

Biceps Brachialis

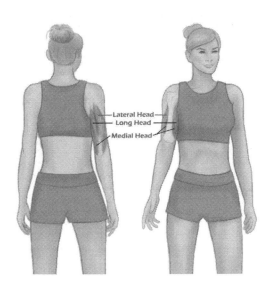

Lateral Head
Long Head
Medial Head

Next is the triceps, which has three heads:

1.   Lateral head

2.   Medial head

3.   Long head

Here's how they look:

As you can see, these parts combine to form the distinctive "horseshoe" that can become quite pronounced when properly developed.

The triceps does the opposite job of the biceps, pushing your forearm away from your upper arm.

You can also see that the lateral head is the largest of the three. This is why it both develops the fastest and most determines the overall look of your triceps. That said, if you want maximum arm definition, you want to make sure all three heads are well developed.

THE BEST BICEPS EXERCISES YOU CAN DO

Barbell Curl

E-Z Bar Curl

Alternating Dumbbell Curl

Dumbbell Hammer Curl

Chin-Up

Short and sweet. You don't need to do fifty types of curls to build strong biceps.

THE BEST TRICEPS EXERCISES YOU CAN DO

Close-Grip Bench Press

Seated Triceps Press

Dip

Lying Triceps Extension ("Skullcrusher")

Triceps Pushdown

You're going to get the most out of triceps exercises that emphasize the lateral and medial heads. These are exercises that have your arms at your side with an overhand (palm-down) grip, like the close-grip bench press, dip, and pushdown.

You don't want to neglect exercises that emphasize the long head, though, which have your arms overhead, like the seated triceps press and lying triceps extension.

That's why you'll be doing a bit of both in your triceps training in *Thinner Leaner Stronger*.

SHOULDERS

Your shoulders consist of several muscles, and the three most prominent are the *deltoids*:

1. Anterior (front) deltoid
2. Lateral (side) deltoid
3. Posterior (rear) deltoid

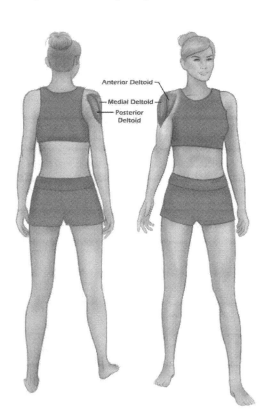

Here's how they look:

The deltoids raise the arm to the front of the body (front delt), the side of the body (side delt), and behind the body (rear delt).

As you can see, there are also smaller muscles that enable the ball-shaped head of the arm bone to spin and roll in the socket of the shoulder blade. These are known as the *rotator cuff muscles*.

When people talk about developing their shoulders, they're usually referring to their deltoids. These are the big, visible muscles, and they're what we'll be focusing on in *Thinner Leaner Stronger*.

Exercises done specifically for the rotator cuffs can be supportive but aren't particularly necessary if you have healthy, functional shoulders, and also don't contribute much to your shoulders' overall strength and look.

THE BEST SHOULDER EXERCISES YOU CAN DO

Overhead Press

Military Press

Seated Dumbbell Press

Arnold Dumbbell Press

Dumbbell Front Raise

Dumbbell Side Lateral Raise

Dumbbell Rear Lateral Raise (Bent-Over or Seated)

Barbell Rear Delt Row

As you can see, I'm a fan of shoulder pressing. As with the chest, you just can't beat heavy pressing for developing your shoulders.

If all you do is press, however, your front deltoids will probably develop faster than your middle and rear deltoids. This is why a good shoulder training routine includes exercises to target each of the three deltoids.

Also, in case you're wondering, although I'm a big believer in the overhead press, I don't include it in *Thinner Leaner Stronger* because it's a rather technical movement that is more suited to experienced weightlifters, and it often requires in-person coaching to get right.

Instead, I'm going to have you do seated dumbbell shoulder pressing, which is easier to learn and execute and still highly effective at developing your shoulder muscles.

If, in time, you want to learn how to overhead press, you can easily incorporate it into your workouts.

CHEST

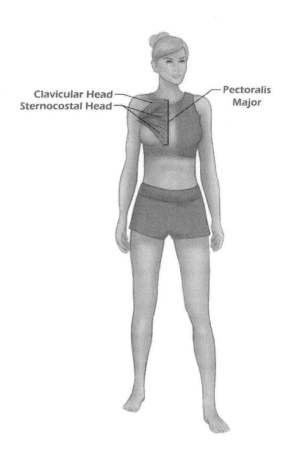

Clavicular Head
Sternocostal Head

Pectoralis
Major

The main muscle of your chest is the pectoralis major. Here's what it looks like:

Its main function is to bring the upper arm across the body, and unlike most other muscles, its fibers aren't all aligned in the same direction.

As you can see in the image, the pec major has two heads. There's a *sternocostal head*, which attaches the sternum (breastbone) and ribcage to your upper arm, and a *clavicular head*, which attaches your collarbone to your upper arm.

Why is this important? How a muscle attaches to the skeleton influences how it responds to various types of training.

For instance, certain exercises, like the flat and decline bench press, emphasize the larger sternocostal head of the pecs, while others, like the incline and reverse-grip bench press, emphasize the smaller clavicular head.[5]

Many women don't train their chest muscles seriously because they don't want muscular chests. What they're missing, however, is that a "muscular" chest on a woman looks nothing like one on a man.

In women, chest development simply adds tone, shape, and "perkiness" to the entire area, which most women would gladly welcome.

That's why we're not going to neglect your chest in *Thinner Leaner Stronger*.

THE BEST CHEST EXERCISES YOU CAN DO

Barbell Bench Press (Incline and Flat)

Dumbbell Bench Press (Incline and Flat)

Dip

Cable Fly

These are the only exercises you really need to build a strong, defined chest.

Forget pullovers, push-up variations, machines, and every other type of chest exercise out there. They aren't as effective as these foundation-building exercises, and they're most suited to intermediate and advanced weightlifters and bodybuilders who have already developed considerable muscle and strength with heavy pressing.

BACK

There are a number of muscles that make up the bulk of your back:

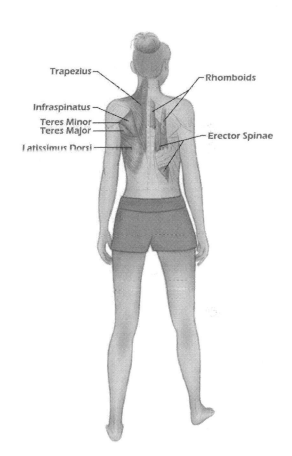

1. Trapezius

2. Rhomboids

3. Latissimus dorsi

4. Erector spinae

5. Teres major

6. Teres minor

7. Infraspinatus

And here's how they look:

Collectively, these muscles are responsible for pulling the upper arms toward the torso; stabilizing the shoulder blades, neck, and spine; and assisting with back extension (moving your chest away from your hips).

Many people undertrain their back muscles because they rarely see them. This can create an imbalanced look (everyone else sees your back) as well as an imbalance between your "push" and "pull" muscles that can lead to poor posture and even shoulder discomfort and injury.

A good rule of thumb is to give your back muscles about as much attention as your chest and shoulder muscles, which is what we're going to do in *Thinner Leaner Stronger*.

THE BEST BACK EXERCISES YOU CAN DO

Barbell Deadlift

Barbell Row

One-Arm Dumbbell Row

Pull-Up

Chin-Up

T-Bar Row

Lat Pulldown (Wide- and Close-Grip)

Seated Cable Row (Wide- and Close-Grip)

Thinner Leaner Stronger gives special love and attention to the barbell deadlift.

It's not only the single best back exercise you can do, but it's also one of the best weightlifting exercises ever invented because it trains just about every muscle in your body.

If you can't deadlift due to injury or other issues, don't worry—you can still do great. If a workout calls for a deadlift, simply replace it with one of the other exercises on the list that you can do.

The barbell row, one-arm dumbbell row, T-bar row, and pull-up are all top choices, which is why you'll be doing a lot of each in *Thinner Leaner Stronger*.

. . .

Gaining muscle and strength doesn't require that you constantly "challenge" your body with new and exotic exercises.

In fact, this is a rather poor strategy because the more often you make changes to the exercises you do, the harder it is to become proficient at any of them. This slows down your progress.[6]

A much better approach is sticking with a relatively small number of highly effective exercises that allow you to safely overload your muscles with heavier and heavier weights over time, and then doing just that.

I've just laid out those exercises for you, and in the next chapter, we're going to drill down into three that are the most important ones you can do.

KEY TAKEAWAYS

- Of the hundreds of resistance training exercises that you can do, a minority stand head and shoulders above the rest, and of those, a handful are the absolute breadwinners.

- Most of the exercises I recommend are compound exercises, which are those that involve multiple joints and muscles.

- Isolation exercises—those that involve just one joint and a limited number of muscles—are included to help develop smaller, stubborn muscle groups like the shoulders and arms and to support the growth of larger muscle groups.

- There are seven major muscle groups that you'll be focusing on in my *Thinner Leaner Stronger* program: legs, glutes, core, arms, shoulders, chest, and back.

- Your legs consist of three major muscle groups: the quadriceps (quads), hamstrings, and calves.

- The squat is the single best leg exercise you can do, but I also think it's smart to include other exercises in your lower-body workouts.

- A good rule of thumb is to always include exercises in your routine that target your hamstrings in addition to your squatting (and other quads-dominant exercises).

- Compound exercises, even when performed with heavy loads, don't involve the "show" muscles of the rectus abdominis, transverse abdominis, and external obliques as much as some people think.

- No matter how much you work on your core or how developed it is, it's not going to look "ripped" until you're around 20 percent body fat or lower.

- There are two major muscle groups in your arms that we're most interested in developing: the biceps and triceps.

- You're going to get the most out of triceps exercises that emphasize the lateral and medial heads. You don't want to neglect exercises that emphasize the long head, though.

- Your shoulders consist of several muscles, and the three most prominent are the deltoids: the anterior (front) deltoids, lateral (side) deltoids, and posterior (rear) deltoids.

- There are also smaller muscles that enable the ball-shaped head of the arm bone to spin and roll in the socket of the shoulder blade, which are known as the rotator cuff muscles.

- If all you do is press, your front deltoids will probably develop faster than your middle and rear deltoids, which is why a good shoulder training routine includes exercises to target each of the three deltoids.

- The main muscle of your chest is the pectoralis major.

- Certain exercises, like the flat and decline bench press, emphasize the larger sternocostal head of the pecs, while others, like the incline and reverse-grip bench press, emphasize the smaller clavicular head.

- In women, chest development simply adds tone, shape, and "perkiness" to the entire area.

- There are a number of muscles that make up the bulk of your back: the trapezius, rhomboids, latissimus dorsi, erector spinae, teres major, teres minor, and infraspinatus.

- A good rule of thumb is to give your back muscles about as much attention as your chest and shoulder muscles.

- The deadlift is not only the single best back exercise you can do, but it's also one of the best weightlifting exercises ever invented because it trains just about every muscle in your body.

- Gaining muscle and strength doesn't require that you constantly "challenge" your body with new and exotic exercises.

A much better approach is sticking with a relatively small number of highly effective exercises that allow you to safely overload your muscles with heavier and heavier weights over time, and then doing just that.

24

THE DEFINITIVE GUIDE TO THE BIG 3

"Courage doesn't always roar. Sometimes courage is the quiet voice at the end of the day saying, "I will try again tomorrow."
—MARY ANNE RADMACHER

Out of all the exercises I recommend, three are particularly special.

They're also particularly challenging, which is why many people neglect or avoid them altogether.

They're known as the "Big Three," and they are as follows:

1. Barbell squat

2. Barbell deadlift

3. Barbell bench press

These exercises have been the staples of strength and bodybuilding programs for over a century now because they involve the most whole-body muscle and safely allow for maximum progressive overload.

The stronger you are on these three exercises, the better you're going to look and feel. It's really that simple. That's why one of your primary goals on my *Thinner Leaner Stronger* program is going to be improving your numbers on these key exercises.

You're also going to learn how to perform them flawlessly, because improper form can dramatically reduce their effectiveness and open the door to injury.

Heavy half reps, for instance, might look neat and feel more difficult than lighter loads moved through full ranges of motion, but research shows they produce less muscle and strength gain.[1]

Heavy partial reps also put much more strain on your joints, tendons, and ligaments—often more than they can safely handle.

Bad form is why these three exercises have been so maligned over the years as harmful to your shoulders, back, and knees. While some people's anatomies don't play well with these exercises, studies show that when performed correctly, they're perfectly safe for most people and maybe even protective against joint pain.[2]

For example, a study conducted by scientists at the Oklahoma Center for Athletes found that powerlifters who were squatting 1.6 times their body weight had better joint stability than college basketball players and recreational runners.[3]

Learning proper form can be difficult, however, because there are many professional opinions as to what a proper squat, deadlift, and bench press look like.

For instance, some well-respected coaches say that your knees should never go past your toes when you squat, that rounding your spine on a deadlift is okay, and that touching the bar to your chest on a bench press is bad for your shoulders.

Others say that it's natural for your knees to push past the toes, that rounding your back while deadlifting is dangerous, and that touching the bar to your chest is perfectly fine and even recommended.

Who's right? How can we know? And why should you listen to me?

Well, I'm going to defer to authority here and cite the methods of the man whose work taught me—and hundreds of thousands of others—how to squat, bench, and deadlift: Mark Rippetoe.

"Rip," as he's known, has been in the strength-training game for nearly four decades now and is the author of the classic bestselling books *Starting Strength* and *Practical Programming*.

Furthermore, while elite athletes of all stripes use Rip's methods, he specializes in helping normal people like you and me who just want to get strong and fit.

In other words, his experience isn't mostly limited to genetic freaks who can do things in the weight room that most of us could only dream of.

So, let's review Rip's techniques for pushing, pulling, and squatting because they've withstood the test of time and proven themselves safe and effective for new and experienced weightlifters alike.

THE BARBELL SQUAT

There's a reason the barbell squat reigns supreme among weightlifting purists.

It requires over 200 muscles in the body to work together to generate a tremendous amount of force, as well as near-perfect form if you're going to ever put up impressive numbers.[4]

And this is why the barbell squat is one of the single best exercises for developing every major muscle group in your body, from beak to butt.

You may have heard, though, that it's also one of the single best ways to destroy your knees.

Specifically, it's often said that heavy squatting damages the tendons, ligaments, and cartilage in the knees, and the more often you squat, the worse it gets.

This is rubbish. Research shows that not only is the squat safe for your knees—it may even improve knee health and reduce your risk of knee injury.[5]

A good example of this comes from a study conducted by scientists at the University of Massachusetts that looked at the forces placed on the knee joints of 12 experienced male powerlifters who squatted between 375 and 650 pounds.[6]

Each of the men performed heavy squats and the researchers measured how much stress it placed on their knees.

The result? Their knee tendons and ligaments never even came close to their breaking points, and in most cases were only pushed to about 50 percent of their maximum strength.

In other words, even when squatting 2.5 times their body weight, the forces placed on the powerlifters' knees were well within healthy levels.

So, you have nothing to fear from the squat—if you do it correctly, that is, which is exactly what you're about to learn.

THE SETUP

The best place to squat is in a power rack or squat rack with the safety bars or arms set to about six inches beneath your knees.

Position the bar on the rack so it cuts across the upper half of your chest. This might feel a bit low, but it's better to be on the low side than tippy-toeing the weight off the rack.

There are two ways to perform the barbell squat:

1. High-bar
2. Low-bar

A high-bar squat has the bar resting directly on the upper traps, whereas a low-bar position has the bar resting between the upper traps and rear deltoids.

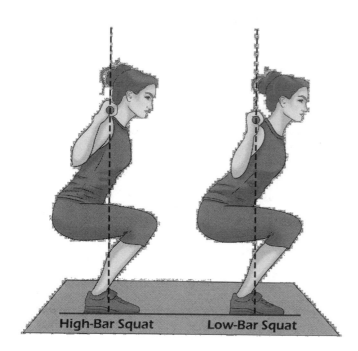

High-Bar Squat   Low-Bar Squat

Here's how they look:

As you can see, your torso remains more upright in the high-bar squat.

Both methods are correct, but most people will find themselves stronger in the low-bar position because it allows you to better leverage your large leg muscles. That said, some people find the low-bar position very uncomfortable for their shoulders or wrists and naturally prefer the high-bar position.

If you're new to the barbell squat, I recommend you start with the low-bar position and only go high bar if it's too uncomfortable.

The barbell squat starts with approaching the weight and getting into position.

To do this, face the bar so you can walk it out backward. Don't ever walk the bar out forward, as trying to rerack it by walking backward is dangerous.

Get under the bar, get it into your preferred position, and place your feet about shoulder width apart, with the toes rotated out by about 20 to 25 degrees (your right foot should be at about 1 o'clock and your left at about 11 o'clock).

Next, place your thumbs on top of the bar and adjust your grip position. A narrow grip is preferable because it helps you maintain upper-back tightness, so get your hands as close together as you can, making sure your shoulder blades are pinched and the weight is solidly on your back muscles, not in your hands or resting on your spine.

Then, unrack the bar, take one or two steps back, and get back into the proper squatting position I've outlined (feet shoulder width apart, toes pointed out), and you're ready to descend.

THE DESCENT

Stand tall with your chest out and take a deep breath of air, pulling it into the bottom of your stomach (as opposed to your chest). Brace your abs as if you were about to get punched.

Pick a spot on the floor about six feet away and stare at it during the entire set. Don't look at the ceiling, as this makes it harder to reach the proper depth, can throw off proper hip movement and chest positioning, and can even cause a neck injury.

Begin the descent by simultaneously pushing your hips back and bending your knees. Don't consciously do one or the other first. You should feel backward motion in your hips and the sensation that you're sitting down between your heels.

Then, sit your butt straight down while keeping your chest up and back straight and tight. Your knees should point at your toes the whole way down (no bowing in!) and move forward for the first third or half of the movement, but no further than just in front of your toes.

Many people tend to want to slide their knees too far forward as they descend, which further loads the quads and puts the knees in a compromised position.

Descending too quickly increases the amount of force placed on your knees, so don't just drop your hips down as quickly as you can.[7] Make sure your descent is controlled.

The bottom of the squat is the point where your thighs are parallel to the ground or slightly lower. Your knees should still be pointing at your toes and over or slightly in front of them, and your back should be straight and at an angle that places the bar over the middle of your feet.

Here's how the bottom position looks:

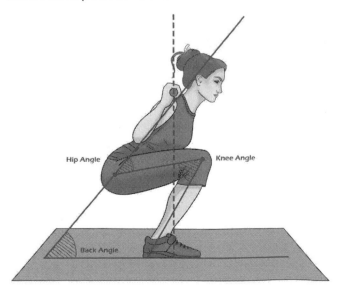

You're now ready to ascend.

THE ASCENT

The key to starting a good ascent is driving through your heels and the middle of your feet, and ensuring that your shoulders move upward at the same rate as your hips.

It also helps to imagine you're gripping the floor with your toes and feet, like an eagle clenching its claws.

As you continue to ascend, drive your hips forward by squeezing your glutes, and push the bar toward the ceiling until you're standing tall.

Begin exhaling once you've passed the hardest point of the ascent (the first couple of feet).

Here's how the sequence looks:

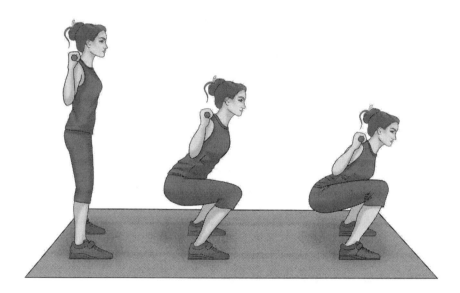

You're now ready for the next rep.

SIX TIPS FOR BETTER SQUATTING

1. If you're having trouble keeping your knees in line with your toes, do the following mobility exercise every day.

Without a bar or weight, squat down to the bottom position, and place your elbows against your knees and touch the palms of your hands together.

Use your elbows to press your knees out and into the proper position (in line with your toes), and hold this position for 20 to 30 seconds, followed by a minute or so of rest. Repeat this several times.

If you do this simple exercise every day, you should notice a marked improvement in your ability to maintain proper knee position when you squat in the gym.

2. Don't squat on a Smith machine unless you have no other choice.

The Smith machine forces you into an unnatural movement pattern that can be very uncomfortable, and research shows it's less effective than the free weight barbell squat.[8]

3. If you can't keep your lower-back in a neutral position as you descend because it begins to round, it's possible that your hamstrings are too tight or your that back isn't strong enough.

This is known as "butt wink," and in many people, it can be resolved through daily hamstring stretching (standing with one leg crossed over the other and then touching your toes, and reversing and repeating, works well).

As your hamstrings loosen, you'll find it much easier to keep your lower-back in a neutral position until you hit the very bottom of the squat, when your pelvis naturally rotates down a little.

Don't stretch before your squatting, though, because this can sap your strength.[9] Save it for after your lower-body workouts, when your muscles are nice and warm.

If you're confident hamstring tightness isn't the problem, it's possible you need to strengthen your back muscles.

In this case, you just need to be more mindful of making sure you don't add weight to the bar until you can maintain a neutral lower-back throughout each rep of each set.

Over time, your weaker back muscles will catch up to your stronger leg and hip muscles.

4. Don't squat with plates or blocks underneath your feet.

This doesn't make the exercise more effective and isn't a worthwhile variation to include in your workouts. That said, by elevating your heels while squatting, you can improve your form and range of motion.

Some people's hips are built in such a way that it makes it harder to safely and comfortably reach the bottom of the squat with good form. By slightly elevating your heels, you can change the mechanics of the squat enough to work around this limitation and perform the movement properly.

The best solution for this is to get a good pair of squat shoes, which have slightly elevated heels.

In fact, you should do this regardless of how comfortably you can squat, because the wrong shoes can make it significantly harder to progress.

Anything with a soft or unstable sole, like running shoes, shouldn't be used when squatting because it doesn't provide a solid, stable base through which you can transfer force into the floor.

Shoes with flat, solid soles and rigid, slightly elevated heels are much better because they allow for maximum force transfer. They also make it easier to maintain your balance as you descend, and they engage your hamstrings and glutes as you ascend.

5. Use the Valsalva maneuver to control your breathing.

The Valsalva maneuver is the process of forcefully breathing out against a closed windpipe. This traps air in your lungs and creates pressure inside your abdomen, known as *intra-abdominal pressure*, which stabilizes your torso against heavy loads.

Research shows that this increased intra-abdominal pressure allows you to lift more weight than you could with continuous breathing, and probably reduces the risk of injury as well.[10]

That's why the Valsalva maneuver is a useful technique for all exercises, not just the squat. Here's how to do it:

1. Take a deep breath of about 80 percent of your maximum lung capacity. Your belly should feel "full" but not so much that you have trouble keeping your mouth closed when the rep gets hard.

2. Press your tongue against the roof of your mouth, and without letting any air escape, try to breathe out. You should feel your abdomen, back, and jaw tighten.

3. Start your descent.

4. Once you're past the "sticking point" (the most difficult point) of the ascent, breathe out as you finish the rep.

5. Repeat for each rep in your set.

An important caveat: the Valsalva maneuver increases your blood pressure more than continuous breathing.

A number of studies show that this isn't inherently dangerous, and holding your breath is instinctive when lifting heavy weights, but if you're hypertensive or have a preexisting heart condition, you should talk with your doctor before using the Valsalva maneuver.[11]

Furthermore, if you use the technique and experience chest pain, dizziness, or other red flags, you should stop using it and talk with your doctor.

6. Use helpful cues as needed.

Cues are short reminders athletes use to draw their attention to particular aspects of their performance, typically whatever they struggle with the most.

Here are some of my favorite cues for good squatting:

- Keep your chest up.
- Throw the bar off your back.
- Grab the floor (with your feet).
- Force your hips under the bar.
- Push the floor apart.
- Bend the bar over your back.

You don't have to memorize these cues or chant them as you squat, but if you're struggling with a particular portion of the movement, one of them may help you correct the issue.

THE BARBELL DEADLIFT

If I could do only one exercise for the rest of my life, it would be the barbell deadlift.

Mark Rippetoe said it best in an article he published on my website Muscle for Life (www.muscleforlife.com/how-to-look-strong-deadlift):

> The deadlift works just about every muscle group you want to develop, from your upper-back muscles down to your calves, and it forces you to get strong the right way, with the bar in your hands balanced on your feet.
>
> If you want to look strong, you have to get strong. And strong you'll get from the deadlift.

Few people argue that the deadlift isn't an effective strength and muscle builder, but some claim it's bad for your joints, and especially your lower-back.

This seems plausible at first glance because it places a lot of stress on the lower-back, but is that actually bad? Let's see what the scientific literature has to say.

The first study we should review was conducted by scientists at the University of Valencia to determine the most effective way to train the paraspinal muscles, which run down both sides of your spine and play a major role in preventing back injuries.[12]

Researchers split 25 people into two exercise groups:

1. Group one performed bodyweight exercises like lumbar extensions, forward flexions, single-leg deadlifts, and bridges.

2. Group two performed two weighted exercises, barbell deadlifts and lunges, using 70 percent of their one-rep max.

Muscle activity was measured using *electromyography*—a technique of measuring and analyzing electrical activity that occurs in the muscles when they contract—and the deadlift most activated the paraspinal muscles, and won by a long shot.

The researchers' conclusion, then, was that the deadlift is a remarkably effective way to strengthen these muscles.

Another insightful study on the matter was conducted by scientists at the University of Waterloo to determine how much strain the deadlift put on the back—the lower-back in particular—and how likely it was to produce injury.[13]

The researchers recruited four elite-level competitive powerlifters and had them do two exercises:

1. Leaning as far forward as possible, bending over from the waist and then returning to an upright posture (fully flexing and extending their backs).

    This allowed the researchers to measure the limits of the powerlifters' natural range of motion.

2. Deadlifting a weight close to their one-rep max, which worked out to 400 to 460 pounds.

The researchers used real-time X-ray imaging (called *videofluoroscopy*) to watch the lifters' spines while they completed both tasks.

Many deadlifting injuries occur because of too much low-back bending, which can pull vertebrae out of position, pinch and compress intervertebral cartilage discs, and strain low-back ligaments.

So the scientists measured each of those things—how much the participants' vertebrae moved, how much their spinal discs were pinched and compressed, and how much their low-back ligaments were stretched.

The examination found that the deadlift was completed within the weightlifters' natural range of motion, and that there were no signs of excessive vertebral shifting, pinching of the intervertebral discs, or pulling of the low-back ligaments.

Thus, the researchers concluded that the deadlift is a fantastic exercise for strengthening your entire back, including your lower-back, and doesn't force an unnatural range of motion or put excess strain on your spine or joints.

As with the other exercises in this chapter, poor form is what has given the deadlift a bad name among some.

For instance, how many people have you seen who round their lower-backs while pulling? This is a major no-no, as it shifts much of the stress away from the powerful erector spinae muscles (which run alongside your spine) to the vertebrae, intervertebral discs, and ligaments.

Perform the lift correctly, however, and you have little to worry about and much to gain. Let's learn how to do that.

THE SETUP

The deadlift starts with the bar on the floor, not on the rack or safety arms or pins.

Walk up to the bar, position your feet so they're slightly narrower than shoulder width apart with your toes pointed slightly out, and move the bar to the point where your shoulders are in line with or even slightly behind it.

This will put the bar somewhere between against your shins and over the middle of your feet. For taller or skinnier people, it'll probably place the bar against their shins. For shorter or thicker people, it'll place it somewhere around the middle of the feet.

Proper bar position is important because it allows for maximum leverage as you pull it up and back. If the bar is too close to your body and your shoulders are too far in front of it, you'll have to move it forward on the way up to get it over your knees. If it's too far from your body, you'll feel like you're going to fall forward and won't be able to drive upward through your heels.

Next, stand up tall with your chest out and take a deep breath of air into your belly (as opposed to your chest), bracing your abs as if you were about to get punched in the stomach.

Then, move down toward the bar by pushing your hips back, just as you do in the squat. Arch your lower-back slightly and keep your shoulders down as you wedge yourself into what's essentially a "half-squat" position.

You should feel considerable tightness in your hamstrings and hips as you get into this position. This is desirable because as soon as your hips rise, your shoulders will be able to follow, and the weight will immediately start coming off the floor.

Don't make the newbie mistake of bringing your hips too low with the intention of "squatting" the weight up. The lower your hips are in the starting position, the more they'll have to rise before you can lift the weight off the floor, which wastes movement and energy.

Next, place your hands on the bar with a double-overhand grip (both palms facing down) just outside your shins, and squeeze it as hard as you can. Keep your shoulders back and down and press your upper arms into your sides as if you were trying to crush oranges in your armpits. Your arms should be completely straight and locked, with enough room on the sides for your thumbs to clear your thighs as you ascend.

Make sure your head is in a neutral position. Don't look up at the ceiling or down at the ground.

Here's how you should look:

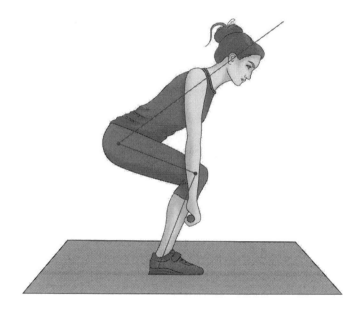

You're now ready to ascend.

THE ASCENT

Start the pull by forcefully driving your body upward and slightly back, onto your heels. Push through your heels, and keep your elbows locked in place and lower-back slightly arched (no rounding!).

Ensure that your hips and shoulders rise simultaneously. Don't shoot your hips up and then use your back like a lever to raise your shoulders. If your hips are moving up, your shoulders should be as well.

The bar should move up your shins, and once it rolls over your knees, push your hips into the bar. As it begins to move up your thighs, you'll feel your hamstrings and hips working hard as you continue to stand.

The entire way up, keep your head in its neutral position in line with your spine, your lower-back slightly arched, and your core tight. Also, try to keep the bar on as vertically straight of a path as possible because any deviations are just going to slow you down and make it harder to maintain good form. The bar shouldn't move noticeably toward or away from you.

At the top, your chest should be up and your shoulders down. Don't lean back, hyperextend your lower-back, or shrug the weight up.

Here's how this movement looks:

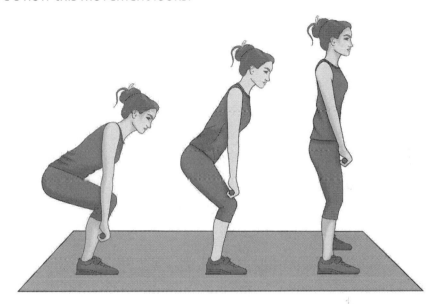

You're now ready to descend.

THE DESCENT

The next half of the deadlift is lowering the weight back down to the floor in a controlled manner. This is basically a mirror image of what you did to stand up.

Begin by pushing your hips back, not bending at the knees, letting the bar slide straight down your thighs. Continue pushing your hips back, lowering the bar in a straight line until it has cleared your knees, and then drop it to the floor.

Your lower-back should remain locked in its neutral position the entire time, and your core should remain tight. Don't try to lower the bar slowly or quietly. The entire descent should take one to two seconds or less.

You're now ready for the next rep.

Many people don't stop to reset in between reps and instead use the tap-and-go transition, which has you maintain tension as you tap the weights to the floor and immediately begin the next rep.

This is fine if you're warming up, but I prefer the stop-and-go method for my hard sets. This method has you fully release the weight to the ground and reset your bottom position—including your breath—before starting the next rep. This is harder than tap-and-go, but that's good, and it's safer as well.

THE ROMANIAN DEADLIFT

As a part of *Thinner Leaner Stronger*, you're going to do one variation of the barbell deadlift: the Romanian deadlift.

At first glance, the Romanian deadlift looks like a lazy or downright dangerous version of the regular deadlift. Ironically, it's not a one-way ticket to snap city but rather one of the single best exercises you can do for developing your hamstrings, glutes, spinal erectors, lats, and even forearms.

The main differences between the Romanian and conventional deadlift are:

1. You can start with the bar in a power rack instead of on the floor (but don't have to).

2. Your legs remain fairly straight, bending only slightly at the knees to lower the bar.

3. You lower the bar to just below your knees or when your lower-back starts to round, and no further.

Why the "Romanian" deadlift, you're wondering?

The story goes that in 1990, a Romanian Olympic weightlifter named Nicu Vlad was in San Francisco demonstrating an exercise that looked like a cross between a stiff-leg and conventional deadlift.

Someone in the audience asked what it was called. He shrugged and said it was just something he did to strengthen his back. The US Olympic weightlifting coach was there and suggested they call it the Romanian deadlift, and it stuck.

Let's go through technique.

THE SETUP

There are two ways to set up for the Romanian deadlift:

1. From the rack
2. From the floor

If you start from the rack, you'll want the bar to be just below where you'll hold it at the top of the movement, or about midthigh.

If you start from the floor, then all you have to do is set up the same way you would for the conventional deadlift.

Most people prefer starting from the rack because it makes it easier to load the bar and doesn't force you to waste energy pulling it off the floor at the beginning of each set.

To set up, walk up to the bar so that it's over the middle of your feet, position your feet about shoulder width apart with your toes pointed slightly out, and grip the bar with a double-overhand grip.

Next, take a deep breath, raise your chest, and press your upper arms into your sides as if you were trying to crush oranges in your armpits.

Lift the bar off the rack (or floor), take a baby step back if you're coming from the rack, and bend your knees slightly. Fix your gaze on a spot about 10 feet in front of you.

You're now ready to descend.

THE DESCENT

To descend, allow your hips to move backward as you lower the bar down the front of your legs.

As the bar drops down in a straight line, keep your knees at more or less the same angle as when you started. Once you start to feel a stretch in your hamstrings, you can allow slightly more bend in your knees.

At this point, the bar should be at knee height or just below.

Don't try to lower the bar to the ground. Doing so forces you to bend your knees even more, which reduces tension on the hamstrings and defeats the purpose of the exercise.

Once you can't go any lower without rounding your lower-back or further bending your knees, you're ready to ascend.

THE ASCENT

Keeping your back and core tight, chest up, and knees slightly bent, drive your hips forward while pulling the bar straight up.

Here's how this movement looks:

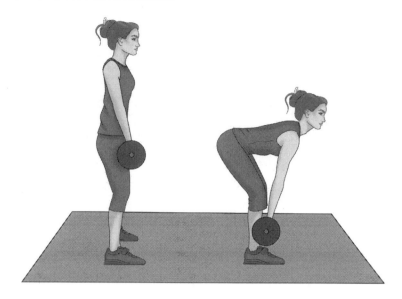

Once you're standing tall, you're ready for the next rep.

SIX TIPS FOR BETTER DEADLIFTING

1. Squeeze the bar as hard as you can.

Try to crush it with your hands. If your knuckles aren't white, you're not squeezing hard enough.

2. Boost your grip.

Grip weakness not only makes the bar harder to hold onto, it shuts down the entire exercise. Once the bar starts rolling out of your hands, you'll grind to a halt.

Your grip will get stronger as you train, but chances are it's going to fall behind the rest of your body in your deadlift and become a limiting factor.

A common workaround is the "mixed grip," which involves alternating one of your hands so it's palm-up. This works well but also has downsides:

1. It makes you tend to rotate your torso toward your palm-down hand, creating a load imbalance between the left and right sides of your body.

2. It places more strain on the biceps of your palm-up arm.[14]

I don't know of any scientific data on how this affects the safety of the exercise, but I'll say this: while biceps tears are rare, when they do happen, it's often from the palm-up biceps during a heavy mixed-grip deadlift.

You can take a simple precaution to make the mixed grip safer—alternate your palm-up hand in individual workouts or between them—but I'd rather you just use a double-overhand grip with straps instead.

Many people shy away from straps because they look at them as a form of "cheating," but this is silly. When used properly, straps allow you to safely pull more weight without any of the downsides of the mixed grip (and its excruciating cousin, the hook grip, which we won't even discuss because of what it does to your thumbs).

To use straps, pick up some simple lasso straps, pull without them until your grip starts to give out (your second or third hard set, for instance), and then use them to finish up. Straps can help with barbell and dumbbell rows, too.

You can also include grip exercises in your routine at any point if you're so inclined. My favorite is the plain ol' barbell hold, which is exactly what it sounds like: holding onto a heavy barbell.

Here's how to do it:

1. Using a squat rack, place the bar at your knees and load it with a weight you can hold for no more than 15 to 20 seconds.

2. Do three sets of 15-to-20-second holds, resting for three minutes between each set.

Do this once or twice per week at the end of workouts, separated by two to three days. You should see marked improvements within your first month or so.

Last but not least, you can also use weightlifting chalk for an easy boost in your grip strength. Chalk helps by absorbing sweat and increasing the friction between your palms and the bar, and you can go with the liquid variety if you don't want to make a mess or your gym doesn't allow it.

3. Use the right shoes.

As with squatting, deadlifting in shoes that have foam or air cushions or gel fillings compromises your stability, power production, and form.

Plus, most athletic shoes aren't made for deadlifting and fall apart after just a few months of regular use. Deadlift in your squat shoes instead, in shoes with flat, hard soles, or in socks.

4. Explode up from the floor.

Don't start the pull slowly. This makes it easier to get stuck. Instead, shoot your body up as quickly as you can by applying maximum force to the ground through your heels.

5. Wear shin guards, knee-length socks, or knee sleeves.

For most people, proper deadlifting form requires pulling the bar up their shins, which starts to tear them up as weights get heavy. ("Are her shins *bleeding*?")

You can wear pants or tights, but they're going to get shredded over time.

This is why I recommend protecting your shins while you deadlift with light-weight shin guards, knee-length socks, or a pair of knee sleeves that you wear below your knees.

6. Use the Valsalva maneuver to control your breathing.

As you learned, this helps stabilize your torso against heavy loads, which helps you safely move more weight. That's why it's useful for all compound exercises.

In the case of the deadlift, you can breathe out after the bar clears the midthighs.

THE BARBELL BENCH PRESS

The barbell bench press is one of the best all-around upper-body exercises you can do, training the pectorals, lats, shoulders, triceps, and even the legs to a slight degree.

It's simple enough, too. You lie on a bench with your feet on the floor, unrack the bar, lower it to the middle of your chest, and press it back up.

There are many ways to do that, though, and unfortunately, many more wrong than right ways.

For instance, you've probably seen at least some of the following at the gym:

- Failing to bring the bar all the way down to the chest
- Bringing the bar down to the collarbone
- Raising the butt off the bench
- Shrugging or rolling the shoulders at the top
- Flaring the elbows out away from the body

And those are all major reasons why the bench press is often bad-mouthed by trainers and gymgoers as damaging to your back and shoulders.

Like many exercises, when performed incorrectly and with too much weight, you can get hurt benching. Do it right, though, and your risk of injury is very low, allowing you to reap all its great benefits safely and healthily.

A study conducted by scientists at the University of Salford is good evidence of this.[15] Researchers found that as long as you follow two pieces of advice, your chances of injury during the bench press will be fairly low:

1. Use a medium grip that's just a little wider than shoulder-width apart.

2. Keep your arms at about a 30-to-60-degree angle relative to your torso.

I've found that about a 45-degree angle works best for me.

Another reason the bench press has copped a bad rap is it's one of the most popular exercises, especially among men.

Many guys simply do too much benching with too much weight and usually with bad form, to boot, and this naturally results in more injuries over time when compared to exercises performed far less frequently with lighter loads.

You're not going to make any of these mistakes. You're going to learn picture-perfect form and do a reasonable amount of bench pressing with a reasonable amount of weight, so your risk of injury will be about as low as possible.

So, let's learn how to bench.

THE SETUP

First, lie down on the bench and adjust yourself so your eyes are under the bar.

Then, raise your chest up and tuck your shoulder blades down and squeeze them together. Think of pulling your shoulder blades into your back pockets. This should produce tightness in your upper-back.

Next, grab the bar with your hands slightly wider than shoulder width apart, about 14 to 20 inches, depending on your build. If you go too narrow, you'll shift the emphasis to the triceps instead of the pecs, and if you go too wide, you'll reduce the range of motion and effectiveness of the exercise and increase the risk of irritating your shoulders.

Hold the bar low in your hands, closer to your wrists than your fingers, and squeeze it as hard as you can. Your wrists should be bent just enough to allow the bar to settle into the base of your palm, but not folded back toward your head.

Here's how this looks:

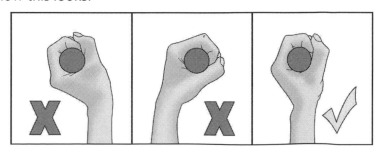

A good way to check your grip width is to have a friend get behind you and check the position of your forearms at the bottom of the movement. You want your forearms to be as close to straight up-and-down vertical as possible, like this:

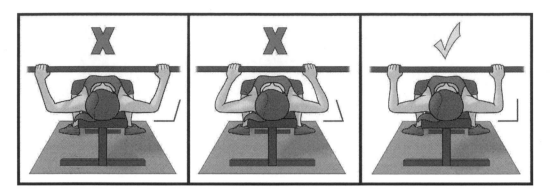

As you can see, the position on the far left is too wide, the middle is too narrow, and the far right is correct.

Don't use a "thumbless" or "suicide" grip (as it's aptly called), where your thumbs are next to your index fingers instead of wrapped around the bar.

When you're going heavy, this grip can make it surprisingly easy for the bar to slip out of your hands and crash down on your chest, or worse, your neck.

Next, slightly arch your lower-back and plant your feet on the ground, directly under your knees, about shoulder width apart.

You don't want your back flat on the bench and you don't want it so arched that your butt is floating above it. Instead, you want to maintain the natural arch that occurs when you push your chest out.

The upper part of your leg should be parallel to the floor, and the lower part should be perpendicular (forming a 90-degree angle). This allows you to push through your heels as you ascend, creating a "leg drive" that'll boost your strength.

Then, unrack the bar by locking your elbows out and moving it off the hooks horizontally until it's directly over your shoulders. Don't try to bring the weight directly from the hooks to your chest, and don't drop your chest and loosen your shoulder blades when unracking.

Finally, with the bar in place, take a deep breath, push your knees apart, and squeeze the bar.

You're now ready to descend.

THE DESCENT

The first thing you should know about the descent is how to tuck your elbows properly.

Many people make the mistake of flaring them out (away from the body), which can cause a shoulder injury. A less common mistake is tucking your elbows too close to your torso, which robs you of stability and strength and can aggravate your elbows.

Instead, you want your elbows to remain at a 30-to-60-degree angle relative to your torso throughout the entire movement. This protects your shoulders from injury and provides a stable, strong position to press from.

Here's a helpful visual:

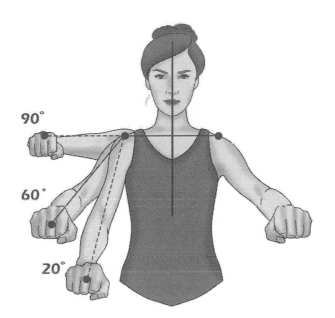

As you can see, in the bottommost position, the arms are at about a 20-degree angle relative to the torso, which is too close. The middle position is the ideal one—about 45 degrees—and the topmost is the undesirable 90 degrees.

Keeping your elbows tucked and in place, lower the bar to the lower part of your chest, over your nipples. The bar should move in a straight line down, not toward your face or belly button.

Once the bar has touched your chest (touched, not bounced off), you're ready to ascend.

THE ASCENT

Although it's called the bench press, it's better to think of it as pushing rather than pressing.

That is, picture that you're pushing your torso away from the bar and into the bench instead of pressing the bar away from your body. This will help you maintain proper form and maximize power.

Keeping your shoulder blades down and pinched, your elbows tucked, your lower-back slightly arched, your butt on the bench, and your feet on the floor, push against the bar to get it off your chest.

You can also utilize the "leg drive" I mentioned earlier by pressing your heels into the floor and spreading your knees as you begin to push the bar. This transfers force up through the hips and back, which helps with form and increases the amount of power you can generate.

The bar should move up in a slightly diagonal path, shifting toward and ending where you began—with it directly over your shoulders, where it's most naturally balanced.

Lock your elbows out at the top of the movement. Don't keep them slightly bent.

You're now ready for the next rep.

Once you've completed your final rep in a set, you're ready to rack the bar. Don't try to press the bar directly into the hooks because if you miss, it's coming down on your face.

Instead, finish your final rep with the bar directly over your shoulders and your elbows locked, and then move the bar horizontally into the uprights.

THE CLOSE-GRIP BENCH PRESS

As a part of *Thinner Leaner Stronger*, you're going to do one variation of the barbell bench press: the close-grip bench press.

As I mentioned earlier, when you narrow your grip on the bar, you place more of the load on the triceps. This is undesirable when you want to focus on your chest, but it's a great way to focus on the triceps.

At bottom, the close-grip bench press is just a regular bench press but with a narrower grip. Other than the grip modification, you should perform the close-grip bench press in exactly the same way as the regular bench press.

For your grip, your hands should be slightly (a few inches) inside your shoulders. Some people place their hands just a few inches apart to try to maximize the triceps' involvement, but this puts the shoulders and wrists in a potentially dangerous position.

If your shoulders or wrists feel uncomfortable at the bottom of the movement (when the bar is touching your chest), simply widen your grip by about the width of a finger on each side and try again. Repeat until it's comfortable.

SIX TIPS FOR BETTER BENCH PRESSING

1. Don't watch the bar as it moves.

Watching the bar will likely vary its angles of descent and ascent, which wastes energy.

Instead, pick a spot on the ceiling to look at during the exercise and see the bar going down and up in relation to it. The goal is to bring the bar up to the same spot in each rep.

2. Try to pull the bar down and apart.

This is an old-school powerlifting tip that has been proven to work in scientific research. The idea is simple:

1. Don't start the descent by letting the bar drop toward your body. Instead, imagine you're pulling the bar down toward your chest in a controlled manner. This will help you maintain the proper body position for generating maximum vertical force.[16]

2. As you descend, try to bend the bar in half or "pull it apart." This requires keeping your shoulder blades in their proper position (pulled in toward each other).

    Applying lateral force in this way also helps you generate more vertical force when you ascend, which is one of the reasons you can move more weight on the barbell bench press than dumbbell press.[17] You can't generate lateral force with dumbbells because they simply move away from each other.

3. Keep your butt on the bench at all times.

If your butt is lifting off the bench, the weight is probably too heavy.

The three points of contact you should always maintain for optimal bench pressing are the upper-back (down on the bench), the butt (ditto), and the feet (always planted on the floor squarely beneath your knees).

4. Don't smash the back of your head into the bench.

This can strain your neck. Your neck will naturally tighten while doing the exercise, but don't forcefully push it down.

5. When you're lowering the weight, think about the ascent.

Visualize the explosive second half of the exercise the entire time, and you'll find it easier to control the descent, prevent bouncing, and even prepare your muscles for the stress of raising the bar.

(This technique works well for all exercises, by the way.)

6. Use the Valsalva maneuver to control your breathing.

As I mentioned previously, I recommend you use the Valsalva maneuver during all your compound exercises, and that includes the bench press.

In this case, you can breathe out after the bar is about four to six inches above your chest.

. . .

Whew!

That was a lot of information to digest, so feel free to reread this chapter and practice the basic movements of the exercises before continuing. Grab a broomstick if you have one handy to use as a bar!

And if you want bonus points, put yourself on camera so you can ensure that what you think you're doing is actually what you're doing.

You should also make sure you download the free bonus material that comes with this book (www.thinnerleanerstronger.com/bonus) because it provides links to in-depth video tutorials for each of these exercises.

If you found anything about my explanations unclear, the videos will fill in the gaps.

KEY TAKEAWAYS

- The barbell squat, barbell deadlift, and barbell bench press have been the staples of strength and bodybuilding programs for over a century now because they involve the most whole-body muscle and safely allow for maximum progressive overload.

- One of your primary goals on my *Thinner Leaner Stronger* program is going to be improving your numbers on these key exercises.

- Bad form is why these three exercises have been so maligned over the years as harmful to your shoulders, back, and knees.

- While some people's anatomies don't play well with these exercises, when performed correctly, they're perfectly safe and maybe even protective against joint pain.

- The barbell squat is one of the single best exercises for developing every major muscle group in your body.

- Not only is the squat safe for your knees—it may even improve knee health and reduce your risk of knee injury.

• The deadlift is a fantastic exercise for strengthening your entire back, including your lower-back, and doesn't force an unnatural range of motion or put excess strain on your spine or joints.

• The Romanian deadlift is one of the single best exercises you can do for developing your hamstrings, glutes, spinal erectors, lats, and even forearms.

• The barbell bench press is one of the best all-around upper-body exercises you can do, training the pectorals, lats, shoulders, triceps, and even the legs to a slight degree.

• The close-grip bench press is just a regular bench press but with a narrower grip, and is a great way to focus on the triceps.

PART 6

DON'T BUY ANOTHER SUPPLEMENT UNTIL YOU READ THIS

25

THE GREAT SUPPLEMENT HOAX

"Your love for what you do and willingness to push yourself where others aren't prepared to go is what will make you great."
—LAURENCE SHAHLAEI

"Pills in a bottle, brother."

I frowned. Was he serious?

"It's pretty slick, right?" Anthony said with a sideways grin.

Anthony had a simple business. His supplement company spent about $2 million per month on pay-per-click advertising and brought in close to $4 million in sales.

What kind of "pills in a bottle" was he selling, exactly?

Anthony didn't know. He couldn't tell me a single ingredient. What he did know, however, is a bottle cost him $3 to produce and sold for $39.99. He also knew that, on average, he got close to $100 out of customers before they finally figured out how to cancel their subscriptions.

Oh, and he also knew that his million-dollar renovation of his multimillion-dollar mansion was coming along splendidly.

When I first entered the fitness industry, I thought Anthony was an anomaly. A bad apple in the orchard. Sadly, I was wrong. People like him are more the rule than the exception.

In fact, the supplement industry is best described by Ben Kenobi's famous words: a wretched hive of scum and villainy.

Seriously. Fake news, fake science, fake products—you can find it all in the supplement racket. It's almost funny … in the not so funny kind of way.

Don't believe me?

In 2015, the New York State Attorney General's office accused four national retailers of selling dietary supplements that were fraudulent and in many cases contaminated with unlisted ingredients.[1]

The authorities said they had run tests on popular store brands of herbal supplements at the retailers—Walmart, Walgreens, Target, and GNC—which showed that roughly four out of five of the products contained none of the herbs listed on their labels.

In many cases, the supplements contained little more than cheap fillers like rice and house plants, or substances that could be hazardous to people with food allergies.

According to lab tests obtained by the Michigan law firm Barbat, Mansour and Suciu in 2015, a number of sports supplement brands including Giant Sports, MusclePharm, CVS Health, 4 Dimension Nutrition, NBTY, and Inner Armour were mixing cheap fillers into their protein powders to bring down costs and were falsifying their supplement fact panels to cover their tracks.[2]

Even worse is the supplement company Driven Sports, which was busted in 2013 for putting a methamphetamine-like drug in their popular preworkout supplement "Craze."[3] Apparently meth makes for some pretty intense workouts.

Oh, and their CEO was also previously busted for selling anabolic steroids and illegal weight loss drugs.[4]

Yet another supplement company, USPlabs, was slapped by the FDA in 2013 for selling a preworkout supplement ("Jack3d") spiked with a dangerously powerful stimulant called *DMAA*, and then again in 2015 for selling a fat loss product ("OxyELITE Pro") laced with fluoxetine (Prozac) and drugs that caused liver damage and failure.[5] After making over $400 million from 2008 to 2013, I might add.[6] A genius plan, if you love jail.

The sad lesson I've learned is the majority of supplement companies, especially sports supplement companies, are first and foremost marketing companies.

Most are in the game of, as one supplement company CEO put it to me, "telling people what they want to hear to sell them what they don't need." He thought that was pretty clever.

That's not a hard game to play, either. Anybody can reach out to a contract manufacturer, ask for some off-the-shelf formulations full of useless ingredients, slap some fancy labels on bottles, recruit some steroid-fueled Instagram celebrities to shill for them, and have a shot at moving a lot of product.

A smart marketer once said that you can persuade people of just about anything if you can convince them it has science or history on its side. If you want easy evidence of this, just browse through workout magazines and check out some of the supplement advertisements.

The copy will be loaded with phrases like "science-based," "evidence-based," and "clinically dosed," and for good reason—they work. Most people don't really know what these buzzwords mean or how to validate the claims, but the connotations and promises are enough to drive billions of dollars per year in sales.

At first glance, it sounds like a scientist's wet dream for companies to care so much about the love and passion they put into their research. The fantasy evaporates when you look a little closer, however.

Most supplement companies don't want to be backed by science, they want to *appear* to be backed by science. To them, science is a family of slogans to sling around for more revenue, and while these companies' errors, inaccuracies, and exaggerations are sometimes honest mistakes, they're more often deliberate deceptions.

This is easy to do because the supplement industry is completely unregulated, so anyone can fraudulently appeal to science with virtual impunity. And when there are millions and millions of dollars on the line, you'd better believe that many supplement marketers are willing to cut every corner they can.

An illustrative example of this is the controversy surrounding the supplement β-Hydroxy β-Methylbutyrate (HMB), a natural substance derived from the amino acid leucine.

According to a study conducted by scientists at the University of Tampa, people supplementing with HMB gained triple the amount of lean mass as those taking a placebo, lost over twice as much body fat, gained far more strength, and were significantly less sore from their workouts.[7]

In other words, according to this research, HMB was about as effective for muscle gain and fat loss as anabolic steroids.[8]

Sorry to interrupt, but do you smell something? You do too? What is that?

Let's follow the money to find out. Who funded this study? The company Metabolic Technologies, which owns several patents related to HMB. Oh, and look at that, three of the study's authors worked there as well.

Could that stench be a steaming pile of conflict of interest?

Several other studies on HMB have reported similarly astounding benefits, but it's hard to get excited when you learn they were conducted by Steven Nissen, who owns Metabolic Technologies.[9]

Even more telling is that quite a bit of unbiased research has been conducted on HMB with very different results. For instance:

- A study conducted by scientists at Massey University found that HMB supplementation improved lower-body strength but had negligible effects on body composition.[10]

- A study conducted by scientists on the Singapore Sports Council found that HMB supplementation had no effect on strength or body composition.[11]

- A study conducted by scientists at the University of Memphis found that HMB supplementation didn't reduce catabolism or enhance body composition or strength.[12]

Researchers from Massey University also conducted a review of HMB research and concluded the following:

> Supplementation with HMB during resistance training incurs small but clear overall and leg strength gains in previously untrained men, but effects in trained lifters are trivial. The HMB effect on body composition is inconsequential.[13]

This little anecdote teaches us a very valuable supplementation lesson: if a supplement sounds too good to be true, it probably is. If even a minority of these products worked half as well as their advertisements claimed, we'd all be fitness models by now.

Why all the skulduggery and shenanigans?

Filthy lucre, of course. Morals can become surprisingly supple and relativistic when plied with cash ("What's right and wrong anyway?"). When you're presented with an unethical opportunity to make millions of dollars fast, you learn who you really are. And many pill and powder pushers are frauds to their bones.

All this is why most workout supplements are completely bogus and can't deliver a fraction of the results they promise. They are, for lack of a better term, worthless crap. And some are even dangerous.

This shell game will continue until something is done about it, and for my part, I don't want to wait and see if the FDA is ever going to get serious about cracking down.

We consumers hold more power than we think. Our dollars determine everything. If we keep giving them to these shady operators, we're giving them permission to keep exploiting us.

If we don't, however—if we withhold our money and demand change—we can send a powerful message to the entire industry: shape up or ship out.

When you take a supplement, you're putting your health in the hands of complete strangers who work in an industry overflowing with cash and crooks. This is why many people have decided to stay away from supplements altogether, which is a perfectly reasonable position considering what I've just told you.

It's too bad though because not all supplements are junk. There *are* safe, natural supplements that can help you gain muscle, lose fat, and get healthy faster.

No, they're not going to transform your body or life, but high-quality, unbiased research shows they *can* give you a slight edge in your journey to a fitter and healthier you.

The trick, then, is knowing which supplements are actually worth buying and which aren't, and that's exactly what you're going to learn in the next chapter.

26

THE SMART SUPPLEMENT
BUYER'S GUIDE

> *"In this age, which believes that there is a short cut to everything,
> the greatest lesson to be learned is that the most difficult way is,
> in the long run, the easiest."*
>
> —HENRY MILLER

Supplements aren't nearly as important as some people would have you believe. The right ones can help speed up your results, but even then, they're *supplementary*, not vital.

So the first thing you need to know is you don't need supplements. Absolutely none are necessary for reaching your health and fitness goals.

That said, you should consider including several supplements in your regimen because sound scientific research has proven they can help you build muscle and lose fat faster, boost workout performance and postworkout recovery, and improve your general health and well-being.

For instance, research shows that creatine, beta-alanine, and citrulline absolutely can help you gain muscle and strength faster, synephrine and yohimbine can help you burn more fat, and vitamin D and fish oil can improve your health and well-being in many ways.[1]

On the other hand, a number of popular supplements you've probably heard of or even tried are proven duds.

For example, branched-chain amino acids are often claimed to increase muscle growth, but a growing body of evidence shows they don't.[2]

Garcinia cambogia is one of the (if not *the*) most popular weight loss supplements of all time, but several studies show that while it may work in rats, it's a complete flop in humans.[3]

The same goes for the go-to supplement for boosting testosterone, *Tribulus terrestris*—it simply doesn't work, period.[4]

It would take an entire book to break down everything you see on the shelves of your local supplement store, so instead, I want to focus on the six types of supplements that are going to be most beneficial for you:

1. Protein powder

2. Fish oil

3. Vitamin D

4. Multivitamin

5. Fat burner

6. Muscle builder

With these six supplements, you can positively and significantly impact just about every meaningful aspect of your physiology, including muscle growth, fat loss, inflammation, heart health, mood, brain and gut health, insulin sensitivity, energy levels, immunity, and more.

We're going to review each of these types of supplements broadly in this chapter, and then, in chapter 30, talk specifics (products and protocols).

Let's start at the top.

PROTEIN POWDER

Whey and casein and soy, oh my!

The selection of protein powders on the market can be overwhelming. There are dozens of popular brands and scores of popular products.

Which should you buy, and why?

Should you choose an animal-based protein powder like whey, casein, or egg? Or maybe a plant-based protein powder like rice, soy, hemp, or pea will be best for you? Or a blend, maybe?

Well, a good protein powder meets a few criteria:

1. It doesn't have to taste like a milkshake, but it should taste good and mix well.

If you have to choke it down, you're going to have trouble sticking with it.

2. It should have a good macronutrient profile.

It should provide the most protein for the fewest calories and be as low in carbs and fat as possible.

3. It should have a good amino acid profile and be absorbed well by the body.

This determines how useful it really is for our purposes.

4. It should be affordable and offer good value in terms of cost per serving.

I also believe it's beneficial to choose a protein powder that doesn't contain artificial sweeteners, food dyes, or other junk, simply because it helps reduce our overall exposure to these chemicals, which may not be as entirely harmless as we've been told.[5]

There are several types of protein powders that pass this test. Let's learn a bit about each (as well as two popular choices that don't pass the test).

THE SCOOP ON WHEY PROTEIN

Whey protein is Grand Poobah of protein powders, and for good reason.

It provides you with a lot of protein per dollar, it tastes good, and its amino acid profile is particularly suited to muscle building.

What is it, though, and what makes it special?

Whey is a translucent liquid that's left over after curdling and straining milk to make cheese. It used to be considered a worthless byproduct of dairy processing, but eventually its high-protein content was discovered.

Scientists also discovered that whey is rich in the amino acid leucine, which plays a vital role in stimulating protein synthesis.[6] This put whey at the top of the list for bodybuilders.

What's more, whey is quickly digested, which means it causes a dramatic spike in amino acids in the blood when eaten.[7] This makes it ideal for postworkout supplementation, and research suggests it may stimulate more immediate muscle growth than slower-burning proteins like casein or egg.[8]

In short, whey is an excellent all-around choice for protein supplementation. What type of whey protein should you buy, though? You have three to choose from:

1. Whey concentrate

Whey concentrate is the least processed form of whey protein. It ranges from 25 to 80 percent protein by weight, depending on the quality, and contains dietary fat and lactose.

2. Whey isolate

Whey isolate is a form of whey protein processed to remove the fat and lactose. It's at least 90 percent protein by weight.

3. Whey hydrolysate

Whey hydrolysate is whey protein (concentrate or isolate, but usually isolate) specially processed to be more easily digested and absorbed.[9]

Whey isolate and hydrolysate are often marketed as superior to whey concentrate in all respects, but this isn't true. Isolate and hydrolysate do have advantages—more protein by weight, no lactose, better mixability and digestibility, and some would say better taste—but as far as bottom-line results go, whey concentrate works just fine.[10]

That said, choosing the cheapest whey you can find, which will always be a concentrate, isn't always a good idea. A quality whey concentrate is somewhere around 80 percent protein by weight, but inferior concentrates can be as low as 25 percent protein by weight.[11]

The general rule with whey protein is you'll get what you pay for. If a product costs a lot less than the going rate for whey, it's probably because it's made with low-quality ingredients.

High prices aren't always indicative of high quality, however.

Disreputable supplement companies will often add small amounts of whey isolate and hydrolysate to a base of low quality concentrate to create a "blend," and then call special attention in their packaging and advertising to just the isolate and hydrolysate.

To protect yourself as a consumer, always check ingredient lists, serving sizes, and amounts of protein per serving before buying a protein powder.

First, look at the ingredients list because ingredients are listed in descending order according to predominance by weight. This means there's more of the first ingredient than the second, more of the second than the third, and so on.

Therefore, if a protein powder bills itself as a whey isolate but has whey concentrate as the first ingredient, it contains more whey concentrate than anything else and may in fact be mostly concentrate and contain very little isolate.

Worse are "whey" protein powders that list milk protein (a very cheap alternative) before any form of whey.

You should also look at the amount of protein per scoop relative to the scoop size, because a large discrepancy between the two is a red flag that something isn't right.

For instance, if a serving weighs 40 grams but contains just 22 grams of protein, don't buy the product unless you know that the other 18 grams consist of stuff you want.

A high-quality whey protein is easy to spot:

1. Whey concentrate, isolate, or hydrolysate is the very first ingredient.

If you see anything other than one of those three ingredients in the number one spot, find another product.

2. The serving size is relatively close to the amount of protein per serving.

It'll never match because even the "cleanest" protein powders have sweeteners, flavoring, and other minor but requisite ingredients in addition to the protein powder itself.

THE SCOOP ON CASEIN PROTEIN

Like whey, casein protein comes from milk. Unlike whey, however, casein digests slowly, resulting in a steadier, more gradual release of amino acids into the blood.[12]

There's an ongoing debate as to whether whey or casein is better for gaining muscle, but here's what most reputable experts agree on:

- Whey's rapid digestion and abundance of leucine makes it a great choice for postworkout nutrition.

- Casein may or may not be as good for postworkout nutrition as whey.[13]

- Casein is just as good as whey for general supplementation needs.[14]

- You can speed up muscle recovery by having 30 to 40 grams of a slow-burning protein like casein (or low-fat cottage cheese or Greek or Icelandic yogurt) before bed.[15]

As far as types of casein protein go, you have two choices:

1. Calcium caseinate

2. Micellar casein

Calcium caseinate is a form of casein processed to improve mixability.

Micellar casein is a higher quality form produced in a way that preserves the small bundles of protein (micelles) that are responsible for its slow-digesting properties and often destroyed during traditional manufacturing processes.

This is why research shows that micellar casein is digested slower than calcium caseinate, making it especially beneficial for prebed use.[16]

Similar to whey, when buying a casein protein, you should look at the amount of protein per scoop relative to the scoop size, because a large discrepancy indicates something isn't right.

THE SCOOP ON EGG PROTEIN

Did you know that you can buy egg protein powder? Many people don't, but you can, and it's perfectly viable for two reasons:

1. It has a high *biological value,* or BV.[17]

This is a measurement of how efficiently the protein is absorbed and utilized by your body.

As you can imagine, high-BV proteins are best for building muscle, and animal research suggests that egg protein is as effective as whey protein for this purpose.[18]

Human research also shows that egg is highly effective at stimulating protein synthesis.[19]

2. It has very little fat and carbohydrate.

Egg protein powder is made from egg white, so it's naturally more or less carb- and fat-free. That means more macros for your food!

As far as types of egg protein go, you can choose powdered or liquid; either is fine.

Also, in case you're wondering, egg protein contains no cholesterol, so you can supplement with it in addition to any whole eggs you eat (if that's something you're concerned about).

THE SCOOP ON SOY PROTEIN

While studies show that soy is an all-round effective source of protein, it's also a source of ongoing controversy, and especially among men.[20]

According to some research, soy foods can have feminizing effects in men due to estrogen-like molecules in soybeans called *isoflavones.*[21]

According to other studies, however, neither soy nor isoflavones can alter fertility or male hormones at normal levels of intake.[22]

Fortunately, as a woman, none of that matters to you. For you, soy protein is a perfectly good vegan source of protein comparable to whey in terms of quality and effectiveness.[23]

You have two types of soy protein to choose from:

1. Soy isolate
2. Soy concentrate

Concentrate generally lacks the isoflavones due to how it's processed, while the isolate contains the isoflavones. Both are fine choices.

THE SCOOP ON RICE PROTEIN

You may not think much of the protein found in rice or even know it contained any protein, but it makes for quite the protein powder.

Rice protein has a high BV of about 80 percent (similar to beef's) and a robust amino acid profile very similar to soy's, which is why research shows that it's an effective muscle builder.[24]

It also has a mild taste and pleasant texture and mouthfeel, making it an all-around winner for plant-based protein supplementation.

As far as forms go, rice protein isolate is really the only game in town. If you want to make it even better, you can mix it with the next option.

THE SCOOP ON PEA PROTEIN

Pea protein is the real unsung hero of plant proteins. I mean, when's the last time you heard a meathead say that he's eating a lot of peas to help bulk up?

Well, he could because pea protein has a high BV (about the same as rice's) and, like whey, a large amount of leucine.[25] That's why studies show that pea protein is indeed effective in promoting muscle gain.[26]

Pea protein is often combined with rice protein because they taste great together and have complimentary amino acid profiles, combining into something chemically similar to whey. In fact, this mix is often referred to as the "vegan's whey."

Pea protein powder comes in two forms:

1. Pea protein concentrate
2. Pea protein isolate

Both pea protein concentrate and isolate are created by drying and grounding peas into a fine flour, mixing it with water, and removing the fiber and starch, leaving mostly protein with a smattering of vitamins and minerals.

Whether the final product is considered a concentrate or isolate just depends on how much of the nonprotein elements are removed. Pea protein isolate needs to be 90-plus percent protein by weight, whereas pea protein concentrate can be anywhere from 70 to 90 percent protein by weight.

This is why I prefer isolate over concentrate (less carbohydrate and fat).

THE SCOOP ON HEMP PROTEIN

Hemp protein is highly nutritious but only about 30 to 50 percent protein by weight, which means it comes with quite a bit of carbs and fat.

Furthermore, hemp protein isn't absorbed nearly as well as soy, rice, or pea protein and is lower in essential amino acids, making it even less useful as a protein supplement.[27]

That's why I look at hemp protein powder more as a whole food than a protein supplement, and why I don't recommend it purely for protein supplementation.

THE SCOOP ON COLLAGEN PROTEIN

Collagen protein is all the rage at the moment, thanks mostly to slick marketers and prominent diet and health influencers.

Unfortunately, it doesn't even deserve a spot on the stage, let alone the spotlight.

As you know, the amount of essential amino acids a protein provides is very important, especially for improving body composition.

Collagen protein scores very low in this regard because while it's abundant in the amino acids glycine, proline, hydroxyproline, and alanine, it's low in the essential amino acids leucine, isoleucine, and valine, which are most related to muscle building.[28]

It's also low in sulphur, which is involved in a number of bodily functions such as blood flow, energy production, and protecting cells from oxidative damage.[29]

One thing collagen protein does have going for it, however, is the high amount of glycine, which can improve the quality of your skin, hair, and nails. That said, glycine is dirt cheap, and you can buy it alone (and in bulk) if you want to supplement with it.

FISH OIL

Fish oil is exactly what it sounds like: oil obtained from fish. Popular sources of fish oil are salmon, herring, mackerel, sardines, and anchovies.

The reason fish oil supplements exist is they're a very good source of two nutrients mentioned earlier in this book: eicosapentaenoic acid (EPA) and docosahexaenoic acid (DHA).

We recall that EPA and DHA are known as omega-3 fatty acids and that our bodies can't produce them, which is why they're also known as essential fatty acids.

Unfortunately, studies show that the average person's diet provides just one-tenth of the EPA and DHA needed to preserve health and prevent disease.[30] This is a serious concern because studies show that inadequate EPA and DHA intake can increase the risk of a number of health conditions, including heart disease, Alzheimer's, and cancer.[31]

Thus, when EPA and DHA intake is too low, increasing it can benefit you in many ways, including:

- Improved mood (lower levels of depression, anxiety, and stress)[32]
- Better cognitive performance (memory, attention, and reaction time)[33]
- Reduced muscle and joint soreness[34]
- Improved fat loss[35]
- Prevention of fat gain[36]
- Faster muscle gain[37]

Fatty fish isn't the only way to get more EPA and DHA in your diet. Grass-fed meat, free-range eggs, and vegetable oils are other options, but none are ideal.

Omega-3 levels are much lower in meat and eggs than fish, and vegetable oils don't contain EPA and DHA but instead the fatty acid alpha- linolenic acid (ALA), which the body then converts into EPA and DHA.[38]

Research shows that this conversion process is very inefficient, however, so you would have to eat large amounts of ALA regularly to supply your body with enough EPA and DHA.[39] This is why vegans often have omega-3 fatty acid deficiencies.[40]

There are three forms of fish oil supplements on the market today:

1. Triglyceride
2. Ethyl ester
3. Reesterified triglyceride

A triglyceride is a molecule that consists of three fatty acids and one molecule of glycerol, a colorless, odorless substance found in fats and oils. The triglyceride form of fish oil is its natural (unprocessed) state.

An ethyl ester fish oil is created by processing natural triglycerides to replace the glycerol molecules with ethanol (alcohol). This removes impurities and increases the amount of EPA and DHA in the oil.

The reesterified triglyceride form is similar to the natural form and is created by using enzymes to convert the ethyl ester oil back into triglyceride oil.

Of these three forms, you'd probably assume that a natural triglyceride supplement is your best choice. Not necessarily.

While natural triglyceride fish oils are absorbed well by the body, they can have much higher levels of contaminants than ethyl ester and reesterified triglyceride oils (due to the low level of processing).[41]

Furthermore, natural triglyceride fish oils are lower in EPA and DHA per gram than ethyl ester and reesterified triglyceride oils, which means you have to take more to achieve the desired results. This can be expensive both in terms of dollars and calories.

Ethyl ester fish oils are the most popular, but that's not because they're the best. They're just the cheapest to produce, which comes with significant downsides.

First, studies show that this form of fish oil isn't absorbed well by the body.[42] It also releases ethanol (alcohol), which needs to be processed by the liver.[43] This can cause various side effects, including burping, flu-like symptoms, upset stomach, strange tastes in your mouth, and skin rash.[44]

Ethyl ester fish oils also oxidize (go bad) more quickly and easily than triglyceride oils.

As you can tell, I'm no fan of ethyl ester fish oils and don't recommend them.

In case you're wondering how to tell whether a fish oil is an ethyl ester product, check the label. If it doesn't specifically state the form of the oil, assume it's ethyl ester. Companies that pay more for the superior, more expensive triglyceride forms call it out in their marketing to increase salability.

And that leaves reesterified triglyceride oil, which is becoming the "gold standard" of fish oil supplements for several reasons:

- High bioavailability[45]
- High concentrations of EPA and DHA
- Low levels of toxins and pollutants
- Resistance to oxidation[46]
- None of the alcohol-related side effects associated with ethyl ester oils

Not many companies sell reesterified triglyceride oils because they're the most expensive to produce, but I think they're well worth the premium.

VITAMIN D

Not too long ago, vitamin D was simply known as the "bone vitamin," and even today many physicians still believe it's essential only for bone health.

Recent research shows otherwise, though. Nearly every type of tissue and cell in the body has vitamin D receptors, including your heart, brain, and even fat cells, and vitamin D plays a vital role in a large number of physiological processes.[47]

Furthermore, studies show that vitamin D also regulates genes that control immune function, metabolism, and even cell growth and development.[48]

This is why insufficient vitamin D levels is associated with an increased risk of many types of disease, including osteoporosis, heart disease, stroke, some cancers, type 1 diabetes, multiple sclerosis, tuberculosis, and even the flu.[49]

Our bodies can't produce enough vitamin D to maintain adequate levels, either, so we have to obtain it from diet, sun exposure, or supplementation.[50]

There are small amounts of vitamin D in various foods like beef liver, cheese, and egg yolks, which have anywhere from 10 to 60 IU (international units) per ounce, and slightly larger amounts in fatty fish like salmon, tuna, and mackerel, which have anywhere from 50 to 150 IU per ounce. Cod liver oil is by far the best food source with over 1,300 IU per tablespoon.

Vitamin D is also added to various "fortified" foods like milk, breakfast cereals, orange juice, and margarine, but getting enough vitamin D through these foods alone isn't feasible if you're trying to follow a sensible meal plan.

When our skin is exposed to UVB rays, which are emitted by the sun, they interact with a form of cholesterol in the body to produce vitamin D. The more skin that's exposed to the sun, and the stronger the sun's rays, the more vitamin D you produce.

For instance, research shows that with 25 percent of our skin exposed, our bodies can produce upwards of 400 IU of vitamin D in just three to six minutes of exposure to the 12 p.m. Florida summer sun.[51]

Depending on your diet and latitude, that means you'd need to spend anywhere from 15 to 60 minutes sunbathing per day to maintain sufficient levels. And you might be simply out of luck in the winter.

All this is why I prefer vitamin D supplementation. It's cheap, effective, and gives you maximum flexibility in your diet.

MULTIVITAMIN

Our bodies need a variety of vitamins and minerals to support all the vital growth and repair processes that keep us alive and functioning.

Ideally, we'd get everything we need from the food we eat, but due to the nature of the average Western diet, most people tend to be deficient in a number of key nutrients.

For example, according to research conducted by scientists at Colorado State University and published in 2005, at least half the US population failed to meet the recommended dietary allowance (RDA) for vitamin B-6, vitamin A, magnesium, calcium, and zinc, and 33 percent of the population didn't meet the RDA for folate.[52]

A more recent study conducted by scientists at Tufts University and published in 2017 found that more than 30 percent of the US population was deficient in calcium, magnesium, and vitamins A, C, D, and E.[53]

Research also shows that average vitamin K intake levels may be suboptimal as well.[54]

Enter the multivitamin supplement. The idea of taking a supplement that can plug any nutritional holes in our diets and mitigate the harmful effects of some of our less-than-healthy habits is great in theory, but most multivitamins fall short of this mark (let alone surpass it).

Instead of doing the hard work of determining optimal dosages of the essential vitamins and minerals for their target publics, most supplement companies go with premade formulations provided by manufacturers.

These products are often stuffed with all kinds of micronutrients, regardless of whether we need to supplement with them or not, and in unjustifiably high or low dosages. This is why many multivitamins provide an overabundance of vitamins and minerals that most people aren't deficient in and little or none of what they need most.

For instance, many multivitamins contain large amounts of the microminerals manganese, molybdenum, and boron and vitamins C, E, and A, despite the fact that most people eating halfway decent diets already get plenty of these nutrients and don't need to supplement with them.

In contrast, a good example of something important lacking in most multivitamins is vitamin K, a group of vitamins that plays an important role in bone growth and repair, blood vessel function, cancer prevention, joint health, and more.[55]

And if a multivitamin does include vitamin K, it's almost always a small dose of a form that's present in large amounts in whole foods, known as *vitamin K1*.

The form that should be included is *vitamin K2*, which offers unique health benefits and is much harder to obtain from diet alone. Why is K2 rarely found in multivitamins? Because it's expensive, of course.

Furthermore, many multivitamins provide potentially dangerous superdoses of certain vitamins and minerals.

For example, the amount of vitamin E in many multivitamins can be harmful to your health. Vitamin E is an antioxidant, meaning it helps protect against oxidative damage, and it's often overdosed on the assumption that more antioxidants is always better. This is why both it and vitamin C (another antioxidant) are usually included in multivitamins in sky-high amounts.

Not all antioxidants are similar, however, and regular supplementation of vitamin E above 400 IU per day is now suspected to increase the risk of all-cause mortality (death from all causes).[56]

To make matters worse, very few multivitamins contain anything worthwhile in addition to the vitamins and minerals.

Call me cynical, but am I supposed to get excited over a 100 milligram "proprietary blend" of fruit and vegetable powders? Some probiotics that are undoubtedly dead and, even if they weren't, wouldn't do anything anyway? A few enzymes or amino acids that I don't need to supplement with? Herbs that purport to help "detox" my body (which no supplement can do)?

So, in the final analysis, I'd rather people just eat a healthy amount and variety of fruit and vegetables than waste money and pin false hopes on a multivitamin that's very unlikely to benefit them in any meaningful way.

FAT BURNER

I probably don't need to say this by now, but I'm going to do it anyway:

No amount of weight loss pills and powders are going to make you lean.

Trust me. If you're trying to lose fat, pill popping, even to excess, is not going to be enough. There just aren't any safe, natural "fat-burning" compounds powerful enough to cause meaningful weight reduction on their own.

Furthermore, you shouldn't be surprised at this point to learn that most weight loss supplements on the market, including some of the most popular ones, are flops.

For example:

- According to a meta-analysis conducted by scientists at the University of Exeter, the best you can hope for with *Garcinia cambogia* is a few extra pounds of weight loss over a few months, and even that is less likely than no additional weight loss whatsoever.[57]

- According to another meta-analysis conducted by the same scientists, green coffee extract may be able to help you lose weight slightly faster only when taken in high enough doses, but the scientific jury is still out and the case isn't looking good.[58]

- *Conjugated linoleic acid* (CLA) is a bit of a mystery as studies show it can help some people lose fat, fail to help others, and even cause fat gain in some cases.[59]

How? Why? What will it do for you? Nobody can say yet.

- Animal research shows that raspberry ketones have anti-obesity effects in mice, but we have no valid human research to see how they affect us.[60]

Now the good news:

If you know how to drive fat loss with proper dieting and exercise, there are a few supplements that can accelerate the process.

Based on my experience with my own body and having worked with thousands of people, I feel comfortable saying that a proper fat loss supplementation routine can increase fat loss by about 30 to 50 percent with few if any side effects.

That is, if you can lose 1 pound of fat per week through proper diet and exercise (and you can), you can lose 1.3 to 1.5 pounds of fat per week by adding the right supplements into the mix.

Another big benefit of taking the right fat loss supplements is that they're especially effective for reducing "stubborn fat," which is belly, hip, and thigh fat for most women.

What are these "right" supplements, how do they work, and how can we use them safely and effectively?

Let's find out, starting with everyone's favorite.

CAFFEINE

Caffeine does a lot more than give you an energy high.

Studies show that it also:

- Decreases perceived effort (makes exercise feel easier)[61]
- Makes you more resistant to fatigue[62]
- Increases power output[63]
- Increases muscle endurance[64]
- Increases strength[65]
- Increases anaerobic performance[66]
- Boosts fat loss[67]

Caffeine can also reverse the muscle weakness many people experience when they train in the morning.[68]

Most of caffeine's benefits are a byproduct of its ability to increase the amount of catecholamines (chemicals that trigger fat burning) in your blood, which also raises your basal metabolic rate.

For instance, research shows that in most people, a relatively small dosage of 200 milligrams of caffeine increases BMR by about 7 percent for three hours.[69] If you have caffeine two or three times per day, then, this can add up to an additional 150 to 200 calories burned.

You should also know that your body begins building a tolerance to caffeine almost immediately, and the higher your tolerance is, the less effective caffeine will be for enhancing performance and fat loss.[70]

Therefore, if you want to get the biggest performance boost out of caffeine, use it just a few days per week before your most difficult workouts (I usually have some before my workouts that involve barbell squatting and deadlifting).

And to get the most fat loss out of caffeine, use it daily for two to three weeks, and then take a week off to "reset" your tolerance and preserve its effectiveness.

YOHIMBINE

Yohimbine is a compound obtained from the bark of the *Pausinystalia yohimbe* tree, and several studies show that it can speed up fat loss.[71]

Like caffeine, it does this by stimulating the production of catecholamines, but unlike caffeine, it can also help you burn more "stubborn fat."

"Stubborn fat?" you might be wondering.

Yep, some fat cells are far more difficult to shrink than others. This isn't a genetic curse. It's simply a physiological mechanism your body uses to defend against low body fat levels.

To trigger fat burning, your body releases catecholamines into your blood, which then "attach" to receptors on fat cells. This causes the release (*mobilization*) of the energy stored within those cells for use.

Fat cells have two types of receptors for catecholamines: alpha- and beta-receptors.[72] To keep this simple, beta-receptors generally speed up fat mobilization, whereas alpha-receptors hinder it.[73] (The physiology is more complex than this, but we don't need to go deeper for our purposes here.)

Thus, the more alpha-receptors a fat cell has, the more "resistant" it is to being mobilized by catecholamines. On the other hand, the more beta-receptors a fat cell has, the more "receptive" it is to the fat-mobilizing molecules.

As you've probably guessed, the areas of your body that get lean quickly have a lot of fat cells rich in beta-receptors, and the areas that take their sweet time leaning out have a large amount of fat cells rich in alpha-receptors.

Another problem with these stubborn fat deposits relates to blood flow.[74]

You may have noticed that fat in areas of your body like the hips and thighs is slightly colder to the touch than fat in other areas of your body, like the arms or chest. This is due to less blood flowing through these cooler areas, and less blood flow means fewer catecholamines, which means even slower fat loss.

So we have two things working against us here: large amounts of fat cells that don't respond well to catecholamines and reduced blood flow that keeps the catecholamines away.

This is why you can steadily lose weight with almost all the fat seeming to come from parts of your body that are already fairly lean. For instance, it's common for women to lose fat from their legs, abs, and arms while their butt, hips, and thighs remain relatively unchanged.

Thus, once you approach about 20 percent body fat, every bit of "stubborn" fat you lose can have a noticeable impact on your physique. At this point, losing just a pound or two of fat from the "right places" can do a lot more in the mirror than several pounds from areas of your body that are already defined.

Now, what does yohimbine have to do with all this?

Studies show that it can speed up stubborn fat loss by attaching itself to, and more or less deactivating, the alpha-receptors on fat cells.[75]

In other words, yohimbine prevents your fat cells' alpha-receptors from putting the brakes on fat burning.

There's a catch, however. Elevated insulin levels completely negate yohimbine's fat loss benefits.[76] That means it's strictly for use while exercising in a fasted state.

SYNEPHRINE

Synephrine is a compound found primarily in the bitter orange fruit, which is why it's often referred to by that name.[77]

It's chemically similar to the ephedrine and pseudoephedrine found in many over-the-counter cold and allergy medications as well as weight loss and energy supplements that contain ma huang.

Consequently, synephrine stimulates the nervous system and increases BMR, and increases the thermic effect of food (the energy cost of digesting and processing what you eat).[78]

There's also evidence that, like yohimbine, synephrine blocks the alpha-receptors on fat cells, which means that it too can speed up stubborn fat loss.[79]

MUSCLE BUILDER

Muscle-building supplements aren't nearly as popular among women as men, so I don't think we need to spend time here debunking testosterone boosters, growth hormone boosters, weight gainers, and the like.

That said, we should discuss one supplement many women use in hopes of building muscle faster—branched-chain amino acids (BCAAs)—and three supplements that are better choices:

1. Creatine

2. Beta-alanine

3. L-citrulline

BRANCHED-CHAIN AMINO ACIDS (BCAAS)

BCAAs are a group of three essential amino acids:

1. Leucine

2. Isoleucine

3. Valine

As you know, leucine directly stimulates protein synthesis. Isoleucine also stimulates it weakly and improves glucose metabolism and uptake in the muscles.[80] Valine doesn't seem to do much of anything for muscle tissue compared to leucine and isoleucine.[81]

BCAA supplements aren't top sellers because they work wonders in the body but rather because they're easy to sell. For example, a number of studies seem to show several impressive benefits, "everyone" into fitness seems to drink them, and they make for some mighty delicious water.

If I wanted to sell you BCAAs, I could point to research that suggests they improve immune function, diminish fatigue, minimize exercise-induced muscle damage, and enhance postworkout muscle growth.[82]

What I wouldn't tell you, however, is the bulk of this research doesn't directly apply to the average healthy, physically active person following a sensible workout routine and high-protein diet.

First off, studies commonly cited as evidence of the muscle-related benefits of BCAA supplementation were done with people who didn't eat enough protein.

For example, one study used by supplement companies to move a lot of BCAA powders was conducted by scientists at the Center for the Study and Research of Aerospace Medicine.[83]

It examined the effects of BCAA supplementation on a group of wrestlers in a calorie deficit, and after three weeks, found that the wrestlers who supplemented with 52 grams of BCAAs per day preserved more muscle and lost a bit more fat than the ones who didn't.

If that's all you were told, you might start reaching for your wallet. Before you do, however, you should know the rest of the story: these wrestlers weighed about 150 pounds on average and were eating a paltry 8-ish grams of protein per day.

As you learned earlier in this book, that's about half as much protein as these athletes should've been eating, so all this study really tells us is BCAA supplementation might mitigate muscle loss when restricting both calories and protein intake. And who knows what to think on the additional fat loss, as there's no plausible mechanism whereby BCAAs can impact this. Color me unimpressed.

Other studies showing various muscle-related benefits of BCAA supplementation are almost always hampered by a lack of dietary controls and low protein intakes. And in almost all cases, the people are exercising in a fasted state, which affects the muscles and body differently than when exercise is done in a fed state.

I think an argument could be made for athletes training several hours per day possibly benefitting from BCAA supplementation, but for the rest of us, it's far more sizzle than steak. We can get all the branched-chain amino acids we need to recover from our training and build muscle from the food we're eating as a regular part of our diets.

In fact, research even suggests BCAAs obtained through food are more conducive to muscle growth than amino acid drinks.[84]

Finally, a recent review of BCAA research that was conducted by scientists at the University of Arkansas found that BCAA supplementation either has no effect on muscle growth or may even decrease it.[85]

Thus, the researchers concluded that "the claim that consumption of dietary BCAAs stimulates muscle protein synthesis or produces an anabolic response in human subjects is unwarranted."

CREATINE

Of all the workout supplements on the market today, creatine stands out as one of the absolute best.

It's the most well-researched molecule in all of sports nutrition—the subject of hundreds of scientific studies—and the benefits are clear:

- It helps you build muscle faster.[86]
- It helps you get stronger faster.[87]
- It improves anaerobic endurance.[88]
- It improves muscle recovery.[89]

And the best part is it does all these things naturally and safely.[90]

What is it, though, and how does it work?

Creatine is a molecule produced in the body and found in foods like meat, eggs, and fish. It's composed of the amino acids L-arginine, glycine, and L-methionine and is present in almost all cells, where it acts as an "energy reserve."

When you supplement with creatine, your total body creatine stores increase, with most going to your muscle cells.[91] And what do you think happens when your muscle cells have significantly higher levels of readily available energy? You got it. Performance is enhanced.

Creatine also enhances muscle growth by increasing the amount of water in muscle cells.[92] This makes muscles bigger, of course, but it also positively impacts *nitrogen balance* (a measure of nitrogen intake minus nitrogen loss, with a positive balance indicating muscle gain) and the expression of certain genes related to muscle building.[93]

Other research suggests that creatine also has anticatabolic effects, which further helps with muscle gain.[94]

Many women shy away from creatine because they've heard it makes you bloated. This used to be a problem years ago, but it has become a nonissue today since processing methods have improved. You shouldn't notice any difference in subcutaneous (underneath the skin) water levels when you supplement with creatine.

Creatine comes in many forms, including creatine monohydrate, creatine ethyl ester, buffered creatine, and others.

We could discuss them one by one, but here's all you really need to know: go with powdered creatine monohydrate. It's the most researched form by which all others are judged, and it's the best bang for your buck.

BETA-ALANINE

Beta-alanine is an amino acid that our body combines with the essential amino acid L-histidine to form a compound molecule called *carnosine*, which is stored in your muscles and brain.

Carnosine does a number of things in the body, including helping regulate acidity levels in our muscles.

When a muscle contracts repeatedly, it becomes more and more acidic. This, in turn, impairs its ability to continue contracting, until eventually it can no longer contract at all. This is one of the ways muscles become fatigued.[95]

Carnosine counteracts this by reducing muscle acidity, thereby increasing the amount of work the muscles can do before becoming fatigued.[96]

This is why a meta-analysis conducted by scientists at Nottingham Trent University found that beta-alanine supplementation results in a slight improvement in endurance when exercise duration is between 60 and 240 seconds.[97]

Several studies also show that beta-alanine can enhance muscle growth.[98]

Scientists aren't sure why just yet, but people who supplement with beta-alanine seem to gain more muscle than those who don't. This effect doesn't appear to be merely a byproduct of improved workout performance, either.

L-CITRULLINE

L-citrulline is an amino acid that plays a key role in the *urea cycle*, the process whereby the body eliminates toxic byproducts of digesting protein and generating cellular energy.

It's called the *urea* cycle because these waste products are converted into a substance called *urea*, which is expelled from the body through urine and sweat.

And in case you're wondering, the "L-" refers to the structure of the amino acid and denotes that it can be used to create proteins (the other type of amino acid is the "D-" form, which is found in cells but not in proteins).

L-citrulline is a popular workout supplement because it can improve both your resistance and endurance training and boost nitric oxide production.

For example, in one study conducted by scientists at the University of Córdoba, people who supplemented with 8 grams of L-citrulline before their chest workouts increased the number of reps they could do by 52 percent and experienced significantly less postworkout muscle soreness.[99]

In another study conducted by scientists at the Biological and Medical Magnetic Resonance Center, 6 grams of L-citrulline per day increased cellular energy production during exercise by 34 percent, resulting in a greater capacity for physical output and intensity.[100]

When you supplement with L-citrulline, your kidneys convert it into another amino acid, L-arginine, and this increases nitric oxide production.[101]

Nitric oxide is a gas produced by the body that widens blood vessels and improves blood flow.[102] By raising nitric oxide production, you can improve exercise performance, lower blood pressure, and even harden erections (give it to your man!).[103]

Ironically, supplementing with L-citrulline accomplishes this better than L-arginine itself because it's absorbed better by the body.

There are two widely available forms of citrulline to choose from:

1. L-citrulline
2. Citrulline malate

The only difference between these two forms is L-citrulline is the pure amino acid, and citrulline malate is L-citrulline combined with *malic acid*, a natural substance found in many fruits.

There isn't much human research available on the potential benefits of supplementing with malic acid, but it has been shown to improve endurance in animal studies.[104] It may offer cardiovascular benefits as well.[105]

Thus, I recommend citrulline malate over L-citrulline for two reasons:

1. It's the form used in most studies that found performance benefits.

2. There's a fair chance malic acid confers additional health and performance benefits.

In other words, there's no downside to citrulline malate, and it may be superior to L-citrulline.

. . .

I wish someone would have taught me what you've just learned back when I started training.

It would've saved me who knows how much time and money I wasted researching and buying worthless pills and powders.

I hope you've found this information not only helpful but relieving, because let's face it: supplementation is a complex and overwhelming subject, and it's all too easy to wind up with cabinets full of expensive bottles and bags of stuff that delivers minimal if any bottom-line results.

If you follow the advice in this chapter, you're not going to be one of these people, because you now know the absolute best choices for gaining more muscle and strength, losing more fat, and improving and maintaining health and vitality.

I should also mention that just because I didn't bring up something here doesn't mean it has no merits. It just means it's not one of the 20 percent of supplements that will provide 80 percent of the benefits we're most after.

If you want to learn more about the science of supplementation and how you can further optimize your mental and physical health and performance, head over to the supplements category of my blog at www.thinnerleanerstronger.com/supplements.

KEY TAKEAWAYS

- Supplements aren't nearly as important as some people would have you believe. The right ones, however, can help speed up your results.

- A good protein powder meets a few criteria:

  It doesn't have to taste like a milkshake, but it should taste good and mix well.

  It should provide the most protein for the fewest calories and be as low in carbs and fat as possible.

  It should have a good amino acid profile and be absorbed well by the body.

  It should be affordable and offer good value in terms of cost per serving.

- Whey protein provides you with a lot of protein per dollar, tastes good, and its amino acid profile is particularly suited to muscle building.

- Whey isolate and hydrolysate do have advantages—more protein by weight, no lactose, better mixability and digestibility, and some would say better taste—but as far as bottom-line results go, whey concentrate works just fine.

- A high-quality whey protein is easy to spot:

  Whey concentrate, isolate, or hydrolysate is the first ingredient.

  The serving size is relatively close to the amount of protein per serving.

- When buying a casein protein, you should look at the amount of protein per scoop relative to the scoop size.

- For women, soy protein is a perfectly good vegan source of protein comparable to whey in terms of quality and effectiveness.

- Rice and pea protein are effective muscle builders.

- Hemp protein isn't absorbed nearly as well as soy, rice, or pea protein and is lower in essential amino acids.

- Collagen protein is low in the essential amino acids leucine, isoleucine, and valine, which are most related to muscle building.

- Fish oil is a very good source eicosapentaenoic acid (EPA) and docosahexaenoic acid (DHA).

- When EPA and DHA intake is too low, increasing it can benefit you in many ways, including improved mood (lower levels of depression, anxiety, and stress), better cognitive performance (memory, attention, and reaction time), reduced muscle and joint soreness, improved fat loss, prevention of fat gain, and faster muscle gain.

- Reesterified triglyceride oil is becoming the "gold standard" of fish oil supplements.

- Insufficient vitamin D levels is associated with an increased risk of many types of disease, including osteoporosis, heart disease, stroke, some cancers, type 1 diabetes, multiple sclerosis, tuberculosis, and even the flu.

- Our bodies can't produce enough vitamin D to maintain adequate levels, so we have to obtain it from diet, sun exposure, or supplementation.

- Ideally, we'd get all the nutrition we need from the food we eat, but due to the nature of the average Western diet, most people tend to be deficient in a number of key nutrients.

- The idea of taking a supplement that can plug any nutritional holes in our diets and mitigate the harmful effects of some of our less-than-healthy habits is great in theory, but most multivitamins fall short of this mark (let alone surpass it).

- I'd rather people just eat a healthy amount and variety of fruit and vegetables than waste money and pin false hopes on a multivitamin that's very unlikely to benefit them in any meaningful way.

- No amount of weight loss pills and powders are going to make you lean.

- Most weight loss supplements on the market, including some of the most popular ones, are flops.

- A proper fat loss supplementation routine can increase fat loss by about 30 to 50 percent with few if any side effects.

- Another big benefit of taking the right fat loss supplements is that they're especially effective for reducing "stubborn fat," which is belly, hip, and thigh fat for most women.

- Caffeine decreases perceived effort (makes exercise feel easier), makes you more resistant to fatigue, increases power output, muscle endurance, strength, and anaerobic performance, and boosts fat loss.

- Caffeine can also reverse the muscle weakness many people experience when they train in the morning.

- Your body begins building a tolerance to caffeine almost immediately, and the higher your tolerance is, the less effective caffeine will be for enhancing performance and fat loss.

- If you want to get the biggest performance boost out of caffeine, use it just a few days per week before your most difficult workouts (I usually have some before my workouts that involve barbell squatting and deadlifting).

- To get the most fat loss out of caffeine, use it daily for two to three weeks, and then take a week off to "reset" your tolerance and preserve its effectiveness.

- Stubborn fat refers to fat cells that are far more difficult to shrink than others. This is why you can steadily lose weight with almost all the fat seeming to come from parts of your body that are already fairly lean.

- Once you approach about 20 percent body fat, every bit of "stubborn" fat you lose can have a noticeable impact on your physique.

- Yohimbine prevents your fat cells' alpha-receptors from putting the brakes on fat burning.

- Elevated insulin levels completely negate yohimbine's fat loss benefits. That means it's strictly for use while exercising in a fasted state.

- Synephrine stimulates the nervous system and increases BMR and the thermic effect of food (the energy cost of digesting and processing what you eat).

- Synephrine also blocks the alpha-receptors on fat cells, which means that it too can speed up stubborn fat loss.

- We can get all the branched-chain amino acids we need from the food we're eating as a regular part of our diets.

- BCAAs obtained through food are more conducive to muscle growth than amino acid drinks.

- Creatine helps you build muscle and get stronger faster and improves both anaerobic endurance and muscle recovery.

- Many women shy away from creatine because they've heard it makes you bloated. This used to be a problem years ago, but it has become a nonissue today.

- Go with powdered creatine monohydrate. It's the best bang for your buck.

- Beta-alanine can improve endurance and enhance muscle growth.

- L-citrulline can improve both your resistance and endurance training and boost nitric oxide production.

- By raising nitric oxide production, you can improve exercise performance, lower blood pressure, and even harden erections (give it to your man!).

- I recommend citrulline malate over L-citrulline.

PART 7

THE *THINNER LEANER STRONGER* PROGRAM

27

YOU PAINT BY THE NUMBERS, YOUR BODY DOES THE REST

"Courage is like a muscle. We strengthen it by use."
— RUTH GORDO

Are you ready for an exact, step-by-step program for eating, exercising, and supplementing that will add lean muscle and melt away handfuls of unwanted fat?

Are you ready to enter a new phase in your personal fitness journey and finally build your best body ever?

And are you ready to do it faster and more enjoyably than you ever thought possible?

If so, I'm excited to officially welcome you to my *Thinner Leaner Stronger* program!

I'm so glad you're here because by the end of this part of this book, you're going to have the complete road map to building a stronger and more beautiful body, and you're going to be ready to put rubber on the road.

Specifically, you're going to get dietary, exercise, recovery, and supplementation guidelines and instructions, as well as foolproof, premade plans and templates you can use to get started right away.

And then, just a few weeks from now, when you start seeing real improvements in how you look, feel, and perform, you're going to realize that the search is finally over.

That you've finally found the answers to your most pressing health and fitness questions. And that you finally understand exactly how to achieve the health and fitness outcomes you desire most.

Imagine how good you're going to feel when you no longer have to fret about your weight or reflection in the mirror.

Imagine how good you're going to feel when your partner, friends, family, and colleagues are constantly complimenting you on your new, toned body.

Imagine how good you're going to feel when you can go to bed every night knowing that you're getting a little stronger, sexier, and healthier every single day.

And imagine how good you're going to feel knowing that you're setting yourself up for a longer life filled with more energy, youthfulness, self-esteem, intimacy, and wellness instead of a shorter one marked by pain, dysfunction, self-doubt, distance, and disease.

That doesn't mean the process isn't going to take time, however.

We live in the Age of Impatience. People want four-hour workweeks, six-minute abs, and 30-second meals. I'm sorry, but you can't lose 20 pounds of fat in 20 days or reshape your butt or flatten your belly in a week.

Transforming your body composition is a rewarding process, but it's probably going to feel slow to you. Many women find they need to lose anywhere from 10 to 15 percent body fat and gain 10 to 15 pounds of muscle to have the bodies they really want. That can take a year or two.

This is why fitness isn't for the weak-minded and weak-willed. You can't slide by on BS. Your body doesn't care about your excuses or justifications. The only way to undo skipped workouts is to put your butt in the gym and do the work. The only way to overcome screwy dieting is to stop screwing up.

If you're going to successfully engineer your lifestyle to help you achieve your biggest goals and dreams, you must learn to love the process and embrace the struggle. If you can do that, then there's nothing that can stop you.

That's what awaits you on *Thinner Leaner Stronger*. That's what I want for you. That's why you need to keep reading.

28

THE *THINNER LEANER STRONGER* DIET PLAN

"To begin is easy, to persist is an art."
—GERMAN PROVERB

What's the easiest way to learn to ride a bike?

Training wheels, right?

Then, once you've built up enough confidence and skill, you can ditch the stabilizers and ride freely.

This is also the best way to learn how to eat and train. You start slow and simple with clear instructions, and once you've logged enough meals and workouts, you can add more moving parts without losing control.

This chapter is going to give you one of those training wheels in the form of simple dietary guidelines that'll help you put everything you've learned into practice, as well as done-for-you meal plans that'll save you the time and trouble of creating your own.

Then, in the next chapter, we're going to bolt on the other training wheel (for working out).

Let's start with answering the first question that determines how to set up your diet:

SHOULD YOU CUT OR LEAN BULK FIRST?

If you're currently unhappy with your body fat percentage and just want to get lean before worrying about gaining significant amounts of muscle definition, you want to cut first.

There's no reason to get fatter (which will happen when you lean bulk properly) just to gain some muscle if that's not your primary concern right now. Start with what's going to keep you most motivated.

Similarly, if you're very overweight, you also want to cut first. This is the healthiest and smartest choice, even if your long-term goal involves gaining a fair amount of muscle tone.

If you're thin and want to focus most on gaining muscle definition and strength, you want to lean bulk first.

And if you're in the middle—if your body fat is in a normal range and you like the idea of having abs but also want more muscle definition—whether you should cut or lean bulk first is dictated by your body fat percentage.

> Not sure what your body fat percentage is?
> Go to www.thinnerleanerstronger.com/bodyfat to find out.

If you're 25 percent body fat or higher, I recommend you start by cutting down to 20 percent for several reasons:

1. You'll be happier with how you look.

We don't have to be ripped year-round, but at least half of the reason why we stick to meal plans and bust our butts in the gym every day is to look good.

Once you get above 25 percent body fat, you're probably going to start feeling overweight, and this can make it harder to stick to your diet and training plans. At some point, you'll start wondering why you're working so hard to look like *that*.

By never letting your body fat percentage go too high, however, you'll find it easier to stay motivated.

2. You'll have an easier time cutting.

Generally speaking, the longer you remain in a calorie deficit, the more likely you are to struggle with muscle loss, hunger, cravings, and the other unwanted side effects of dieting.

Thus, when you allow yourself to gain too much fat, you set yourself up for longer, more difficult cuts. If you always keep your body fat at reasonable levels, however, your cuts will be shorter and more manageable, both physically and psychologically.

3. You'll gain more muscle and less fat when you lean bulk.

As body fat levels rise, insulin sensitivity drops, which hinders muscle protein synthesis and promotes fat gain.[1]

Finally, if your body fat percentage is somewhere between 20 and 25 percent, you should choose to cut or lean bulk based on what's most appealing and motivating to you.

HOW LONG SHOULD YOU CUT AND LEAN BULK?

Once you know where to start with your diet, the next question is how long you should continue for before changing course.

There's no pat answer as to how long you should cut or lean bulk because it depends entirely on how quickly you lose and gain body fat while cutting and lean bulking.

A good rule of thumb is this: Your cut phases should end when you're around 18 to 20 percent body fat (unless you have a special reason to get leaner, don't bother because it's not sustainable for most people), and your lean bulk phases should end when you're around 25 to 27 percent body fat (go any further and you'll regret it once it comes time to cut).

Thus, when cutting, you should generally go for as long as it takes to get to at least 20 percent body fat (unless you want to end sooner for whatever reason), and when lean bulking, for as long as it takes to get to 25 to 27 percent body fat (again, unless you want to end sooner).

Then, when you've cut to around 20 percent body fat, you're ready to lean bulk, and when you've lean bulked to no more than 27 percent body fat, you're ready to cut. Rinse, repeat, and reap the amazing and transformative benefits.

When you get settled into this rhythm of moving between cut and lean bulk phases, you'll probably find that your cuts last 10 to 14 weeks and your lean bulks 12 to 16 weeks.

This is how you get the physique you really want. You simply repeat the process of lean bulking to add muscle and cutting to remove fat until you're thrilled with what you see at 18 to 20 percent body fat.

Then, most women like to enter a maintenance phase where they make slow muscle and strength gains without any noticeable change in body fat percentage.

FIVE TIPS FOR BETTER CUTS

1. Eat plenty of nutritious foods.

As you know, no foods cause weight gain or loss, but some foods are more conducive to weight gain or loss than others.

Generally speaking, foods that are "good" for weight loss are relatively low in calories but high in volume and fiber (and thus are filling).[2]

This is one of the reasons why most fruits and vegetables are so helpful when cutting. They add a significant amount of volume and fiber but not calories to meals, helping you stay fuller longer.

2. Take diet breaks if needed.

A diet break is different than "cheating"—it's a planned break from dieting, and it can last anywhere from a day to a couple of weeks.

Why would you want to do that?

Research shows that when cutting, scheduling periods of planned and controlled increased calorie intake can help you lose fat faster and better maintain your muscle mass and metabolic rate.[3]

It works by giving your body a chance to reverse some of the negative physiological and psychological adaptations that occur while dieting.

In other words, a diet break gives your body a chance to enjoy an increase in energy intake and your mind a chance to relax and stop stressing about food.

You don't have to take diet breaks if you don't want or feel the need to, but if you do, here's how to do it right:

- When on a break, increase your daily calorie intake to your approximate total daily energy expenditure by increasing your carbohydrate intake.

- If you have a high body fat percentage that requires you to diet for more than three months to reach your goal, you can plan a one-week break every six to eight weeks.

- If you need less than three months to reach your goal, then you can probably just suck it up and get it done without any breaks.

  If you want to include one in your cut, however, you can take a one-week break anywhere between the sixth and eighth weeks.

- If you're lean and working to get really lean, you can take a one-week break every four to eight weeks.

- If at any point during a cut, you're feeling especially tired, worn out, or just plain sick of cutting, take a one-week break and then get back to it.

Keep in mind that you *will* gain weight during your diet breaks mostly due to the increased carbohydrate intake, but this doesn't mean you're gaining fat. You're simply holding more water and glycogen in your muscles and liver.

3. Drink plenty of water.

The amount of water you drink isn't going to make or break your fat loss efforts, but drinking enough can help.[4] Research shows that increasing water intake is an effective way to increase fullness, which helps you fight off hunger and stick to your diet.[5]

You may have heard that increasing your water intake can speed up your metabolism as well. Some studies do suggest that drinking water can increase basal metabolic rate because the body has to heat it up to its internal temperature, but at least one study has found no such effects.[6]

So, how much water should you drink?

The National Academy of Medicine recommends drinking between 0.75 and 1 gallon of water per day for adult men and women.[7]

You're going to be exercising regularly, however, and this increases the amount of water your body needs. Specifically, you want to replace all water lost through sweating.[8]

The amount of water lost through exercise can range anywhere from 0.75 to 2 liters per hour depending on intensity and climate and how much you sweat. Ironically, as your fitness improves, your body will lose more sweat during exercise.[9]

Therefore, start with a baseline water intake of about 0.75 to 1 gallon per day, and add 1 to 1.5 liters per hour of exercise, plus a bit more for additional sweating, and you'll be good.

The easiest way to do this is to keep a bottle with you during the day and never allow yourself to go thirsty for too long.

4. Get enough sleep.

A large amount of fat loss occurs while you sleep for two reasons:

1. Your body burns quite a few calories while you sleep.

   A 160-pound person burns about 70 calories per hour while asleep, and much of it comes from body fat.

2. Much of your body's growth hormone is produced while you're sleeping, further stimulating fat loss.[10]

Thus, we shouldn't be surprised that research shows that the amount people sleep has a marked effect on weight loss.

For example, in a study conducted by scientists at the University of Chicago, overweight adults on a weight loss diet were split into two groups:[11]

1. Group one slept 8.5 hours per night.

2. Group two slept 5.5 hours per night.

After 14 days, the 5.5-hour group lost 55 percent less fat and 60 percent more muscle than the 8.5-hour group, and also experienced increased hunger throughout the day.

This correlation has been observed elsewhere as well.

Research conducted by scientists at the National Center for Global Health and Medicine found that shorter sleep duration was associated with increased levels of body fat.[12]

There's also evidence that acute sleep loss causes insulin resistance to a level similar to what's seen in type 2 diabetes, which can increase fat gain.[13]

Sleep needs vary from individual to individual, but according to the National Sleep Foundation, adults need seven to nine hours of sleep per night to avoid the negative effects of inadequate sleep.[14]

5. Don't drink calories.

We recall that caloric beverages don't trigger satiety like food, which makes it easier to overeat.[15]

For instance, a cup of orange juice contains about 100 calories and isn't going to do much to stave off hunger. For the same number of calories, however, you could have an apple, which will.[16]

THREE TIPS FOR BETTER LEAN BULKS

1. Follow a meal plan.

Many people think meal planning is mostly for cutting and tend to wing it when lean bulking. This rarely works well because it often leads to undereating, which hinders muscle growth, or overeating, which accelerates fat gain.

For a maximally effective lean bulk, make a meal plan and stick to it just as you would when cutting.

2. Drink calories if necessary.

If you have to eat a large number of calories every day to gain weight and struggle to do this with whole foods alone (some people do), don't be afraid to drink some of your calories.

Milk and no-sugar-added fruit juices are popular choices.

3. Keep cardio to a minimum.

Remember that the more cardio you do while lean bulking, the harder it's going to be to gain muscle and strength.

Try to do no more than a couple of hours of cardio per week when lean bulking, and stick with walking if you're struggling to make muscle and strength gains.

PREMADE MEAL PLANS FOR CUTTING AND LEAN BULKING

Thanks to part 4 of this book—and chapter 19 in particular—you have everything you need to create your own highly effective meal plans, but if you'd rather short-cut the process and follow a premade meal plan based on your weight and goals, I have good news.

On the following pages, you'll find meal plans that have been designed by my diet coaches according to everything you've learned in this book.

These meal plans can provide you with a simple and sensible starting point for your diet. Then, once you're comfortable with the routine and happy with the results, you can modify your plan, make a new one from scratch, or simply stick with it for as long as it continues to work for you.

Training wheels, remember?

These meal plans are also included in the free bonus material that comes with this book (www.thinnerleanerstronger.com/bonus) as Google Sheets and Excel and PDF files, so you can easily modify and print them.

CUTTING MEAL PLAN FOR A 120-POUND WOMAN						
MEAL	FOOD	AMOUNT	CALORIES	PROTEIN	CARBS	FAT
Breakfast	Egg white	150 grams	78	16	1	0
	Whole egg	50 grams	72	6	0	5
	Strawberry	140 grams	45	1	11	0
	Apple	182 grams	95	0	25	0
Total			290	23	37	5
Workout						
Postworkout Shake	Plain nonfat Greek yogurt	400 grams	236	41	14	2
	Unsweetened rice milk	240 grams	80	1	20	0
	Blueberry	140 grams	113	1	22	2
Total			429	43	56	4
Lunch	Lettuce	30 grams	5	0	1	0
	Skinless boneless chicken breast	120 grams	144	27	0	3
	Beet	50 grams	22	1	5	0
	Tomato	120 grams	22	1	5	0
	Sweet pepper	160 grams	42	2	10	0
	Low-fat balsamic vinaigrette	30 grams	45	0	2	4
Total			280	31	23	7
Dinner	Sirloin, trimmed of visible fat	150 grams	231	32	0	11
	Brussels sprout	100 grams	43	3	9	0
	Asparagus	100 grams	20	2	4	0
	Cauliflower	100 grams	25	2	5	0
	70% to 85% dark chocolate	20 grams	120	2	9	9
Total			439	41	27	20
Daily Total			1,438	138	143	36
Daily Target			1,440	144	144	32

MEAL	FOOD	AMOUNT	CALORIES	PROTEIN	CARBS	FAT
CUTTING MEAL PLAN FOR A 160-POUND WOMAN						
Preworkout Meal	Plain nonfat Greek yogurt	340 grams	201	35	12	1
	Banana	136 grams	121	1	31	0
	Total		322	36	43	1
	Workout					
Postworkout Shake	Plain nonfat Greek yogurt	240 grams	142	24	9	1
	Unsweetened almond milk	240 grams	36	1	3	2
	Blueberry	140 grams	80	1	20	0
	Banana	136 grams	121	1	31	0
	Total		379	27	63	3
Lunch	Skinless boneless chicken breast	200 grams	240	45	0	5
	Fat-free refried bean	130 grams	120	7	22	0
	Reduced-fat cheddar cheese	28 grams	49	7	1	2
	Onion	60 grams	60	19	0	5
	Tomato	120 grams	22	1	5	0
	Salsa	36 grams	10	1	2	0
	Olive oil	10 grams	88	0	0	10
	Total		589	80	30	22
Dinner	Pork chop, trimmed of visible fat	200 grams	254	45	0	7
	Butternut squash	200 grams	90	2	23	0
	Broccoli	100 grams	34	3	7	0
	Cauliflower	100 grams	25	2	5	0
	Butter	10 grams	72	0	0	8
	Total		475	52	35	15
	Daily Total		1,765	195	171	41
	Daily Target		1,760	176	176	39

CUTTING MEAL PLAN FOR A 200-POUND WOMAN						
MEAL	FOOD	AMOUNT	CALORIES	PROTEIN	CARBS	FAT
Preworkout Meal	Egg white	300 grams	156	33	2	0
	Whole egg	100 grams	143	13	1	10
	Onion	60 grams	19	0	5	0
	Sweet pepper	80 grams	21	1	5	0
	Mushroom	40 grams	9	1	1	0
Total			348	48	14	10
Workout						
Postworkout Meal	Plain 2% Greek yogurt	300 grams	219	30	12	6
	Strawberry	200 grams	64	1	15	1
	Blueberry	200 grams	114	1	29	1
Total			397	32	56	8
Lunch	Roasted turkey breast	250 grams	318	67	0	5
	Pea	200 grams	162	11	29	1
	Carrot	200 grams	82	2	19	0
	Olive oil	10 grams	88	0	0	10
Total			650	80	48	16
Dinner	Tilapia	250 grams	240	50	0	4
	Brown rice	120 grams	434	9	91	3
	Broccoli	100 grams	34	3	7	0
	Lemon juice (to taste)	0	0	0	0	0
	Butter	10 grams	72	0	0	8
Total			780	62	98	15
Daily Total			2,175	222	216	49
Daily Target			2,200	220	220	49

Want even more cutting meal plans like these?
Go to www.thinnerleanerstronger.com/cutting.

LEAN BULKING MEAL PLAN FOR A 100-POUND WOMAN						
MEAL	**FOOD**	**AMOUNT**	**CALORIES**	**PROTEIN**	**CARBS**	**FAT**
Preworkout Meal	Egg white	100 grams	52	11	1	0
	Cooked bacon	13 grams	60	6	0	4
	Whole grain bread	28 grams	80	4	14	0
	Jam	20 grams	56	0	14	0
	Butter	5 grams	34	0	0	4
	Total		282	21	29	8
Workout						
Postworkout Shake	Plain nonfat Greek yogurt	170 grams	100	17	6	0
	Unsweetened rice milk	240 grams	113	1	22	2
	Banana	136 grams	121	2	31	1
	Blueberry	148 grams	84	1	22	1
	Total		418	21	81	4
Lunch	Whole wheat pita bread	64 grams	168	6	36	1
	Reduced-fat provolone cheese	14 grams	38	3	1	2
	Roasted turkey breast	100 grams	147	30	1	0
	Reduced-fat mayonnaise	15 grams	50	0	1	5
	Mustard	10 grams	6	0	1	0
	Total		409	39	40	8
Snack	Apple	182 grams	95	0	25	0
	Total		95	0	25	0
Dinner	Sirloin, trimmed of visible fat	100 grams	126	22	0	4
	Brown rice	80 grams	290	6	61	2
	70 to 85% dark chocolate	14 grams	85	1	7	6
	Total		429	29	68	12
	Daily Total		1,705	110	243	32
	Daily Target		1,700	106	234	38

LEAN BULKING MEAL PLANS

LEAN BULKING MEAL PLAN FOR A 120-POUND WOMAN						
MEAL	**FOOD**	**AMOUNT**	**CALORIES**	**PROTEIN**	**CARBS**	**FAT**
Breakfast	Plain nonfat Greek yogurt	240 grams	142	24	9	1
	Banana	136 grams	121	1	31	1
	Raspberry	140 grams	73	2	17	1
	Low-fat granola	30 grams	120	3	24	1
	Total		456	30	81	4
Workout						
Postworkout Meal	Low-fat tortilla	50 grams	160	3	26	4
	Cheddar cheese	30 grams	121	7	1	10
	Skinless boneless chicken breast	100 grams	120	23	0	3
	Fat-free refried bean	150 grams	118	8	20	1
	Salsa	36 grams	10	1	2	0
	Total		529	42	49	18
Lunch	Shrimp	100 grams	85	20	0	1
	Brown rice	70 grams	253	5	53	2
	Broccoli	100 grams	34	3	7	0
	Zucchini	100 grams	17	1	3	0
	Carrot	100 grams	41	1	10	0
	Olive oil	5 grams	44	0	0	5
	Total		474	30	73	8
Dinner	Skinless boneless chicken thigh	100 grams	121	20	0	4
	Barley	60 grams	211	6	47	1
	A1 steak sauce	15 grams	14	0	3	0
	Cauliflower	200 grams	50	4	10	1
	Butter	10 grams	72	0	0	8
	Total		468	30	60	14
Daily Total			1,927	132	263	44
Daily Target			1,920	120	264	43

MEAL	FOOD	AMOUNT	CALORIES	PROTEIN	CARBS	FAT
	LEAN BULKING MEAL PLAN FOR A 140-POUND WOMAN					
Breakfast	Oatmeal	40 grams	152	5	27	3
	Skim milk	240 grams	82	8	12	0
	Brown sugar	15 grams	57	0	15	0
	Strawberry	140 grams	45	1	11	0
	Banana	136 grams	121	2	31	1
	Cinnamon	(to taste)	0	0	0	0
	Total		457	16	96	4
	Workout					
Postworkout Meal	93% lean ground beef	120 grams	182	25	0	8
	White rice	75 grams	267	5	58	0
	Brussels sprout	200 grams	86	7	18	0
	Olive oil	5 grams	44	0	0	5
	Total		579	37	76	13
Lunch	Lettuce	30 grams	5	0	1	0
	Skinless boneless chicken breast	170 grams	204	38	0	4
	Beet	50 grams	22	1	5	0
	Tomato	120 grams	22	1	5	0
	Sweet pepper	160 grams	42	2	10	0
	Low-fat balsamic vinaigrette	30 grams	45	0	2	4
	White bread	80 grams	213	7	40	3
	Total		553	49	62	11
Dinner	Farmed Atlantic salmon	120 grams	250	25	0	16
	Sweet potato	300 grams	258	5	60	0
	Asparagus	150 grams	30	3	6	0
	70 to 85% dark chocolate	20 grams	120	2	9	9
	Total		658	35	75	25
	Daily Total		2,247	137	309	53
	Daily Target		2,240	140	308	50

Want even more lean bulking meal plans like these?
Go to www.thinnerleanerstronger.com/leanbulking.

. . .

You now have all the dietary knowledge and tools you need to start my *Thinner Leaner Stronger* program and build the body of your dreams.

Next up is training, so keep reading!

KEY TAKEAWAYS

- If you're currently unhappy with your body fat percentage and just want to get lean before worrying about gaining significant amounts of muscle definition, you want to cut first.

- Similarly, if you're very overweight, you also want to cut first.

- If you're thin and want to focus most on gaining muscle definition and strength, you want to lean bulk first.

- If you're in the middle—if your body fat is in a normal range and you like the idea of having abs but also want more muscle definition—whether you should cut or lean bulk first is dictated by your body fat percentage.

- If you're 25 percent body fat or higher, I recommend you start by cutting down to 20 percent.

- If your body fat percentage is somewhere between 20 and 25 percent, you should choose to cut or lean bulk based on what's most appealing and motivating to you.

- Your cut phases should end when you're around 18 to 20 percent body fat (unless you have a special reason to get leaner, don't bother because it's not sustainable for most people), and your lean bulk phases should end when you're around 25 to 27 percent body fat (go any further and you'll regret it once it comes time to cut).

- When cutting, you should generally go for as long as it takes to get to at least 20 percent body fat (unless you want to end sooner for whatever reason), and when lean bulking, for as long as it takes to get to 25 to 27 percent body fat (again, unless you want to end sooner).

- You simply repeat the process of lean bulking to add muscle and cutting to remove fat until you're thrilled with what you see at 18 to 20 percent body fat.

- Generally speaking, foods that are "good" for weight loss are relatively low in calories but high in volume and fiber.

- When cutting, scheduling periods of planned and controlled increased calorie intake can help you lose fat faster and better maintain your muscle mass and metabolic rate.

- A diet break gives your body a chance to enjoy an increase in energy intake and your mind a chance to relax and stop stressing about food.

- You'll gain weight during your diet breaks mostly due to the increased carbohydrate intake, but this doesn't mean you're gaining fat.

- Increasing water intake is an effective way to increase fullness, which helps you fight off hunger and stick to your diet.

- Start with a baseline water intake of about 0.75 to 1 gallon per day, and add 1 to 1.5 liters per hour of exercise, plus a bit more for additional sweating.

- A large amount of fat loss occurs while you sleep.

- Sleep needs vary from individual to individual, but most adults need seven to nine hours of sleep per night to avoid the negative effects of inadequate rest.

- Caloric beverages don't trigger satiety like food, which makes it easier to overeat.

- Many people think meal planning is mostly for cutting and tend to wing it when lean bulking. This often leads to undereating, which hinders muscle growth, or overeating, which accelerates fat gain.

- If you have to eat a large number of calories every day to gain weight and struggle to do this with whole foods alone, don't be afraid to drink some of your calories.

- Try to do no more than a couple of hours of cardio per week when lean bulking, and stick with walking if you're struggling to make muscle and strength gains.

29

THE *THINER LEANER STRONGER* TRAINING PLAN

"We who cut mere stones must always be envisioning cathedrals."

—QUARRY WORKER'S CREED

In chapter 21, you learned the following training formula:

2–3 | 8–10 | 9–15 | 2–4 | 3–5 | 1–2 | 8–10

And in this chapter, I'm going to give you an effective training plan patterned on it that will help you lose fat, gain muscle, and get strong.

You could use everything you've learned so far to create your own training plan, of course, but I recommend you follow mine for at least three months before going off on your own.

Workout programming can be difficult because there are several layers that must work together—training phase, training routine, and workout—and a number of interdependent factors to consider, including goals, intensity, frequency, volume, recovery, and others.

It's also very helpful to have a bit of weightlifting experience under your belt before creating training plans so you know firsthand what is and isn't likely to work in actual practice.

If you like my programming and would rather continue with it versus going solo, you'll find an entire year's worth of *Thinner Leaner Stronger* workouts in the free bonus material that comes with this book (www.thinnerleanerstronger.com/bonus).

You can also get all my workouts in my book *The Year One Challenge for Women* (www.thinnerleanerstronger.com/challenge).

So, let's start our review of my *Thinner Leaner Stronger* training program with the first of the three layers I just mentioned: the training phase.

THE *THINNER LEANER STRONGER* TRAINING PHASE

A training phase is a block of training designed to accomplish a specific goal, like increased power, strength, muscle growth, endurance, or recovery.

A training phase generally lasts a number of weeks or even months.

In *Thinner Leaner Stronger*, our primary goal is muscle and strength gain, so there's only one type of phase. It lasts nine weeks and consists of two parts:

1. Hard training

Each phase begins with eight weeks of hard training designed to maximize muscle and strength gain.

2. Deloading or resting

Each phase ends with one week of deloading or resting to facilitate recovery from the previous eight weeks of hard training.

Each year, then, separates roughly into six training phases.

Depending on your goals, progress, and other factors, your training routines can change or not as you move from one training phase to another. For instance, bodybuilders tend to change their routines more often and more significantly than strength athletes.

In *Thinner Leaner Stronger*, your training routines are going to change slightly from phase to phase to expose your muscles to new and different types of movement patterns to more fully develop them.

For example, horizontal and vertical pulling movements train your back muscles slightly differently, and you can alternate between emphasizing one and the other in different training phases to good effect.

As you'll see in my workout routines for you, every one will include at least three sets of heavy squatting, deadlifting, and bench pressing per week, and these exercises will always come first in your workouts.

The reason for this prioritization is simple: no exercises will help you build a lean, muscular, and powerful body more than these, so you want to make sure you're working on them every week.

And you want to do them first in your workouts because they require the most physical and mental energy.

I don't recommend changing anything in the middle of a training phase unless you have to due to injury, traveling, or some other pressing circumstance. Otherwise, stick with the same workouts for eight weeks before making exercise substitutions or rearrangements.

So that's layer one. Let's move on to number two: the training routine.

THE *THINNER LEANER STRONGER* TRAINING ROUTINES

Whereas a training phase delineates the goals and duration of a training block, a training routine delineates what you're going to do in that time to achieve those goals.

Specifically, a training routine indicates how often you're going to train and what you're going to do in each workout.

In *Thinner Leaner Stronger*, you have three training routines to choose from:

1. A five-day routine

2. A four-day routine

3. A three-day routine

Each are weekly (seven-day) routines, so the most weightlifting you can do on the program is five workouts per week. Cardio isn't explicitly included in the routines because it's optional, and how much you do depends on how much time you have to give to it and whether you're cutting, lean bulking, or maintaining.

As far as results go, the five-day routine is better than the four- and three-day routines, and the four-day routine is better than the three-day routine. That doesn't mean you can't do well with the four- or three-day routines, though, because you absolutely can.

You'll probably notice that each of the routines emphasizes the lower body but provides enough upper-body work to ensure it doesn't fall behind in development.

Try not to change routines during individual training phases. Ideally, you'd choose one routine and stick with it for the entire phase. That said, if you'd like to "upgrade" to the four- or five-day routine in the middle of a phase, go for it. Try not to "downgrade" unless you have to.

THE FIVE-DAY ROUTINE

WORKOUT 1

Lower Body (Legs and Glutes)

WORKOUT 2

Push and Core

WORKOUT 3

Pull

WORKOUT 4

Upper Body and Core

WORKOUT 5

Lower Body (Legs and Glutes)

If you have the time and inclination, start here in your first training phase and see how you like it. You can always try the other routines in later phases.

Most people who follow this routine train Monday through Friday and take the weekends off, but you can incorporate your off days however you'd like. The important thing is that you do each of the workouts every seven days and in the order given.

One caveat, however, is you want to include at least one day of rest between workouts 5 and 1, as doing these workouts on back-to-back days is counterproductive. Your leg muscles are the largest muscle group in your body and thus need more time to recover than smaller muscle groups that can survive daily beatings, like the abs or calves.

So, for example, if you need to train on the weekends due to your schedule or lifestyle, you might train Monday (lower body), Tuesday (push and core), and Wednesday (pull), rest Thursday, and then train Friday (upper body and core) and Saturday (lower body), and rest Sunday.

THE FOUR-DAY ROUTINE

WORKOUT 1

Lower Body (Legs and Glutes)

WORKOUT 2

Upper Body and Core

WORKOUT 3

Pull

WORKOUT 4

Lower Body (Legs and Glutes)

The main difference between this four-day routine and the five-day routine is that the push and upper-body workouts are combined into one to ensure we remain focused on the lower body.

Again, you can do these workouts on any days of the week that you like so long as you do each once per seven days and in the order given and include at least one day of rest between workouts 4 and 1.

THE THREE-DAY ROUTINE

WORKOUT 1

Lower Body (Legs and Glutes)

WORKOUT 2

Upper Body and Core

WORKOUT 3

Lower Body and Pull (Legs and Back)

This is your time-proven "push-pull-legs" routine slightly modified to expand the "push" workout into a full upper-body one and to emphasize the lower body (the first workout you do each week will generally be your best, so use it to train the muscle groups you want to develop most).

That's it for the training routines. Next, let's review the third and final layer of the program: the workouts.

THE *THINNER LEANER STRONGER* WORKOUTS

You probably don't need a definition for it, but just for the sake of thoroughness, a workout is an individual training session.

All *Thinner Leaner Stronger* workouts I'm going to provide you with follow the formula you learned in chapter 21:

- 2 to 3 major muscle groups trained
- Warm-up sets as needed
- 8 to 10 reps per hard set
- 9 to 15 hard sets per workout
- 2 to 4 minutes of rest in between hard sets

Furthermore, as I mentioned, it's generally a good idea to do your hardest exercises first in your workouts, followed by the second hardest and so forth, because you always have the most energy and focus in the beginning of your workouts.

Practically speaking, this means starting with your hardest compound exercises and finishing with your easier isolation exercises.

For instance, if a pull workout is going to include deadlifting (and it should), you'd want to do that before barbell or dumbbell rows or anything else. If a lower-body workout includes squats, lunges, and lying leg curls, you'd want to do them in that order.

You also want to do the exercises in a workout one at a time and complete all the hard sets for one exercise before moving on to another, like this:

EXERCISE 1
Hard set 1

Rest

EXERCISE 1
Hard set 2

Rest

EXERCISE 1
Hard set 3

Rest

EXERCISE 2
Hard set 1

Rest

And so on.

If you can't do an exercise in a workout for whatever reason, simply choose an alternative "approved" exercise from chapter 23 to take its place, or do three more sets of an exercise already in your workout.

Now let's get to the actual workouts.

As I mentioned earlier, I've created a year's worth of *Thinner Leaner Stronger* workouts for you to do, but to save space (and trees), I'm going to include just the first training phase here in this chapter.

To get the rest of the workouts, simply download the free bonus material that comes with this book (www.thinnerleanerstronger.com/bonus) or pick up a copy of *The Year One Challenge for Women* (www.thinnerleanerstronger.com/challenge) if you'd prefer the workouts in the form of a digital or hard-copy book.

PHASE 1
THE FIVE-DAY ROUTINE

WORKOUT 1

LOWER BODY (LEGS AND GLUTES)

Barbell Squat: Warm-up and 3 hard sets
Leg Press: 3 hard sets
Romanian Deadlift: 3 hard sets
Hip Thrust: 3 hard sets

WORKOUT 2

PUSH AND CORE

Barbell Bench Press: Warm-up and 3 hard sets
Seated Dumbbell Press: 3 hard sets
Dumbbell Bench Press: 3 hard sets
Dumbbell Side Lateral Raise: 3 hard sets

Crunch: 3 hard sets

WORKOUT 3

PULL

Barbell Deadlift: Warm-up and 3 hard sets
One-Arm Dumbbell Row: 3 hard sets
Lat Pulldown (Wide-Grip): 3 hard sets
Barbell Curl: 3 hard sets

WORKOUT 4

UPPER BODY AND CORE

Seated Dumbbell Press: Warm-up and 3 hard sets
Dumbbell Bench Press: 3 hard sets
Dumbbell Rear Lateral Raise: 3 hard sets
Seated Triceps Press: 3 hard sets
Captain's Chair Leg Raise: 3 hard sets

WORKOUT 5

LOWER BODY (LEGS AND GLUTES)

Barbell Squat: Warm-up and 3 hard sets
Dumbbell Lunge (In-Place): 3 hard sets
Lying Leg Curl: 3 hard sets
Glute Blaster: 3 hard sets

PHASE 1
THE FOUR-DAY ROUTINE

WORKOUT 1

LOWER BODY (LEGS AND GLUTES)

Barbell Squat: Warm-up and 3 hard sets
Leg Press: 3 hard sets
Romanian Deadlift: 3 hard sets
Hip Thrust: 3 hard sets

WORKOUT 2

UPPER BODY AND CORE

Barbell Bench Press: Warm-up and 3 hard sets
Seated Dumbbell Press: 3 hard sets
Dumbbell Side Lateral Raise: 3 hard sets
Seated Triceps Press: 3 hard sets
Crunch: 3 hard sets

WORKOUT 3

PULL

Barbell Deadlift: Warm-up and 3 hard sets
One-Arm Dumbbell Row: 3 hard sets
Lat Pulldown (Wide-Grip): 3 hard sets
Barbell Curl: 3 hard sets

WORKOUT 4

LOWER BODY (LEGS AND GLUTES)

Barbell Squat: Warm-up and 3 hard sets
Dumbbell Lunge (In-Place): 3 hard sets
Lying Leg Curl: 3 hard sets
Glute Blaster: 3 hard sets

PHASE 1
THE THREE-DAY ROUTINE

WORKOUT 1

LOWER BODY (LEGS AND GLUTES)

Barbell Squat: Warm-up and 3 hard sets
Leg Press: 3 hard sets
Romanian Deadlift: 3 hard sets
Hip Thrust: 3 hard sets

WORKOUT 2

UPPER BODY AND CORE

Barbell Bench Press: Warm-up and 3 hard sets
Seated Dumbbell Press: 3 hard sets
Dumbbell Side Lateral Raise: 3 hard sets
Seated Triceps Press: 3 hard sets
Crunch: 3 hard sets

WORKOUT 3

LOWER BODY AND PULL (LEGS AND BACK)

Barbell Squat: Warm-up and 3 hard sets
Barbell Deadlift: Warm-up and 3 hard sets
One-Arm Dumbbell Row: 3 hard sets
Lat Pulldown (Wide-Grip): 3 hard sets
Barbell Curl: 3 hard sets

THE *THINNER LEANER STRONGER* WORKOUT PROGRESSION

In chapter 21, you learned about double progression—the system of working to increase reps with a given weight until reaching a "reps-for-sets" target, and then increasing the weight.

Many weightlifting and strength-training programs use the double progression model because it's simple, "newbie friendly," and effective. Many advanced weightlifters and strength athletes use it too because of how well it works.

For those reasons, we're going to use double progression in *Thinner Leaner Stronger*, and here's how to implement it:

When you get 10 reps for one hard set, you immediately move up in weight by adding 5 pounds to the bar or moving up to dumbbells that are 5 pounds heavier (per dumbbell).

Remember the example of how this works?

Let's say you're squatting in the 8-to-10-rep range, and on your first (or second) hard set in the workout, you get 10 reps of 100 pounds. You then immediately add 5 pounds to the bar (not in your next workout), rest a few minutes, and get 8 or 9 reps on your next hard set.

Great! The progression has succeeded, and you now work with 105 pounds in your current and future workouts until you can squat it for one hard set of 10 reps. Then, you'd move up in weight again, and so on.

What if you only get 5 or 6 reps with the new, heavier weight before your form starts breaking down? What if the progression doesn't succeed?

In this case, you should drop the weight back to the original, lighter load (100 pounds in our example) and work there until you can squat it for *two* hard sets of 10 reps (in the same workout).

Then, you should immediately move up to the heavier weight again on your next hard set (even if that's in your next workout) and try again.

If you do that and *still* can't get at least 7 reps, go back to the lighter weight and work with it until you can do *three* hard sets of 10 reps (in the same workout). At this point, your progression should succeed.

Also, if you get 10 reps in your first set after moving up in weight, then you get to move up again!

And what should you do if you get 10 reps on your third and final hard set for an exercise in your workout? You should increase the weight on your first hard set of your next performance of that exercise.

Finally, if your gym doesn't have 2.5-pound plates, then you can add 10 pounds to the bar when you move up in weight.

HOW TO TRAIN YOUR CORE CORRECTLY

You may be wondering what's meant by a hard set on a core exercise like the crunch or captain's chair leg raise.

Are you supposed to add weight or resistance to these exercises? Should anything change in terms of progression, rest, rep tempo, or the like?

Let's clarify everything exercise by exercise.

CAPTAIN'S CHAIR LEG RAISE

This exercise is normally unweighted, but you can add weight by holding a dumbbell in between your feet as you raise and lower them.

Here's how I like to approach this exercise:

1. Start unweighted.

2. Take all hard sets to technical failure.

3. Once you can do at least 30 reps before failing, turn it into a weighted exercise by snatching a dumbbell in between your feet. Start with 10 pounds.

4. Once you do 30 reps with 10 pounds, go up by 5 pounds.

5. Continue progressing in this way.

If you reach the point where adding more weight becomes awkward, then it's time to switch to a different exercise, like the hanging leg raise.

HANGING LEG RAISE

This exercise is a harder variation of the captain's chair leg raise, and I recommend going about it in the same way.

LYING LEG RAISE

This exercise is similar to the previous two but doesn't require any equipment.

Once you can do at least 50 reps in a single hard set before reaching technical failure, start doing weighted captain's chair or hanging leg raises instead.

CRUNCH

This is a staple ab exercise that should be done unweighted and to technical failure in each hard set.

Once you can do at least 50 reps in a single hard set before reaching technical failure, start doing weighted sit-ups or cable crunches instead.

CABLE CRUNCH

This is a weighted exercise and one of my favorites for developing the rectus abdominis (the most prominent "ab muscles") in particular.

Most women don't do weighted ab work because they're afraid it's going to widen their waists and make them look "blocky." This is just a myth.

Doing too much weighted work for your oblique muscles, which sit on either side of your waist, can cause this, but weighted training for your rectus abdominis won't.

More importantly, if you want clear-cut ab definition, it's going to require highly developed rectus abdominis muscles. And what's the most effective way to develop a muscle? Heavy resistance training, of course.

This is why I recommend the 8-to-10-rep range for all hard sets of cable crunches and increasing the weight in 5- or 10-pound increments.

Furthermore, you should treat this exercise exactly the same as any other resistance training exercise—your goal is to get stronger over time, you rest a couple of minutes in between sets, you use a 1-1-1 rep tempo, and so on.

WEIGHTED SIT-UP

This weighted exercise allows you to effectively train your abdominal muscles with free weights.

As previously noted, I recommend you work up to 50 unweighted crunches before moving on to weighted sit-ups.

As with the cable crunch, work in the 8-to-10-rep range on this exercise and increase the weight in 5- or 10-pound increments.

As with the cable crunch, you should treat this exercise exactly the same as any other resistance training exercise—your goal is to get stronger over time, you rest a couple of minutes in between sets, you use a 1-1-1 rep tempo, and so on.

Also, you may see some people hold the weight behind their necks while doing this exercise. This can work with light weights but becomes uncomfortable and even dangerous with heavier weights, so keep the weight on your chest instead.

PLANK

This is another effective unweighted exercise for training the back and core muscles.

Start by holding a hard set for as long as you can before reaching technical failure. Then, try to increase the amount of time you can hold the plank position by five seconds per workout.

Once you can do at least one two-minute hard set of the basic plank, you can increase the difficulty by making two small adjustments:[1]

1. Instead of positioning your elbows directly under your shoulders, extend them three to six inches in front of your shoulders.

2. Instead of relaxing your glutes, flex them as if you were doing a hip thrust.

Once you can do one two-minute hard set of the modified plank, start doing a more difficult exercise instead, like the cable crunch, abdominal rollout, or weighted sit-up.

ABDOMINAL ROLLOUT

The abdominal rollout is a classic unweighted ab exercise that deserves a place in your repertoire.

Start this exercise on your knees, and once you can do at least 30 reps before reaching technical failure, increase the difficulty by remaining on your feet, like a plank.

Once you can do at least 30 reps on your feet before reaching technical failure, start doing weighted sit-ups or cable crunches instead.

THE *THINNER LEANER STRONGER* DELOAD WEEK

Some people say deloading by reducing workout volume (number of hard sets) is better than reducing intensity (load) and vice versa.

I'm in the middle (I think both can work fine), but I lean toward deloading volume for two reasons:

1. Studies show that reducing volume instead of intensity is more effective for decreasing fatigue, which is the main goal of a deload.[2]

2. Research shows that reducing volume instead of intensity is more effective for maintaining performance.[3]

This makes it easier to pick up where you left off when you get back to your hard training.

So, here's what I recommend for your deload weeks while on *Thinner Leaner Stronger*:

WORKOUT 1

DELOAD LEGS

Barbell Squat: Warm-up and 3 sets of 5 reps
with last hard- set weight

Romanian Deadlift: 3 sets of 5 reps with last hard-set weight

Hip Thrust: 3 sets of 5 reps with last hard-set weight

WORKOUT 2

DELOAD PUSH

Barbell Bench Press: Warm-up and 3 sets of 5 reps
with last hard-set weight

Seated Dumbbell Press: 3 sets of 5 reps
with last hard-set weight

Dumbbell Side Lateral Raise: 3 sets of 5 reps
with last hard set weight

WORKOUT 3

DELOAD PULL

Barbell Deadlift: Warm-up and 3 sets of 5 reps
with last hard-set weight

Barbell Row: 3 sets of 5 reps with last hard-set weight

Lat Pulldown (Wide-Grip): 3 sets of 5 reps with last hard-set weight

Put at least one day in between each of these workouts.

Everything about the workouts remains the same as your hard-training workouts with the exception of progression, as there's no progression in your deload workouts (because you don't do any hard sets and, instead, do just five reps with your normal hard-set weight).

CAN YOU DO CARDIO ON YOUR DELOAD WEEK?

Sure.

That said, remember the goal is to significantly decrease the amount of stress on your joints, ligaments, nervous system, and muscles. As you can imagine, doing too much high-intensity cardio won't help with that.

So do as much walking and light physical activity as you'd like, but limit HIIT and similar activities to an hour or so for the week and you should be fine.

WHAT SHOULD YOU DO WITH YOUR DIET WHEN DELOADING?

If you're cutting, you can maintain your current calorie intake while deloading, unless you feel the need for a diet break, in which case you can increase your intake to your approximate total daily energy expenditure.

If you're lean bulking, you can maintain your current calorie intake or reduce it to your approximate TDEE if you'd like a break from all the food.

SHOULD YOU JUST TAKE A WEEK OFF INSTEAD?

Maybe.

To find out, try a deload week and write down how you feel coming back to your hard training and how the first week goes. The next time around, do the same with a rest week (i.e., a week off).

Going forward, pick whichever seems to best suit your body.

It's also helpful to plan your deloads or rest weeks to coincide with trips, holidays, vacations, or any other upcoming disruptions to your routine. This way, you don't have to interrupt any of your hard training.

FINDING YOUR STARTING WEIGHTS (WEEK ONE)

It's all well and good to know that you should put enough weight on the bar to do your hard sets in the 8-to-10-rep range, but how do you determine this when you're starting out?

Finding your starting weights is mostly a matter of trial and error. You start light on an exercise, try it out, and increase the weight for each successive hard set until you've dialed everything in.

Thus, the goal of your first week is to learn your weights for all the exercises you'll be doing in that phase.

You might find that the bar alone (45 pounds) feels quite heavy on some exercises (barbell squat, for instance) and may even be too heavy for others (bench press, for example).

Don't be discouraged by this. It's completely normal. You'll gain strength quickly, and before you know it, you'll be adding weight to the bar.

In cases where the bar is too much, you have two options:

1. You can switch to a dumbbell variation of the exercise until you're strong enough for the bar.

2. You can use a fixed-weight straight bar instead, which allows for less than 45 pounds.

For instance, if the bar is too heavy for the bench press (you can't get at least six to seven reps with it), you can do the dumbbell bench press instead or use a fixed bar lighter than 45 pounds.

You might also find your starting weights quickly and easily and feel comfortable diving right into proper hard sets in your first workouts. If that's the case, then be my guest!

TO GET A SPOT OR NOT?

Most exercises don't benefit from spotting, and even those that do can be performed safely without assistance. That said, having a spotter does provide two advantages:

1. It encourages you to go for that extra rep or two you might not want to try otherwise.

    As you know, you don't need to take sets to technical failure, but you need to come close most of the time. That can be scary when you have a heavy bar on your back and your legs are on fire.

    A spotter can give you the confidence boost you need to power through those last couple of reps.

2. It can (strangely) increase your strength.

    This sounds silly until you experience it for yourself. You'll be struggling, and the moment your spotter puts their fingers underneath the bar, you suddenly find the strength to shoot it up.

So don't be afraid to ask someone in the gym for a spot on exercises like the bench press and squat if it'll help you progress more comfortably.

Just make sure they know the golden rule of good spotting: so long as you're keeping the weight moving, you don't want their help.

You want to move the weight without assistance if possible, so they shouldn't touch the bar or assist unless they're absolutely needed.

. . .

And just like that, your second training wheel is firmly in place, and you're about ready to start your journey toward a thinner, leaner, and stronger you!

Before I send you on your way, however, let's talk supplementation and make sure you know exactly what you are and aren't going to take while on the program, and how to get the most out of your supplementation regimen.

KEY TAKEAWAYS

- A training phase is a block of training designed to accomplish a specific goal, like increased power, strength, muscle growth, endurance, or recovery.

- In *Thinner Leaner Stronger*, your training routines are going to change slightly from phase to phase to expose your muscles to new and different types of movement patterns to more fully develop them.

- I don't recommend changing anything in the middle of a training phase unless you have to due to injury, traveling, or some other pressing circumstance.

- Whereas a training phase delineates the goals and duration of a training block, a training routine delineates what you're going to do in that time to achieve those goals.

- As far as results go, the *Thinner Leaner Stronger* five-day routine is better than the four- and three-day routines, and the four-day routine is better than the three-day routine.

- Try not to change routines during individual training phases.

  That said, if you'd like to "upgrade" to the four- or five-day routine in the middle of a phase, go for it. Try not to "downgrade" unless you have to.

- It's generally a good idea to do your hardest exercises first in your workouts, followed by the second hardest and so forth, because you always have the most energy and focus in the beginning of your workouts.

- You also want to do the exercises in a workout one at a time and complete all the hard sets for one exercise before moving on to another.

• If you can't do an exercise in a workout for whatever reason, simply choose an alternative "approved" exercise from chapter 23 to take its place, or do three more sets of an exercise already in your workout.

• When you get 10 reps for one hard set, you immediately move up in weight by adding 5 pounds to the bar or moving up to dumbbells that are 5 pounds heavier (per dumbbell).

• If your gym doesn't have 2.5-pound plates, you can add 10 pounds to the bar when you move up in weight.

• Doing too much weighted work for your oblique muscles can make your waist look "blocky," but weighted training for your rectus abdominis won't.

• The goal of a deload week is to significantly decrease the amount of stress on your joints, ligaments, nervous system, and muscles.

• Reducing volume instead of intensity is more effective for decreasing fatigue and maintaining performance.

• Do as much walking and light physical activity as you'd like during your deload week, but limit HIIT and similar activities to an hour or so for the week.

• If you're cutting, you can maintain your current calorie intake while deloading, unless you feel the need for a diet break.

• If you're lean bulking, you can maintain your current calorie intake while deloading or reduce it to your approximate TDEE if you'd like a break from all the food.

30

THE *THINER LEANER STRONGER* SUPPLEMENTATION PLAN

Now that we have the most important aspects of my *Thinner Leaner Stronger* program buttoned up—the diet and training—let's go over supplementation.

As we discussed in chapter 26, this element of the program is wholly optional and not terribly important as far as results go.

Most of what you're going to accomplish is going to come from the work you do in the kitchen and gym. Supplements can only give you a slight edge in losing fat, building muscle, and getting healthy.

That said, if you have the budget, supplementation (with the right supplements) is worthwhile because its advantages compound over time.

In other words, the minor improvements supplementation can provide in fat burning, muscle building, and general health and physiological function can add up to significant upswings over the course of months and years.

A few chapters ago, you learned about six worthwhile types of supplements you can include in your regimen:

1. Protein powder
2. Fish oil
3. Vitamin D
4. Multivitamin
5. Fat burner

6. Muscle builder

And in this chapter, I'm going to show you how to use each most beneficially.

Also, in the spirit of full disclosure, I want you to know that the specific products I recommend are not just what I personally use but are from my own supplement line.

If your eyes are starting to roll ("Oh great, here comes the sales pitch ..."), I totally understand, but let me explain.

Over the years, I've always struggled to find high-quality supplements and companies I could actually trust.

And so I wondered, should I "scratch my own itch" and create the supplements that I myself have always wanted? Would anyone else want them as well?

This wasn't an easy decision. I've made my bones as an author and educator. I've sold over a million books, published over a million words of free content on my blogs and hundreds of episodes of my podcast, and worked with thousands of people of all ages and circumstances. And most people think that's awesome. Go me.

What would happen if I were to start selling supplements, though?

As you can imagine, I feared that no matter how good my products might be or how honestly or fairly I might try to offer them, many of my readers and followers would assume the worst, reach for their pitchforks and torches, and try to run me off the internet.

And so I was on the horns of a dilemma.

On one hand, I saw an opportunity to do things very differently in the supplement space and create 100 percent natural, science-based, and safe supplements that really work.

On the other hand, doing so would mean getting into the 20-ton-turd salad that is the supplement industry and trying to convince people I wasn't a lying scammer like everyone else.

And so after much deliberation and many sacrificial offerings to the gods of commerce and capitalism, I decided to go with my gut and throw my hat in the ring.

I started a supplement company called Legion Athletics (www.legionathletics.com) and wasn't sure what to expect.

Would people have enough faith in me and appreciate the products and what makes them special? Would it be a flash in the pan, or would it have staying power?

Well, that was 2014 and I'm glad I made that leap of faith, because Legion is now a thriving business with over 200,000 customers from all over the world who have left thousands and thousands of glowing reviews all over the internet.

One of the primary reasons Legion is going gangbusters is our commitment to complete transparency, from formulating to scientific research, marketing and advertising, labeling, and more.

As you probably gathered from part 6 of this book, I'm an extremely skeptical person and consumer and, quite frankly, would assume that a supplement company is guilty until proven innocent. I've approached Legion with that mentality.

In other words, I've approached it from the angle of, What would it take for someone like me to buy supplements from Legion? What would I need to see to be convinced?

I'd want to know several things:

1. I'd want to know who came up with the formulations and what their credentials are.

Again, we're talking about our health here, so I'd want to know a bit about the person or persons I'm trusting mine to.

2. I'd want to know exactly what's in the products.

I'd want to know every active and inactive ingredient, and the doses of every active ingredient in particular to ensure it's not "pixie dusted" with tiny, ineffective amounts of ingredients.

3. I'd want to see science-based explanations of how the products are supposed to work.

I wouldn't want flashy ads with hulking bodybuilders barking buzzwords at me.

I'd want to understand why ingredients were chosen and what they're supposed to do in the body, and I'd want to see all the relevant scientific research to back that up.

4. I'd want to see formal proof that the products are legitimate.

I trust product labels about as much as I do mainstream news reports, so I'd want to see certificates of analysis confirming the labels are 100 percent accurate.

5. I'd want to see what other people are saying about the products.

That means independent online reviews, reviews from verified purchasers and customers, and opinions from respected industry leaders.

If a supplement company could satisfactorily check all five of those boxes, I'd probably be willing to give them a try. Otherwise, hard pass.

If you're like me, then I think you're going to really like what I'm doing with Legion because it lives up to all those standards, and more.

Simply put, Legion outclasses everything on the market and is the yardstick by which all other supplement companies can be measured.

The bottom line is I'm not just looking to build a supplement company. I'm looking to build a culture that people like you appreciate and want to be a part of.

I believe in respecting customers, telling things like they are, and delivering what I promise. I believe honesty and integrity sell better than cutting corners and relying on ridiculous advertisements and lies.

I don't just want to sell pills and powders, I want to change the supplement industry for the better.

So, with that out of the way, let's get to learning how to get the most out of each of the six types of supplements I recommend.

PROTEIN POWDER

Most people like to take a scoop of protein powder before and after workouts because it's quick and convenient, and then again during the day as a snack (midafternoon is popular). This is reasonable.

However, some people get most of their daily protein from powders, which I don't recommend.

There's a limit to how much protein powder you should have every day because too much can cause negative side effects like nutritional deficiencies and gastrointestinal (GI) distress.

One of the main benefits of protein powder is that it's mostly protein (it contains very little carbohydrate or dietary fat). This is great for your macros but not so great for the nutritional quality of your diet because many whole-food sources of protein are also great sources of vitamins, minerals, and other micronutrients.

For instance, eggs are one of the most nutrient-rich foods you can eat, legumes are chock-full of prebiotic fiber and microminerals, and meat contains beneficial compounds like L-carnitine, CoQ10, iron, and creatine, all of which are missing from most protein powders.

Therefore, if you're getting too many of your daily calories from protein powder (30 percent or more) and not ensuring your remaining calories are extremely nutrient dense, you're likely to develop nutritional gaps in your diet that can cause health problems over time.

Eating too much protein powder—especially in one sitting—can also cause gas, bloating, and cramping.

We can only have so much protein powder in a day before something just doesn't feel right, especially when it comes to milk-derived powders like whey and casein. Tolerance varies from person to person, but for me, any more than 70 to 80 grams of whey or casein in a day will upset my stomach.

Powders are also digested faster than whole-food proteins, so if you gulp down a large amount of protein powder, some of the protein molecules can make their way into the large intestine only partially digested, resulting in GI distress.

This problem is unique to protein powder because of how easy it is to eat.

Foods that require chewing are more filling than powders, making them harder to overconsume. A protein shake with a couple of chicken breasts' worth of protein can be downed in a matter of seconds, though, placing an immediate and intense demand on your digestive system.

Whey protein can be particularly troublesome in this regard, as many people can't comfortably digest a hefty dose of dairy protein in one sitting. This is less of an issue with whey isolate protein, which doesn't contain lactose, but it can still occur.

So, all things considered, here are my recommendations for protein powder intake:

1. Don't get more than 30 percent of your daily calories from protein powders.

2. Don't have more than 40 to 50 grams of protein from powder in one sitting.

As far as specific products go, I alternate between three protein powders produced by Legion:

1. My 100 percent whey isolate protein, Whey+ (www.legionathletics.com/whey)

2. My 100 percent vegan protein, Thrive (www.legionathletics.com/thrive)

3. My 100 percent micellar casein protein, Casein+ (www.legionathletics.com/casein)

FISH OIL

Research shows that a combined intake of 500 milligrams to 1.8 grams of EPA and DHA per day is adequate for general health, but additional benefits are seen up to a combined intake of as much as 6 grams per day.[1]

For physically active people, 2 to 4 grams per day is a sensible recommendation.

Take your fish oil with meals, and if you're going to take more than 2 grams per day, split it up into two doses separated by several hours (breakfast and dinner, for instance). This maximizes absorption and effectiveness.

Also, remember that I recommend a natural or reesterified triglyceride fish oil (the latter being my favorite), not an ethyl ester product.

To prevent the nasty fish oil burps so many people complain about, you can store the pills in the freezer and take them with food.

As far as specific products go, I take a high-potency 100 percent reesterified triglyceride fish oil produced by Legion called Triton (www.legionathletics.com/triton).

VITAMIN D

According to the National Academy of Medicine, 600 IU of vitamin D per day is adequate for ages 1 to 70 (and 800 IU per day for 71-plus), but these numbers have been severely criticized by scientists who specialize in vitamin D research.[2]

These scientists call attention to the over 125 published studies that indicate such recommendations are too low and likely lead to deficiencies.

A committee of the US Endocrine Society convened in 2011 to review the evidence and concluded that 600 to 1,000 IU per day is adequate for ages 1 to 18, and 1,500 to 2,000 IU per day is adequate for ages 19 and up.[3]

So, assuming you're 18 or older, I recommend you start at 2,000 IU per day, and then, if you're experiencing any symptoms of low vitamin D levels, get blood tested for your *25-hydroxyvitamin D* levels (the usable form of vitamin D your body creates) to ascertain your status and adjust your intake accordingly.

As far as specific products go, I take a vitamin D supplement produced by either NOW Foods or Jarrow.

MULTIVITAMIN

Steer clear of multivitamins that claim to provide 100 percent of everything you need in just one pill per day.

They're generally low quality, down-market supplements that mostly contain things you don't need to supplement with and very little of what you probably do need.

Most good multivitamins have you take at least a few pills per day, because that allows for optimal dosages of a wide variety of micronutrients.

Multivitamins should also be taken with food, ideally a meal containing a bit of dietary fat, as this helps with nutrient absorption.[4]

As far as specific products go, I take a multivitamin produced by Legion called

Triumph (www.legionathletics.com/triumph) that contains 21 vitamins and minerals as well as 14 additional ingredients proven to enhance health, performance, longevity, and more.

FAT BURNER

In chapter 26, we discussed several natural ingredients proven to accelerate fat loss:

1. Caffeine
2. Yohimbine
3. Synephrine

Let's look at how to use each safely and effectively.

CAFFEINE

The dosage of caffeine seen in most weight loss studies ranges from 2 to 6 milligrams per kilogram of body weight per day.

Personally, I take about 4 milligrams per kilogram of body weight per day in the *anhydrous* ("containing no water") form when cutting.

As you know, one downside of caffeine as a weight loss aid is that it loses its effectiveness over time as your body becomes desensitized to it.

The best way to prevent this is to limit your intake. Here's what I recommend:

- Have at least some of your caffeine before your training unless you have a good reason not to (training later in the day, for instance).

- If you're not sure of your caffeine sensitivity, start with 3 milligrams per kilogram of body weight per day, and work up from there.

- Keep your daily intake at or below 6 milligrams per kilogram of body weight per day.

- Do one to two low-caffeine days and one no-caffeine day per week.

A low day should be half your normal intake, and a no day means less than 50 milligrams of caffeine. (One or two cups of tea would be fine, but no coffee, preworkout drink, caffeine pills, etc.)

As far as specific products go, I get most of my caffeine from my bestselling preworkout supplement Pulse (www.legionathletics.com/pulse), which contains an effective dosage of caffeine along with five other natural ingredients that improve mood, sharpen mental focus, boost strength and endurance, and reduce fatigue.

YOHIMBINE

Research shows that 0.2 milligrams of yohimbine per kilogram of body weight per day is sufficient for fat loss purposes and that taking it 15 to 30 minutes before exercise is particularly effective.[5]

Yohimbine can make some people jittery and anxious, though, so I recommend you start with 0.1 milligrams per kilogram of body weight to assess tolerance. If you feel fine, then increase to 0.2 milligrams per kilogram of body weight.

Furthermore, yohimbine can raise blood pressure, so if you have high blood pressure, I don't recommend you use it.[6]

As far as specific products go, when cutting, I take a preworkout fat burner produced by Legion called Forge (www.legionathletics.com/forge), which contains an effective dosage of yohimbine along with two other ingredients that help preserve lean mass and workout quality while dieting.

SYNEPHRINE

Effective dosages of synephrine range from 25 to 50 milligrams and can be taken anywhere from one to three times daily, depending on individual tolerance.

Research also shows that pairing synephrine with caffeine further speeds up fat loss.[7]

As far as specific products go, when cutting, I take a fat burner produced by Legion called Phoenix (www.legionathletics.com/phoenix), which contains an effective dosage of synephrine along with eight other ingredients that help boost metabolic rate, enhance fat burning, and reduce appetite.

MUSCLE BUILDER

As we've covered, there are three muscle-building supplements worth including in your regimen:

1. Creatine monohydrate
2. Beta-alanine
3. Citrulline malate

Let's review each.

CREATINE MONOHYDRATE

Studies show that supplementing with 5 grams of creatine monohydrate per day is optimal.[8]

When you start taking creatine monohydrate, you can "load" it by taking 20 grams per day for the first five to seven days and see benefits sooner.[9]

That said, loading creatine can upset some people's stomachs, so I don't generally recommend it unless you don't mind "risking" a bit of GI distress.

I also recommend you take your creatine monohydrate with your postworkout meals for two reasons:

1. Research shows that taking creatine with a moderate amount of protein and carbohydrate increases its effectiveness.[10]

2. Studies show that taking creatine after a workout is slightly more effective for increasing strength and muscle gain than taking it before.[11]

As far as specific products go, I take a postworkout supplement produced by Legion called Recharge (www.legionathletics.com/recharge), which contains an effective dosage of creatine monohydrate along with two other ingredients that boost postworkout recovery and reduce muscle soreness.

BETA-ALANINE

Effective dosages of beta-alanine range from 2 to 4.8 grams per day, with 4.8 grams being slightly more effective than 2 grams.

It's also generally thought that people doing higher-volume weightlifting programs may benefit most from larger doses of beta-alanine.

This is because carnosine stores are depleted during muscle contractions, so naturally, the more you contract your muscles, the more carnosine your body uses. Although plausible, this theory hasn't been demonstrated in scientific research yet.

As far as specific products go, I get my beta-alanine from the preworkout supplement produced by Legion, Pulse (www.legionathletics.com/pulse), which contains an effective dosage of beta-alanine (and more).

CITRULLINE MALATE

For improving exercise performance, research shows that you should take 6 to 8 grams of citrulline malate per day.[12]

Unlike creatine and beta-alanine, citrulline malate's performance-enhancing effects don't accumulate over time, but instead only last several hours. This is why

I recommend you take it 30 to 45 minutes before exercise (resistance training or cardiovascular).

As far as specific products go, I get my citrulline malate from the preworkout supplement produced by Legion, Pulse (www.legionathletics.com/pulse), which contains an effective dosage of citrulline malate (and more).

SUPPLEMENTATION WHEN CUTTING

When cutting, consider taking all the supplements listed in this chapter for the following reasons:

- The protein powder will help you hit your protein targets more easily.
- The fish oil, vitamin D, and multivitamin will provide your body with vital nutrients (which will be scarcer due to calorie restriction).
- The fat burners will help you lose fat faster.
- The muscle builders will help you retain or even gain lean mass.

I take all these supplements when cutting (and more), and it helps make for maximally productive and painless fat loss.

SUPPLEMENTATION WHEN LEAN BULKING

When lean bulking, consider taking all the supplements listed in this chapter except the fat burners (with the exception of caffeine—this can be taken when lean bulking).

Some people like to take a number of fat burners when lean bulking in hopes of gaining less fat, but this doesn't really make sense.

The primary mechanism through which these supplements work is increasing your metabolic rate, which simply means you'll need to eat more food to maintain a calorie surplus (which will still result in some fat gain).

Furthermore, some fat burners reduce your appetite, which is also counterproductive when lean bulking.

So aside from caffeine, save the fat burners for when you're cutting.

SUPPLEMENTATION WHEN MAINTAINING

Similar to lean bulking, when maintaining, consider taking all the supplements listed in this chapter but the fat burners (again, with the exception of caffeine).

That said, you can temporarily include fat burners in your regimen if you're going into a "minicut" (two to four weeks) after a holiday, vacation, or just-for-fun bout of overeating.

. . .

That's a wrap on supplementation!

If you plan to use supplements to get fit faster, take a break now to order what you'll need.

Then, when you're ready to continue, we're going to tie off a couple of remaining loose ends—tracking progress and breaking through weight loss plateaus—and then get you started on the program!

Let's go!

KEY TAKEAWAYS

- Supplements can only give you a slight edge in losing fat, building muscle, and getting healthy.

- I've always struggled to find high-quality supplements I could trust, so I started my own supplement line called Legion Athletics (www.legionathletics.com).

- There's a limit to how much protein powder you should have every day because too much can cause negative side effects like nutritional deficiencies and gastrointestinal (GI) distress.

- Whey protein can be particularly troublesome in this regard, as many people can't comfortably digest a hefty dose of dairy protein in one sitting. This is less of an issue with whey isolate protein, which doesn't contain lactose, but it can still occur.

- Here are my recommendations for protein powder intake:

  Don't get more than 30 percent of your daily calories from protein powders.

  Don't have more than 40 to 50 grams of protein from powder in one sitting.

• A combined intake of 500 milligrams to 1.8 grams of EPA and DHA per day is adequate for general health, but additional benefits are seen up to a combined intake of as much as 6 grams per day.

For physically active people, 2 to 4 grams per day is a sensible recommendation.

• Take your fish oil with meals, and if you're going to take more than 2 grams per day, split it up into two doses separated by several hours (breakfast and dinner, for instance).

• 600 to 1,000 IU of vitamin D per day is adequate for ages 1 to 18, and 1,500 to 2,000 IU per day is adequate for ages 19 and up.

Assuming you're 18 or older, I recommend you start at 2,000 IU per day, and then, if you're experiencing any symptoms of low vitamin D levels, get blood tested for your *25-hydroxyvitamin D* levels and adjust your intake accordingly.

• Most good multivitamins have you take at least a few pills per day, because that allows for optimal dosages of a wide variety of micronutrients.

• Multivitamins should be taken with food, ideally a meal containing a bit of dietary fat, as this helps with nutrient absorption.

• The dosage of caffeine seen in most weight loss studies ranges from 2 to 6 milligrams per kilogram of body weight per day.

• One downside of caffeine as a weight loss aid is that it loses its effectiveness over time as your body becomes desensitized to it.

The best way to prevent this is to limit your intake. Here's what I recommend:

Have at least some of your caffeine before your training unless you have a good reason not to (training later in the day, for instance).

If you're not sure of your caffeine sensitivity, start with 3 milligrams per kilogram of body weight per day, and work up from there.

Keep your daily intake at or below 6 milligrams per kilogram of body weight per day.

Do one to two low-caffeine days and one no-caffeine day per week.

• 0.2 milligrams of yohimbine per kilogram of body weight per day is sufficient for fat loss purposes, and taking it 15 to 30 minutes before exercise is particularly effective.

• Yohimbine can make some people jittery and anxious, so I recommend you start with 0.1 milligrams per kilogram of body weight to assess tolerance. If you feel fine, then increase to 0.2 milligrams per kilogram of body weight.

- Effective dosages of synephrine range from 25 to 50 milligrams and can be taken anywhere from one to three times daily, depending on individual tolerance.

- Supplementing with 5 grams of creatine monohydrate per day is optimal.

- Effective dosages of beta-alanine range from 2 to 4.8 grams per day, with 4.8 grams being slightly more effective than 2 grams.

- People doing higher-volume weightlifting programs may benefit most from larger doses of beta-alanine.

- For improving exercise performance, research shows that you should take 6 to 8 grams of citrulline malate per day, and 30 to 45 minutes before exercise.

- When cutting, consider taking all the supplements listed in this chapter.

- When lean bulking, consider taking all the supplements listed in this chapter except the fat burners (with the exception of caffeine—this can be taken when lean bulking).

- When maintaining, consider taking all the supplements listed in this chapter but the fat burners (again, with the exception of caffeine).

31

THE RIGHT AND WRONG WAYS TO TRACK YOUR PROGRESS

The brilliant 19th century physicist and engineer Sir William Thomson said when you can measure something and express it in numbers, you know something about it, and when you can't, your knowledge is lacking.

This insight is applicable to many things in life, including exercise and diet.

Only when you can measure your progress (or lack thereof) and express it in real numbers can you know whether you're headed in the right direction. If you don't have any consistent, objective way to measure it, however, then you're going blind, hoping for the best.

This is one of the major reasons why so many people fail to achieve their fitness goals. If you don't track your progress correctly, it doesn't matter how well you understand everything in this book—you *will* end up in a rut, and probably sooner rather than later.

There are three elements to tracking progress:

1. Body composition
2. Diet
3. Exercise

In my *Thinner Leaner Stronger* program, however, you're only going to need to track your body composition and exercise. By following structured meal plans, you don't have to *track* anything in your diet—you just have to eat according to the plan.

Calorie and macro tracking only become necessary when you're making food decisions on the fly, which can work but is best suited to more experienced dieters.

So, let's learn how to track your body composition and exercise correctly.

HOW TO TRACK YOUR BODY COMPOSITION

Tracking your body composition is a vital part of your fitness journey.

Even when you do everything right, it can take longer than you might realize to see marked changes in your appearance. And when the squishy parts don't transform as quickly as you'd like, it's easy to lose heart. It can feel like all that work in the kitchen and gym is more or less for naught.

If you learn to track your body composition properly, you can avoid this problem because you'll always know exactly what is or isn't happening with your physique, and you'll be able to adjust your diet and exercise accordingly.

It's pretty easy, too. There are just three steps:

1. Weigh yourself daily and calculate weekly averages.
2. Take weekly body measurements.
3. Take weekly progress pictures.

If that sounds like a lot of work, don't worry, it's not. It doesn't take more than five minutes a week, and you'll probably come to enjoy it. Games are more fun when you keep score, and quantifying your progress is how you keep score in the "building a better body" game.

Furthermore, if your numbers aren't moving in the right direction, you want to know as soon as possible so you can take corrective actions.

Let's review each of the steps.

1. WEIGH YOURSELF DAILY AND CALCULATE WEEKLY AVERAGES.

Your weight can fluctuate on a daily basis due to fluid retention, glycogen levels, and bowel movements (or the lack thereof), so you can expect regular ups and downs.

That's why I recommend weighing yourself every day and then calculating averages every seven days.

Here's an example of how this might look:

Monday: 153 pounds
Tuesday: 152 pounds

> Wednesday: 154 pounds
>
> Thursday: 154 pounds
>
> Friday: 151 pounds
>
> Saturday: 152 pounds
>
> Sunday: 151 pounds
>
> Total weekly weigh-ins: 1,067 pounds
>
> Average daily weight: 1,067 pounds / 7 days = 152.4 pounds

This method of tracking your weight keeps you focused on the bigger picture instead of fussing over meaningless day-to-day variances, which can cause unnecessary frustration and confusion.

If your average weight is going up, you're gaining weight. If it's going down, you're losing weight. Simple and clean.

The procedure here is easy:

1. Weigh yourself first thing in the morning, naked and after the bathroom and before eating or drinking anything.

2. Then, every seven days, add up your last seven weigh-ins and divide by seven to get your average daily weight for the last week.

3. Record your averages somewhere easily accessible, like an Excel or Google Sheet or the notepad app in your phone.

If you want to take your weight-tracking game a step further, you can graph the numbers in Excel or Google Sheets.

As you're well aware, your weight can shoot up a few pounds during your period, so I recommend you watch the averages of the weeks before and after your period weeks to track your progress.

2. TAKE WEEKLY BODY MEASUREMENTS.

Even when tracked properly, your weight alone doesn't always tell you how your body composition is changing. That is, it doesn't tell if you're gaining or losing muscle or fat—just that you're gaining or losing something.

"Newbie gains" also render body weight less important. If you're new to weightlifting and have fat to lose, you can expect to gain muscle and lose fat at the same time.

That means your weight may not change as much as you'd expect. I've seen some pretty dramatic one- and even two-year female transformations where body weight only changed by 5 to 10 pounds.

All this is why you should record at least one body measurement every week in addition to your weight: your waist circumference.

The size of your waist is a reliable indicator of fat loss or gain, so by keeping an eye on it, you can quickly assess whether you're gaining or losing fat.

So take this measurement once per week, when you calculate your average body weight, and watch it over time.

To take this measurement, wrap a tape measure around your bare stomach, right at your navel. Make sure the tape measure is parallel to the floor (not slanted) and snug to your body, but not so tight that it compresses the skin. Exhale while taking the measurement, and don't flex or suck your stomach in.

Make sure you measure in the same spot every time so your readings stay consistent.

Hip circumference is another measurement some women like to take because it too is another reliable marker of fat loss or gain.

If you want to take it, do so when you measure your waist (once per week).

To take this measurement, wrap a tape measure around the widest point between the top of your hip bone and the bottom of your butt. This spot can vary from person to person depending on body composition, but it's generally right above your "naughty bits."

Make sure you measure in the same spot every time so your readings stay consistent.

And if you're the type of person who loves tracking data and quantifying things, here are two more measurements you can take:

- Your upper-leg circumference

  To take this measurement, wrap a tape measure around the widest part of one of your leg's thigh and hamstrings. Then do the same for your other leg.

  Take these measurements every week with your other weekly measurements, and make sure you measure in the same spots every time.

- Your flexed arms

  To take this measurement, flex one of your arms and wrap a tape measure around the largest part (the peak of your biceps and middle of your triceps). Then do the same for your other arm.

Take these measurements every week with your other weekly measurements, and make sure you measure in the same spots every time.

3. TAKE WEEKLY PROGRESS PICTURES.

For some people, taking pictures is even better than taking measurements because numbers are great and all, but ultimately what we care about most is what we see in the mirror.

So even if you don't like what you see right now, do take your "before" pictures because you're going to love watching how your body is going to change over the next weeks and months.

And some time from now, you're going to be downright shocked at how much your physique has improved!

To watch your transformation unfold, take progress pictures every week when you take your weekly measurements.

Here's how to do it right:

- Take pictures from the front, side, and back.

- Show as much skin as you feel comfortable with. The more the better because it gives you the best idea of how your body is changing.

- Use the same camera, lighting, and background for each picture. If you aren't able to do this, make sure the pictures are clear.

- Take the pictures at the same time every day, preferably in the morning, after using the bathroom and before breakfast.

- Take both flexed and unflexed pictures, as this lets you see how your muscles are developing.

I also recommend saving all your progress photos in an individual album on your phone or computer so as time goes on, you can easily scroll through them.

HOW TO TRACK YOUR EXERCISE

Tracking your workouts—and your resistance training workouts in particular—is just as important as tracking your body composition. It's the only way to ensure you're progressively overloading your muscles over time.

At first, your strength will shoot up by leaps and bounds, but in time, it'll slow to a crawl. From that point forward, you'll have to work harder and harder to continue gaining reps and adding weight to the bar.

Keeping tabs on your progress gets hazy if you don't have a training journal. Unless you're a memory athlete, you won't remember exactly what you did in your previous workouts and thus won't know what to aim for each week.

Remember that once your "newbie gains" are spent, a successful workout is one where you beat your last performance of it by even a little—a rep or two with the same weight on just one exercise, for instance.

This is how you build muscle and strength—one rep at a time.

That's why every time you step up to a barbell or dumbbell, you want to know exactly what you're going for, not wondering what you did the last time.

For instance, if you know your first hard set of squats in your previous lower body workout was 135 pounds for 8 reps, all you should have on your mind in this next workout is hitting 9 or 10 reps with that weight.

Remember, studies even show that visualizing yourself doing this before stepping under the bar can boost your strength and increase your chances of getting it done (mind over matter for the win!).[1]

If you don't keep a training journal, your workouts get sloppy and eventually turn into lifting random amounts of weight for random numbers of reps each week.

This may produce satisfactory results when you first start out, but it won't cut it in the long run. You need to work off of real data to achieve impressive long-term results.

So to track your *Thinner Leaner Stronger* workouts, you have several options:

1. Pen and paper
2. App
3. Excel or Google Sheet
4. Workout journal

Let's look at each.

PEN AND PAPER

This is the simplest way to plan and track your workouts. All you need is a notebook and pen, and in it, you write out the workouts you'll be doing and then record what you actually do in each as you go.

For *Thinner Leaner Stronger*, this means writing out the exercises and number of hard sets for each workout you'll be doing each week of your upcoming training phase, and then recording the weight and reps used for those exercises as you do the workouts.

Here's a simple way to lay this out:

WEEK 1

Workout 1

Monday 7/23/2018

LOWER BODY (LEGS AND GLUTES)

Barbell Squat
Warm-up sets:
Hard set 1:
Hard set 2:
Hard set 3:

Leg Press
Hard set 1:
Hard set 2:
Hard set 3:

Romanian Deadlift
Hard set 1:
Hard set 2:
Hard set 3:

Hip Thrust
Hard set 1:
Hard set 2:
Hard set 3:

And then, when you do this workout, you'd fill it out, like this:

Barbell Squat
Warm-up sets: *55 (pounds) x 10 (reps), 55 x 10, 75 x 4*
Hard set 1: *110 x 10*
Hard set 2: *120 x 8*
Hard set 3: *120 x 7*

Leg Press
Hard set 1: *145 x 10*
Hard set 2: *155 x 8*
Hard set 3: *155 x 8*

Romanian Deadlift
Hard set 1: *95 x 8*

Hard set 2: *95 x 8*
Hard set 3: *95 x 8*

Hip Thrust
Hard set 1: *135 x 10*
Hard set 2: *145 x 8*
Hard set 3: *145 x 7*

You can also make notes if you feel particularly strong or weak on a given set or exercise, if you experienced an ache or pain, if you didn't sleep well the night before, etc.

These notes can help you better understand your workout numbers when you're looking back to review your progress.

Then, when you go to do your workouts again the following week, you can look back at what you did the previous times around to see what you'd like to achieve in this week's performance.

For instance, in the workout example just listed, you moved up to 120 pounds on your squat and got two sets for eight and seven reps, respectively.

Therefore, the next time you do this workout, you could strive to get two or even three sets of eight reps (or more) with 120 pounds, which would be an improvement.

Many people like to record their daily and weekly body measurements in their notebooks as well for an extra boost of motivation.

APP

There are literally hundreds of apps for tracking your workouts. I never quite liked any of the ones I've used in the past, so I made my own and use it to plan and track all my training.

It's called Stacked, it's 100 percent free, and whether you're a beginner or an experienced weightlifter, it'll help you better plan and do your workouts, accurately measure and monitor your body composition, and see and analyze your training progress.

Go to www.getstackedapp.com now to check it out.

EXCEL OR GOOGLE SHEET

For me, this is a close second to an app and even preferable for more advanced programming that requires a bit more planning and math.

As far as formatting goes, I've always created a new spreadsheet (workbook, technically) for each training phase and then listed each week's workouts in individual worksheets (named accordingly, Week 1, 2, 3, etc.) in the same basic manner as I would with a pen-and-paper notebook.

For *Thinner Leaner Stronger*, this would mean creating one spreadsheet (workbook) per phase with nine worksheets containing the workouts for each week (ending with the ninth deload week).

Then, to do a workout, you load the spreadsheet on your phone and follow along, entering your numbers as you go. Google Sheets is especially nice for this because it's free and easy to load and edit on your phone (just get the app).

WORKOUT JOURNAL

There are just as many blank workout journals as there are apps, but I've never used one, so I don't have anything in particular to recommend.

That said, as I mentioned earlier, I do have a journal specifically for *Thinner Leaner Stronger* called *The Year One Challenge for Women* (www.thinnerleanerstronger.com/challenge).

It has a year's worth of workouts neatly organized and laid out, so all you have to do is follow and fill out the workouts one by one, week by week, phase by phase.

. . .

If you've brushed over this chapter because you're itching to get started and I've caught your eye here, please take 10 minutes or so to go through it in detail.

Much of your future success or failure is going to hinge on how well you track your progress.

If you don't track your body composition correctly, you'll probably fail to register the positive or negative changes occurring and wind up confused, anxious, and demotivated.

If you don't track your workouts correctly, you'll probably fall into a rut of doing the exact same thing every workout and stop progressing, which is just as discouraging.

Plus, tracking your body composition and workouts just makes the whole program more fun. Make it a game! It's exciting to see real numbers changing for the better and to review old records from time to time and see just how far you've come.

KEY TAKEAWAYS

• If you don't track your progress correctly, it doesn't matter how well you understand everything in this book—you *will* end up in a rut, and probably sooner rather than later.

• There are three elements to tracking progress: body composition, diet, and exercise.

• There are just three steps to tracking your body composition:

Weigh yourself daily and calculate weekly averages.

Take weekly body measurements.

Take weekly progress pictures.

• Your weight can fluctuate on a daily basis due to fluid retention, glycogen levels, and bowel movements (or the lack thereof), so you can expect regular ups and downs.

• If your average weight is going up, you're gaining weight. If it's going down, you're losing weight.

• As you're well aware, your weight can shoot up a few pounds during your period, so I recommend you watch the averages of the weeks before and after your period weeks to track your progress.

• "Newbie gains" render body weight less important. If you're new to weightlifting and have fat to lose, you can expect to gain muscle and lose fat at the same time, which means your weight may not change as much as you'd expect.

• The size of your waist is a reliable indicator of fat loss or gain. Take this measurement once per week, when you calculate your average body weight, and watch it over time.

• If you're the type of person who loves tracking data and quantifying things, here are two more measurements you can take: your upper-leg circumference and your flexed arms.

• Take these measurements every week with your other weekly measurements, and make sure you measure in the same spots every time.

• Take progress pictures every week when you take your weekly measurements.

• Tracking your workouts—and your resistance training workouts in particular—is just as important as tracking your body composition. It's the only way to ensure you're progressively overloading your muscles over time.

• Every time you step up to a barbell or dumbbell, you want to know exactly what you're going for, not wondering what you did the last time.

• To track your *Thinner Leaner Stronger* workouts, you have several options: pen and paper, app, Excel or Google Sheet, and workout journal.

• Pen and paper is the simplest way to plan and track your workouts. All you need is a notebook and pen, and in it, you write out the workouts you'll be doing and then record what you actually do in each as you go.

• There are hundreds of apps for tracking your workouts, but I never quite liked any of the ones I've used in the past, so I made my own and use it to plan and track all my training.

It's called Stacked. Go to www.getstackedapp.com now to check it out.

• An Excel or Google Sheet is a close second to an app and even preferable for more advanced programming that requires a bit more planning and math.

• I have a workout journal specifically for *Thinner Leaner Stronger* called *The Year One Challenge for Women* (www.thinnerleanerstronger.com/challenge).

32

HOW TO BREAK THROUGH
WEIGHT LOSS PLATEAUS

"Hard choices, easy life. Easy choices, hard life."
—JERZY GREGOREK

What's the most common gripe among dieters everywhere?

Easy: not losing weight.

They feel like they're doing everything right and following all the rules, yet the scale flashes the same scowling, mocking number at them every morning.

You've probably experienced this yourself.

This plight extends to our more "enlightened" perspective of monitoring body composition as well—you can carefully apply everything you've learned in this book and suddenly stop losing fat.

In fact, you can count on this happening.

Fortunately, while the human metabolism is incredibly complex, breaking through weight and fat loss plateaus isn't. You simply need to widen the gap between energy in and energy out.

To do this, you first need to ensure you're accurately measuring and recording everything you're eating and drinking. Remember in chapter 7 where you learned how easy it is to mess up calorie counting if you're not paying enough attention to the details?

You also need to ensure you're not making any of the cheating mistakes we discussed in chapter 20.

Once you're certain you're not making any energy-balance blunders, the easiest way to break through a weight or fat loss plateau is to eat less. That said,

I recommend "maxing out" on exercise first because this is better for staving off the negative side effects associated with calorie restriction.[1]

In short, I'd rather you move more before eating less.

There isn't a clear scientific answer as to how much exercise you can do while dieting before it becomes unhealthy and counterproductive, but it's more than many people think.

I've worked and spoken with many thousands of people, and here's what I've learned: 4 to 5 hours of weightlifting and 1.5 to 2 hours of high-intensity cardio per week will maximize fat loss while minimizing unwanted side effects.

And that's exactly what I recommend you work up to as your exercise "ceiling" when you're cutting.

What happens when you exceed those numbers and exercise even more?

Some people's bodies are particularly resilient and do fine with more exercise, but in my experience, many don't. If you take it much further than I recommend, it's more likely that hunger and cravings will kick into overdrive, sleep quality will decline, energy levels will plummet, and your mood will sour.

Once you've reached your exercise limit and it appears you're no longer losing fat, it's usually due to one of the two following scenarios:

1. Fat loss is being obscured by fluctuations in water weight or bowel movements.

   Water retention can vary wildly when you're cutting. Sometimes you can go for two or even three weeks without losing weight and suddenly, overnight, drop several pounds through frequent urination (the "whoosh effect" bodybuilders often talk about).

   This overnight "flush" often occurs after a cheat meal or diet break because increasing calories (and carbs in particular) can significantly decrease cortisol levels, which in turn reduces water retention.[2]

   Stool retention can also play tricks on you, obscuring both weight and fat loss by increasing body weight and bloating.

   All this is why it's smart to wait two or three weeks before reducing your calories when you've hit your exercise ceiling and your weight or fat loss has stalled.

2. Fat loss has slowed to a crawl due to the natural metabolic adaptations that occur while cutting.

   As time goes on, what started out as a 20 or 25 percent calorie deficit can shrink to a much smaller one that no longer results in appreciable fat loss.

So if you've reached your exercise limit and failed to lose any weight or fat in at least two to three weeks, the next move is to eat less and to do it gradually, not drastically.

Specifically, you should cut your daily food intake by about 100 calories every 14 days by reducing your carbohydrate intake (don't reduce your protein or fat).

How low you can ultimately go will depend on your body, but a good rule of thumb is to stop cutting calories when you've reached about 90 percent of your BMR.

And then, don't remain there for more than a couple of weeks before calling it quits on the cut.

What should you do if you've been slightly below your BMR for a couple of weeks but still haven't reached your desired body fat percentage?

Your best bet in this case is to bring your calories back to your total daily energy expenditure for four to six weeks to allow your body to normalize itself, and then start cutting anew.

. . .

Weight loss plateaus are nothing to be afraid of or worried about.

They're an inevitable consequence of proper dieting, and they're easily conquered by making minor adjustments to your meal and exercise plans and staying the course.

That's all there is to it.

KEY TAKEAWAYS

• While the human metabolism is incredibly complex, breaking through weight and fat loss plateaus isn't. You simply need to widen the gap between energy in and energy out.

• To do this, you first need to ensure you're accurately measuring and recording everything you're eating and drinking.

• You also need to ensure you're not making any of the cheating mistakes we discussed in chapter 20.

• Once you're certain you're not making any energy-balance blunders, the easiest way to break through a weight and fat loss plateau is to eat less.

That said, I recommend "maxing out" on exercise first because this is better for staving off the negative side effects associated with calorie restriction.

• 4 to 5 hours of weightlifting and 1.5 to 2 hours of high-intensity cardio per week will maximize fat loss while minimizing unwanted side effects.

• Once you've reached your exercise limit and it appears you're no longer losing fat, it's usually due to one of the two following scenarios:

Fat loss is being obscured by fluctuations in water weight or bowel movements.

Fat loss has slowed to a crawl due to the natural metabolic adaptations that occur while cutting.

• If you've reached your exercise limit and failed to lose any weight or fat in at least two to three weeks, cut your daily food intake by about 100 calories every 14 days by reducing your carbohydrate intake (don't reduce your protein or fat).

• A good rule of thumb is to stop cutting calories when you've reached about 90 percent of your BMR.

• If you've been slightly below your BMR for a couple of weeks but still haven't reached your desired body fat percentage, bring your calories back to your total daily energy expenditure for four to six weeks to allow your body to normalize itself, and then start cutting anew.

PART 8

THE BEGINNING

33

THE *THINNER LEANER STRONGER* QUICKSTART GUIDE

This is it—the moment you've been waiting for.

You've read, digested, and absorbed hundreds of pages of diet, exercise, and supplementation principles, strategies, and tactics.

As a result, you've probably gained a whole new perspective on diet, exercise, and fitness and hopefully feel more prepared than ever to transform your body.

And that means you're ready to start my *Thinner Leaner Stronger* program.

To make things as smooth as possible for you, I'm going to give you a comprehensive checklist that'll take you by the hand and get you up to speed fast.

This quickstart guide is broken down into eight major steps:

1. Buy your supplies.
2. Join or set up a gym.
3. Take your first measurements and pictures.
4. Create your first meal plan.
5. Create your workout schedule.
6. Prepare for your first week.
7. Do your first week.
8. Get ready for your next week (and beyond!).

Each of these steps has several substeps, including optional ones, which aren't necessary for following the program but are recommended for reasons you've learned about in this book.

Once you've done those eight things, you'll officially be on your way, so let's get to it!

1. BUY YOUR SUPPLIES

You don't need much in the way of gear and gadgets to follow *Thinner Leaner Stronger*, but you do need a few items, and you should consider picking up a few others as well.

You can find links to my specific product recommendations in the free bonus material that comes with this book (www.thinnerleanerstronger.com/bonus).

1. Buy a digital food scale and learn to use its basic functions, like switching between units and taring, because you need to be precise with your food intake.

2. OPTIONAL: Buy plastic containers to store your meals.

Any kind will do, but they should be BPA-free and microwave safe and have see-through lids and compartments. You can also get small containers for snacks, glass ones instead of plastic, and mason jars for salads (that's right, entire salads, Google it!).

3. Buy a measuring tape and, if you don't have one, a digital bathroom scale.

4. OPTIONAL: Buy the supplements you're going to use (if any).

5. OPTIONAL: Buy a pair of workout gloves if you want to protect your hands.

6. OPTIONAL: Buy a pair of squat shoes for better squatting and deadlifting.

7. OPTIONAL: Buy a pair of lasso straps for better pulling.

8. OPTIONAL: Buy a pair of shin guards or a few pairs of knee-high socks for bloodless (literally) deadlifting.

9. OPTIONAL: Buy equipment for your home gym.

2. JOIN OR SET UP A GYM

Many women are turned off by gyms, and understandably so.

Between the chorus of sweaty, smelly guys grunting, groaning, and gawking; the gaggles of wannabe Instagram celebrities busily snapping selfies; and the pack of stony-faced bodybuilders laying claim to every machine in the joint, there are plenty of reasons to feel about as comfortable in a gym as you would going for a swim in the Ohio River.

I want you to be able to tune all that out, though, and to see the gym through another lens—one I describe in my book *The Little Black Book of Workout Motivation* (www.workoutmotivationbook.com):

> The gym is a lot more than a place to move, grunt, and sweat.
>
> It's a microcosm where we can make contact with the deeper parts of ourselves—our convictions, fears, habits, and anxieties. It's an arena where we can confront these opponents head-on and prove we have what it takes to vanquish them.
>
> It's a setting where we can test the stories we tell ourselves. It calls on us to demonstrate how we respond to the greater struggles of life— adversity, pain, insecurity, stress, weakness, and disadvantage—and, in some ways, who we really are. In this way, the gym is a training and testing ground for the body, mind, and soul.
>
> The conflicts we learn to endure in the gym empower us in our daily lives as well. The concentration, discipline, and resilience carry over. The way to do anything is, at bottom, the way to do everything.
>
> The gym is also a source of learning because it calls on us to constantly attempt new things. It's a forum where questions are at least as important as answers, and it cultivates what scientists call a "growth mindset" by teaching us that our abilities can be developed through dedication and hard work—a worldview that's essential for great accomplishment.
>
> The gym is practical, too, not idealistic. It's a laboratory open to all ideas and methodologies, and it gives clear, unqualified feedback on them: either they work or they don't.
>
> In short, the gym can be so much more than merely a place to work out. It can be a refuge from the chaos around us, a world of our own that we create to satisfy dreams and desires.

So, if you're on the fence about joining a gym, don't let yourself be talked or intimidated out of it. Take heart in the fact that you now know more than, well, probably everyone there, and before long, don't be surprised if people start coming to *you* for advice.

Plus, you have nothing to be self-conscious about. What many women don't realize about gyms is at least 90 percent of the people there are so intently focused on themselves that they give barely a glance to anyone around them.

Assuming I've sold you on taking the plunge, the most important things to consider when picking a gym are:

1. Does it have the equipment you'll need to do your workouts?

Just about any gym that's well stocked with free weights and machines will do.

So long as it has a few bench presses and squat racks, a full set of dumbbells, and several basic machines—and allows deadlifting (important point!)—you're golden.

2. Is it close enough that you won't have any trouble going consistently?

I've found that if going to the gym requires more than about 40 minutes of total driving, compliance tends to suffer.

So, if you can, find a gym that's close to your home or office.

3. Does it fit your budget?

As with most things, you get what you pay for. Don't spend more on a gym than you can afford, but it's a good idea to invest a little money in going to one that's clean and has nice equipment, friendly staff, and other perks like showers, towels, cardio machines (if you want to do your cardio there), etc.

Most entry-level gym memberships will cost you anywhere from $10 to $50 per month, depending on where you live. Higher-tier gym memberships will cost anywhere from $100 to $300 per month.

For entry-level gyms, your best bets are going to be Gold's Gym, 24 Hour Fitness, LA Fitness, and Anytime Fitness. For premium gyms, Equinox and Life Time Fitness are great choices.

Your other option is a home gym, and this comes with pros and cons in terms of cost effectiveness, convenience, and privacy.

On the pro side:

- You can't beat the convenience of working out in your own home, and this may make it easier to stick to the program.

- You can train whenever you want and don't need to work around holiday hours or other schedule irregularities.

- You never have to wait for someone to finish using equipment.

- You can blare your favorite music, decorate the walls however you like, and more or less turn it into your own little fitness playground.

- You save the time and money you'd have to spend commuting to and paying for a gym.

- You don't have to worry about guys ogling you or sweating all over the equipment.

And on the con side:

- You're going to pay a couple thousand dollars for nice and new equipment, which doesn't include shipping or installation fees.

  That's two years (give or take) of membership dues at a higher-end gym that costs $100 per month, like Equinox or Life Time Fitness.

- You're going to be fairly limited in the exercises you can do, and if you want to do cardio on a machine, you'll need to buy that too.

- You may enjoy your workouts less since you'll likely be alone while you train.

- You have to maintain, repair, and replace your equipment.

- You may get distracted by chores, kids, pets, your spouse or partner, etc.

Personally, I like to train at a commercial gym. It's slightly less convenient, but it allows me to do many different exercises, it helps me focus entirely on my training, I like meeting new people there, and I don't have to worry about waking up the kiddos when deadlifting.

That said, I do have a set of adjustable dumbbells and an exercise bike at home for whenever I want to sneak in some cardio and curls.

If you're going to be working out at home, then you need at least a few pieces of equipment. Here are the main ones:

POWER RACK

A power rack, also called a squat rack, is a sturdy metal frame usually about eight feet tall, four feet wide, and three to six feet long with adjustable hooks to hold a barbell and safety bars to allow for safe solo weightlifting.

Many power racks also have pegs to hold weight plates.

This is what you'll use for the squat, bench press, pull-up, and chin-up.

BARBELL

Many of the exercises in the program are going to require a barbell, so it's worth investing in a good one.

WEIGHT PLATES

You'll want to get at least two 2.5-, 5-, 10-, 25-, and 45-pound plates when you set up your home gym. You can buy more as you get stronger (most people like to add extra 10- and 45-pound plates).

Make sure you get round plates and not multi-sided ones, which shift out of position when you deadlift.

ADJUSTABLE DUMBBELLS

Adjustable dumbbells allow you to do just about any dumbbell exercise, and are much more space efficient than normal dumbbells.

BENCH

You'll need a padded, adjustable bench with wheels that can be set completely flat or upright.

This allows you to do your seated isolation exercises, and when combined with a power rack, allows you to do both flat and incline bench and dumbbell presses.

DEADLIFT PLATFORM

A deadlift platform is a metal frame that sits on the ground and holds thick tiles of rubber.

As the name suggests, a deadlift platform allows you to deadlift without damaging the floor or your equipment or making too much noise.

It's also useful for barbell rowing for the same reasons.

You don't *need* a deadlift platform, but it'll let you descend faster while deadlifting and barbell rowing, which means you won't have to waste energy slowly lowering the weights.

You may want to add a dip station as well, which allows you to do both dips and leg raises.

There are countless other tools, toys, and machines you can buy, but you'll be able to do almost all the exercises in *Thinner Leaner Stronger* with this setup.

There are a few exercises you won't be able to do, like the lat pulldown, cable fly, seated cable row, and leg press, but you can substitute them for other "approved" exercises you can do. Simply go back to chapter 23 to find alternative exercises.

All told, you'll probably need $1,000 to $3,000 (depending on what type of equipment you want) and 100 to 200 square feet to put it together. For reference, the average two-car garage is 676 square feet.

In terms of where to set up your home gym, I recommend you pick a room that has a concrete floor, like a garage or unfinished basement.

I also recommend you set up your home gym on the first floor or in the basement because working out on an upper floor—and deadlifting in particular—can scare others in the house or even damage your floor.

3. TAKE YOUR FIRST MEASUREMENTS AND PICTURES

Remember the importance of taking measurements and pictures?

If you want a refresher, go back to chapter 31. Here's a summary of what you should do:

1. Take the following body measurements first thing in the morning, nude, after using the bathroom, and before eating or drinking anything:

    - Weight
    - Waist circumference
    - Hip circumference
    - OPTIONAL: Upper-leg circumference
    - OPTIONAL: Flexed arms

    Record your numbers in your phone, workout journal, or app, or somewhere else you prefer.

2. Take flexed and unflexed pictures from the front, back, and sides, and store them in an album or folder you can easily find.

    Remember to show as much skin as you feel comfortable with. The more the better because it'll give you the best idea of how your body is changing.

4. CREATE YOUR FIRST MEAL PLAN

If you haven't done this already, it's time to use your newly acquired meal-planning skills!

You can go back to chapters 17 and 19 if you want to do an in-depth review of how to calculate calories and macros and create a meal plan, but here's a simple checklist to get you through it:

1. Calculate your daily calorie target based on your goals.
2. Calculate your daily macronutrient targets based on your goals.

3. Load the meal-planning template in the free bonus material that comes with this book (www.thinnerleanerstronger.com/bonus), open up Excel or Google Sheets, or get a paper or notebook and pen.

4. Create a list of your preferred foods and recipes.

5. Familiarize yourself with the nutritional facts of your food choices using CalorieKing, SELF Nutrition Data, or the USDA Food Composition Databases.

6. Remove from your list any foods or recipes that are too high calorie or macronutritionally imbalanced to fit your needs.

7. Set up your pre- and postworkout meals first.

8. Add your primary sources of protein to the rest of your meals.

9. Add your fruits and vegetables.

10. Add any additional carbs and caloric beverages that aren't dessert or junk.

11. Tweak your protein intake as needed.

12. Add additional fat as needed.

13. Add treats if desired.

Remember that you want to be within 50 calories of your target intake when cutting and within 100 calories when lean bulking and maintaining.

5. CREATE YOUR WORKOUT SCHEDULE

Life is hectic and it always feels like there's never enough time in the 24 hours we get each day.

As I say in my book *The Little Black Book of Workout Motivation* (www.workout-motivationbook.com):

> Who has the time for half of all the stuff we want to do? I'm sorry that life isn't gift wrapping a chunk of your days so you can train in Zen-like comfort and solitude. Join the club. Face the fact that you're going to die with a long to-do list. Make damn sure "start training" isn't on that list.

What we're really talking about here is *priorities*. We have to make our fitness a top priority and only then will we be able to "find the time" to get our workouts in.

Thankfully, we don't need to find *that* much time to make it all work. As you'll recall from chapter 29, you have three *Thinner Leaner Stronger* workout routines to choose from:

1. A five-day routine

2. A four-day routine

3. A three-day routine

Each are weekly (seven-day) routines, so the most weightlifting you can do on the program is five workouts per week. Cardio isn't explicitly included in the routines because it's optional, and how much you do depends on how much time you have to give to it and whether you're cutting, lean bulking, or maintaining.

As far as results go, the five-day routine is better than the four- and three-day routines, and the four-day routine is better than the three-day routine. That doesn't mean you can't get great results with both the four- and three-day routines, though. You absolutely can.

So, decide now which routine you're going to follow, and then choose which days you're going to lift weights on. If you're going to do cardio workouts as well, decide how you want to fit those into your weekly schedule.

Here's what your week might look like if you were to do the five-day routine plus two cardio workouts:

- Monday: Lower Body (Legs and Glutes)
- Tuesday: Push and Core
- Wednesday: Pull and Cardio
- Thursday: Upper Body and Core
- Friday: Lower Body (Legs and Glutes)
- Saturday: Cardio
- Sunday: Rest

Here's what your week might look like if you were to do the four-day routine plus two cardio workouts:

- Monday: Lower Body (Legs and Glutes)
- Tuesday: Cardio
- Wednesday: Upper Body and Core
- Thursday: Pull
- Friday: Lower Body (Legs and Glutes)
- Saturday: Cardio
- Sunday: Rest

And here's what your week might look like if you were to do the three-day routine plus two cardio workouts:

- Monday: Lower Body (Legs and Glutes)

- Tuesday: Cardio

- Wednesday: Upper Body and Core

- Thursday: Cardio

- Friday: Lower Body and Pull (Legs and Back)

- Saturday: Rest

- Sunday: Rest

6. PREPARE FOR YOUR FIRST WEEK

1. Decide when to start *Thinner Leaner Stronger*.

Mondays work best for most people as this leaves the weekend to prepare meals (if necessary).

2. Pick a day to prepare all your meals for your first week.

If you want to learn more about effective meal prepping, go to www.thinnerleanerstronger.com/mealprep.

3. Create a grocery list for everything you'll need to follow your meal plan for the first week, and then add any other items you need to buy.

4. Go grocery shopping. Buy what's on your list and nothing else.

5. OPTIONAL: Sort any snacks, treats, or calorie-dense foods you'll be tempted to overeat (nuts, dried fruit, chocolate, etc.) into smaller containers or bags.

6. Clean any tools or surfaces you'll need to prepare your meals (knives, countertops, pans, etc.).

7. Wash and chop all the foods you're going to cook.

8. Cook all your meals and store them in containers.

9. Make sure you have any supplements you're going to be taking.

10. Ensure you know exactly what you're supposed to do in your first week of workouts and that you have a way to track them (Excel or Google sheet, journal, app, or notepad).

11. Watch the form videos for all the exercises you're going to be doing in your first week, and practice the Big Three with a broomstick until you feel comfortable with the basic movements.

Remember, links to videos showing proper form can be found in the free bonus material that comes with this book (www.thinnerleanerstronger.com/bonus).

You may want to save the PDF with links to these videos on your phone so you can pull them up in the gym as needed.

12. OPTIONAL: Announce on social media that you're starting *Thinner Leaner Stronger*, tag me (@muscleforlifefitness on Instagram and @muscleforlife on Twitter), and add the #thinnerleanerstronger hashtag.

13. OPTIONAL: Join my Facebook group and introduce yourself to this community of positive, supportive, like-minded people who are striving to become the best they can be.

You can find it at www.facebook.com/groups/muscleforlife.

7. DO YOUR FIRST WEEK

In chapter 29, you learned that week one is for finding your starting weights on all the exercises you'll be doing in your first training phase.

This is mostly a matter of trial and error. You start light on an exercise, try it out, and increase the weight for each successive hard set until you've dialed in everything.

You might find that the bar alone (45 pounds) feels quite heavy on some exercises (barbell squat, for instance) and may even be too heavy for others (bench press, for example).

Don't be discouraged by this. It's completely normal. You'll gain strength quickly, and before you know it, you'll be adding weight to the bar.

In cases where the bar is too much, you have two options:

1. You can switch to a dumbbell variation of the exercise until you're strong enough for the bar.

2. You can use a fixed-weight straight bar instead, which allows for less than 45 pounds.

For instance, if the bar is too heavy for the bench press (you can't get at least six to seven reps), you can do the dumbbell bench press instead or use a fixed bar lighter than 45 pounds.

You might also find your starting weights quickly and easily and feel comfortable diving right into proper hard sets in your first workouts. If that's the case, then be my guest!

As far as your diet goes, follow your meal and supplementation plans as closely as possible. Don't make on-the-fly food substitutions; try not to undereat, overeat, or eat "off-plan" foods or meals, treats, or even condiments; and take your supplements at the same time every day (so you don't forget and establish the habit).

Also, remember to weigh yourself daily so you can calculate your average daily weight at the end of the week.

8. GET READY FOR YOUR NEXT WEEK (AND BEYOND!)

With your first week in the books, it's time to congratulate yourself for work well done and prepare for the following week (and exciting journey ahead!).

That means adjusting your meal plan as needed, repeating your grocery shopping and meal prepping, taking new measurements and pictures, calculating your average daily weight for the previous week, and ensuring you have your next week's workouts penciled into your schedule.

Then, week after week, you simply repeat this routine, keeping a close eye on how your body is responding and modifying your diet and exercise accordingly.

. . .

And just like that, you're going to be on your way to the best shape of your life.

Keep eating, training, and supplementing according to everything you've learned in this book, and it won't be a matter of *if* but only *when*.

That's not all, either. If you're like the thousands of women I've spoken and worked with over the years, *Thinner Leaner Stronger* is going to give you a lot more than a new body. It's going to give you a new lease on life.

You're going to feel strong, sexy, and competent, and it's going to shine through in everything you do, both inside and outside the gym. People are going to start noticing and asking what the heck you're doing. You might not even believe the results yourself!

All that and more will be yours, and sooner rather than later.

Before you rush off to begin, however, make sure to read the next and final part of this book, because I have a little more to share that will help speed you on your journey!

34

FROM HERE, YOUR BODY WILL CHANGE

"One is not born, but rather becomes, a woman."
—SIMONE DE BEAUVOIR

So ... I guess this is it, right? We've reached the end.

No way.

You're in a process now—and yup, it has already begun—of proving to yourself that you can transform your body faster than you ever thought possible.

In just your first three months of following my *Thinner Leaner Stronger* program, you're going to know with absolute certainty that you're on the fast track to the body of your dreams. Your self-confidence and self-esteem are going to surge, and people are going to start noticing the sparkle in your eyes.

No matter how "ordinary" you might think you are, I promise that you have what it takes to create an extraordinary body. Don't be surprised when your new-found positivity and pride start touching other areas of your life as well, inspiring you to reach for other goals and improve yourself in other ways.

As I say in my book *The Little Black Book of Workout Motivation* (www.workout-motivationbook.com), if you have the power to change your body, you have the power to change your life.

From here, all you have to do is walk the path I've laid out for you, and soon, you're going to look in the mirror and think, "I'm glad I did," not "I wish I had."

My goal is to help you reach your goals, and I know that if we work together as a team, we can and will succeed.

So, if you're ready to begin, fire up your favorite social media networks, an-nounce that you're starting *Thinner Leaner Stronger*, tag me (my information follows), and add the #thinnerleanerstronger hashtag.

Why do this? you're wondering. Three reasons:

1. It's a powerful way to "precommit" to your journey and thereby strengthen your resolve.

2. I'd love to e-meet you and keep tabs on your progress (and feature you on my website once you're ready, if you'd like!).

3. By adding the hashtag, other women looking for *Thinner Leaner Stronger* inspiration will be able to find you and follow your transformation. Who knows who you might help motivate!

You can also search this hashtag on any social media platform and see what others who are on the program are doing and sharing.

Here's how we can connect:

- Facebook: www.facebook.com/muscleforlifefitness
- Instagram: www.instagram.com/muscleforlifefitness
- YouTube: www.youtube.com/muscleforlifefitness
- Twitter: www.twitter.com/muscleforlife

I also want to invite you again to join my Facebook group because it's a community of thousands of positive, supportive, like-minded people who are striving to become the best they can be.

People who can answer your questions, push you forward, cheer your victories, and soothe your setbacks, and for whom you can do the same in return.

In short, this group is an ecosystem that exists to make personal transformation easier. Here's where you can find it:

www.facebook.com/groups/muscleforlife

All you have to do is visit that URL and click the "+ Join Group" button. One of my team members will approve your application, and then you're ready to go.

If you want to write me, my email address is mike@muscleforlife.com. Keep in mind that I get a lot of emails every day, so it may take a week or so for me to get back to you.

Also, if you've enjoyed this book and are better off in any way after reading it, please pass it on to someone you care about. Let them borrow your copy, or, better yet, get them their own as a gift and say, "I love and appreciate you and want to help you live your best life, so I got you this. Read it."

And if there are any men in your life who could use some help getting into shape, tell them about my book *Bigger Leaner Stronger*. Or just get it for them— they won't take it the wrong way!

My personal mission is to get this information into as many hands as possible, and I simply can't do that without your help. So please spread the word.

Thank you so much, and I hope to hear from you soon.

35

FREQUENTLY ASKED QUESTIONS

*"Even if you fail at your ambitious thing, it's very hard
to fail completely. That's the thing people don't get."*
—LARRY PAGE

It has been several years since I published the first edition of *Thinner Leaner Stronger*, and as of this writing, it has sold over 250,000 copies.

That's incredibly humbling, and it has allowed me to speak with a *lot* of women who have asked a lot of good questions about how to get in the best shape of their lives.

(In fact, my inbox currently has over 100,000 emails sent and received from men and women around the world.)

By this point in the book, we've covered all the most important questions, but there are still a few that might be stuck in your craw (or soon will be!) that didn't have an obvious place in this book.

Let's tackle them here.

Q: I can't find time to exercise but want to get in shape. What should I do?

A: I don't know anybody who can *find* time to exercise. I've never had anyone tell me, "Mike, I have too much free time these days. I think I'll spend a few hours in the gym every day to get in shape. What should I do while I'm there?"

It's always the opposite. Most of us lead busy, hectic lives and feel we don't have time for anything new. But in almost all cases, that just isn't true.

As much as some people would like to think they're too busy to exercise, when they analyze in detail how they actually spend their every waking minute every day, they discover how it could be worked out (no pun intended). And especially when they realize how little time it really takes to get fit!

The reality is people who have successfully transformed their bodies have the same 24 hours in a day as you and the rest of us, and they still have lives to live.

They still have to go work, spend time with their loved ones, maintain some semblance of a social life, and remember to decompress and have some fun now and then. The only difference is they've decided exercise is important enough to be in the plan.

For some, that means watching less TV or giving it up altogether. For others, it means waking up an hour earlier than normal a few days per week to get into the gym. For others still, it means handing the kids over to the husband after dinner when necessary.

My point is: if you really want to carve out an hour a few days per week to train, I'm positive you can.

Q: I'm in my 30s/40s/50s-plus. Can I do this program?

A: Absolutely.

Every week I get emailed by at least a few people asking if it's too late to build muscle and get fit.

Most are very pleasantly surprised when I explain that it's definitely *not* too late, and that I'm regularly working with guys and gals in their 40s, 50s, and even 60s who are building their best bodies ever.

How should people in their 40s and beyond go about building a great body, though? Certainly they can't eat and train like the 20-year-olds, right?

You might be surprised to learn that not nearly as much changes as people think.

One of the first things I refer people to who are worried about age squashing their dreams of being fit is a study conducted by scientists at the University of Oklahoma, which had 24 college-aged (18 to 22) and 25 middle-aged (35 to 50) men follow the same weightlifting routine for eight weeks.[1]

Researchers then analyzed everyone's body composition and found that the middle-aged men had gained just as much muscle as their college-aged counterparts had. Strength gains were very similar as well.

In my experience, this is equally true for women. Middle age isn't a physiological strikeout, even when compared to your 20s. You can do just fine.

People in their 60s and beyond aren't left out of the party, either. Studies show that they too can gain significant amounts of muscle and strength, and more importantly, that training and developing their muscles is a great way to fight the "dwindling health spiral" normally associated with aging.[2]

There are two other age-related myths I'd like to debunk. The first is the claim that your metabolism craters as you get older. This is *very* fake news.

Research shows that the average adult's metabolism slows by just 1 to 3 percent per decade and that the primary reason for this is muscle loss, not genetic programming.[3]

Therefore, if you maintain your muscle as you age, you maintain your metabolism. And if you add muscle to your frame, you can increase it.[4]

Why do so many people gain weight as they get older, then?

For most, it's mainly a matter of lifestyle. They were far more active when they were younger, which allowed them to eat far more food without gaining any weight to speak of. Now, however, they're mostly sedentary, which makes it very easy to overeat.

So, unless you've lost significant amounts of muscle over the years from things like frenzied starvation dieting or excessive cardio, your metabolism is just fine. And even if you have made those mistakes, you can correct them now with proper diet and training.

The second myth is the old saw about your hormones imploding as you get older.

It was once believed that the hormonal disturbance associated with aging was inevitable. We now know this isn't true. Research shows that lifestyle factors are equally causative of hormonal changes as aging itself, if not more so.

For example, here's a short list of the biggest lifestyle factors that can disrupt estrogen, progesterone, follicle-stimulating hormone, sex hormone binding globulin, and more:

- Weight gain[5]
- Stopping exercise[6]
- Chronic illness[7]
- Sleeping too little[8]
- Moderate alcohol consumption[9]

These are all under your control. Your hormone health truly is in your hands.

For example, studies show that there are plenty of ways to naturally improve your hormone profile, including staying lean, doing regular resistance training, and maintaining good sleep hygiene.[10]

You'll also be happy to know you don't need stellar hormone levels to get fit. If you're willing to work hard, you can have below-average hormones and a far-above-average physique.

All that said, there are several key differences between college-aged and middle-aged bodies that make fitness a little harder as you get older.

Research shows that after about age 50, your muscles recover slower from exercise and that you begin to lose muscle over time (if you don't do anything to stop it).[11]

Your tendons and ligaments also become stiffer and recover slower, which can increase the risk of injury.[12]

Overall, though, the science is clear: you can stay in remarkably good shape well into old age if you stay active and take care of your body, and that's just as true for women as it is for men.[13]

How do you do that, though? You just have to make some adjustments to your training protocols and take some extra measures to ensure adequate recovery.

Let's go over the major points here.

Be a stickler for form (especially if you're new to weightlifting).

The older you get, the less shenanigans you can get away with in your weightlifting.

Lumbar rounding in your deadlifts … knee bowing in your squats … elbow flaring in your bench pressing … it all increases the risk of injury at any age, but it becomes more dangerous as the years go by.

This is one of the reasons why I put a lot of emphasis on learning and using proper form from day one, regardless of age or fitness level.

It's also why I'm not willing to sacrifice form to hit PRs and chest bump with my buddies. I'm willing to give sets everything I've got, but if I'm going for a big pull and feel my lower-back rounding, I drop the weight. If I'm squatting and deep into my set, I simply can't keep my shoulders rising with my hips, I set the weight down on the safety arms.

I'm not a competitive powerlifter or strength athlete. I like lifting heavy things and being strong, but I like staying healthy and injury-free more. I suspect you're in the same boat.

Make sure you take at least one day off the weights each week. Two is better.

Don't underestimate how taxing heavy weightlifting is on your body. Even the young'uns can't do it every day, week after week, without eventually running themselves into the ground.

Train hard six or seven days per week, and physical fatigue will start accumulating. Your sleep will deteriorate. Your workouts will suffer. You'll continue feeling worse and worse until you rein it in and give your body more time to rest.

That's why a big part of proper recovery is taking time off the weights every week and resisting the urge to replace weightlifting with some other form of intense physical exercise or activity.

Depending on your goals, that may mean you have to eat less than you'd like on your rest days. That's just part of the game.

Don't fall into the trap of using exercise as a way to eat more and more food. That's a one-way street to overtraining, not to mention life and psychological imbalances.

Forcing yourself to do excessive amounts of exercise just so you can gorge on food is a terrible use of time and great way to develop anxiety or even eating disorders.

Rest or deload more frequently.

Even when you're properly managing your workout volume and intensity and taking a couple of days off each week, your body eventually needs a bigger break. And the older you are, the sooner that time comes.

Specifically, what I've found is while guys and gals in their 20s can go anywhere from 12 to 15 weeks or longer before needing additional recovery time, people in their 40s and 50s need it more frequently, sometimes as often as every 4 to 6 weeks.

There are many factors that determine how long you'll be able to go before needing additional rest—age, training programming and history, genetics, sleep hygiene, diet, etc.—but it's pretty easy to discover for yourself.

As you continue to train and progress, you'll start noticing symptoms like worse sleep, lower energy levels, aches and pains, and less interest in training. Deload the following week, and they should disappear.

Many people mistake these symptoms as mental obstacles to push through and try to fight fire with fire. It doesn't go well. Listen to your body, play the long game, and play it intelligently.

Q: What should I do when I'm on or about to get on my period?

A: You don't have to change anything.

Most women doing my *Thinner Leaner Stronger* program follow the same meal and exercise plans throughout their menstrual cycles without a problem.

That said, research suggests that when cutting, you may be able to lose slightly more weight if you modify your diet to coincide with the different phases of the menstrual cycle.[14]

As your cycle progresses, your body becomes more efficient at burning fat and less efficient at burning carbs. When cutting, some women like to use this to their advantage by decreasing carbohydrate and increasing dietary fat intake during the last two weeks of their cycles (two weeks before their next periods). Protein intake shouldn't change, however.

Many women also experience cravings in the week or so preceding their periods. A simple way to deal with this is adjusting your meal plan to include more treats if needed.

Finally, you may find that you don't have quite as much energy immediately before and during your period. Schedule deloads and rest weeks during these times whenever possible.

Q: I'm pregnant or nursing. Can I do this program?

A: Definitely!

In fact, research shows that women who stay active and follow a healthy diet during pregnancy are at a lower risk of excessive gestational weight gain and conditions such as gestational diabetes, preeclampsia, preterm birth, varicose veins, and deep vein thrombosis.[15]

During most of your pregnancy, you can eat and exercise more or less exactly as laid out in this book. That said, there are some things you should keep in mind.

First, regarding your diet:

1. Don't try to lose weight during your pregnancy.

This can compromise the health of your baby. It's better to limit excessive weight gain during pregnancy and then focus on losing weight afterward.

2. You don't need to eat much more than when you're not pregnant.

The National Institutes of Health recommends that you eat maintenance calories during your first trimester, add 340 calories to your daily intake (total daily energy expenditure + 340) during the second trimester, and add another 110 calories to your daily intake (TDEE + 450) during the third trimester.[16]

3. You want to keep eating mostly whole, minimally processed, nutritious foods.

It's fine to sneak in a few more treats here and there, but you should still get at least 80 percent of your calories from healthy foods.

As far as training goes, you can follow any of the *Thinner Leaner Stronger* workout routines while pregnant, but you should make the following modifications:

1. Stay at least three to four reps short of technical failure for all your sets.

Research shows that strength training appears to be just as safe as cardio during pregnancy, but it's probably not a good idea to push your physical limits while pregnant.[17]

2. Do at least 30 minutes of exercise per day.

Recommendations vary, but most medical institutions agree that this is a good minimum.[18] A simple way to hit this number is to go on an easy walk on the days you don't lift weights.

3. Don't use the Valsalva maneuver or do direct core or ab exercises.

There's no evidence the Valsalva maneuver is dangerous, but it's not worth the risk until we know more about how this might affect pregnant women.[19]

Core and ab exercises may increase the risk of diastasis recti and pelvic floor issues, so it's best to avoid these exercises during and immediately after pregnancy.

Q: I have pelvic floor or diastasis issues. What should I do?

A: Diastasis recti is a condition in which the connective tissue between the two vertical walls of the rectus abdominis becomes overstretched, causing an abnormal amount of separation between them.

Research shows that about 60 percent of women experience diastasis recti after pregnancy and about 30 percent still have it a year after giving birth.[20]

A similar and related problem is stretching in the pelvic floor muscles, which are the muscles that surround the base of the pelvis and the vagina.

These muscles can become stretched during pregnancy, which some experts believe can lead to back pain, incontinence, and prolapse (a condition in which an organ in your pelvis, like your uterus, bladder, or rectum, slips into the vaginal canal and feels like it's going to "fall out").

There's no official diagnosis for "pelvic floor issues," so there's no way to know how common it is.

There are many theories on what you can do to fix diastasis recti and pelvic floor problems, and both do seem to be largely correctable.

One of the most promising solutions is an exercise program created by scientists at Weill Cornell Medical College targeted at strengthening the transverse abdominis and muscles of the pelvic floor.

In one 12-week experiment of theirs, this program reduced diastasis recti in all 63 of the participants.[21]

This routine has been adapted into a series of workouts called *Every Mother* (www.every-mother.com) that you can do if you're dealing with diastasis recti or pelvic floor issues.

Most experts also agree that you should avoid core and ab exercises during and immediately after pregnancy, as well as exercises that have you on all fours or on your back after your first trimester.

Q: If I cut first will I sacrifice my newbie gains?

A: To some degree, yes.

If you start the program with cutting, you're going to gain less muscle and strength during that period than you would by starting with lean bulking or maintaining.

That said, thanks to newbie gains, you can still gain a significant amount of muscle and strength while cutting when you start out—far more than later, when you're a more experienced weightlifter.

Then, when you've completed your first cut, you can switch to lean bulking or maintaining and reap more muscle-building benefits from whatever is left of your "honeymoon phase."

Q. How do I switch from cutting to maintaining or lean bulking?

A. To go from cutting to maintaining, simply increase your calories to about 90 percent of your average TDEE (as calculated per the methods in chapter 17), and set up your macros for maintenance (30 percent protein, 45 percent carbohydrate, and 25 percent dietary fat).

You can expect to gain weight for the first week or two mostly due to the increase in carbohydrate intake, not body fat. After that your weight should stabilize.

To go from cutting to lean bulking, first increase your calories to about 90% of your average TDEE and set up your macros for maintenance. Then, after three or four weeks of this, increase your calories to 110 percent of your average TDEE and switch to lean bulking macros (25 percent protein, 55 percent carbohydrate, and 20 percent dietary fat).

Q: I travel a lot. Can I follow this program?

A: Yes, but it'll require some forethought.

First, you'll want to book hotels that are close to adequate gyms (hotel gyms suck), and you'll want to plan ahead to determine when you'll work out (early in the morning or after dinner works best for most people).

Second, you have three options for your diet:

1. You can make a meal plan of simple foods that you can pick up at a local grocery store and store and prepare in your hotel room.

Good choices include salad, deli meat, rotisserie chicken, fruit, nuts, and the like. A grocery delivery service like Instacart (www.instacart.com) can be incredibly helpful here.

2. You can track food intake on the go with an app like MyFitnessPal.

3. You can eat according to your appetite and do your best to keep your calorie and macro intakes in check.

If you travel a lot and still want to make good progress, options one and two are your best bets. Option three works fine for the occasional short trip but not for regular travelers.

Q: I'm not getting very sore. Is that a problem?

A: I used to think that perpetual muscle soreness was a price you had to pay to build muscle.

In time, I almost thought of this as a badge of honor. ("Damn straight I have to walk down stairs backwards! My legs are going to be HUGE!")

I assumed a major reason we trained our muscles was to damage them, which resulted in soreness. Therefore, considerable soreness meant considerable damage that would hopefully lead to considerable muscle gain, right?

Not quite.

Research shows that muscle damage may contribute to muscle growth but isn't a requirement.[22] This is why workouts that produce large amounts of muscle soreness won't necessarily result in muscle growth, and workouts that produce very little soreness can result in significant muscle growth.[23]

For instance, an hour of downhill running can produce a tremendous amount of muscle soreness in your legs, but it isn't going to do much toward building strong, toned leg muscles.[24]

Similarly, modifying your workouts to produce more muscle damage can cause significantly more muscle soreness, but doesn't necessarily result in more muscle growth.[25]

Several other observations provide more evidence of the disconnect between muscle soreness and muscle building:

- People who train infrequently build far less muscle but experience far more muscle soreness than those who train more frequently.

- Muscle soreness generally decreases as training frequency increases, which can accelerate muscle growth.

- Muscles like the shoulders and calves generally don't get very sore from training but can grow substantially.

Further complicating matters is the fact that the degree of muscle soreness you experience after workouts isn't a reliable indicator of the degree of muscle damage caused.[26]

In other words, a high or low amount of muscle soreness doesn't necessarily reflect a high or low amount of muscle damage.

To quote scientists at Yokohama City University who examined the relationship between strength training and muscle soreness:

> Because of generally poor correlations between DOMS [delayed onset muscle soreness] and other indicators, we conclude that use of DOMS is a poor reflector of eccentric exercise-induced muscle damage and inflammation, and changes in indirect markers of muscle damage and inflammation are not necessarily accompanied with DOMS.[27]

That is, damaged muscles won't necessarily hurt, and muscles that hurt aren't necessarily much damaged.

The physiology of these phenomena isn't fully understood yet, but one study conducted by scientists at Concordia University found that at least some of the pain we're feeling in muscle soreness stems from the connective tissue holding muscle fibers together, not from the actual fibers themselves.[28]

Therefore, what you think is "muscle soreness" is at least partially (if not mostly) "connective tissue" soreness.

And while we're on the topic of muscle soreness, we might as well tackle another common question:

Can you train muscles that are still sore from a previous workout?

Yes, you can.

Despite what you've probably heard, training sore muscles doesn't necessarily hinder recovery and prevent muscle growth.[29]

That said, regardless of the presence or absence of muscle soreness, intense workouts do cause muscle damage that must be repaired before the muscles are ready for another round.

That's one of the reasons why training too intensely too frequently can impair your progress.

Q: Should I exercise when I'm sick?

A: No. At least not intensely.

I totally understand the desire to exercise when sick. Once you've established a good workout routine, skipping days can be harder than going to the gym even when you're not feeling well.

Force yourself to rest, though, because your normal workouts are only going to make things worse by temporarily depressing immune function.[30]

That said, animal research shows that light exercise (20 to 30 minutes of light jogging on a treadmill) while infected with the influenza virus boosts immune function and speeds recovery.[31] Similar effects have been seen in human studies as well.[32]

Human research also shows that light exercise like walking or jogging doesn't impair immune function or prolong or worsen infections.[33]

So if you're going to do any exercise while under the weather, make it 20 minutes or so of very light cardio (you should never get too winded to speak comfortably).

Q: I only have dumbbells. Can I do the program?

A: Kind of.

You can't do the program exactly as I've laid it out because there are no great dumbbell substitutions for some of the exercises, but you can still use a lot of what you've learned to create effective dumbbell workouts.

To do this, you have the dumbbell exercises I've provided you with, but those won't be enough for all the major muscle groups. Here's a more extensive list of dumbbell and bodyweight exercises to choose from:

LEGS

Goblet Squat

Dumbbell Squat

Dumbbell Romanian Deadlift

Dumbbell Lunge (Walking or In-Place, Forward or Reverse)

Nordic Hamstring Curl

GLUTES

Dumbbell Hip Thrust

Dumbbell Glute Bridge

Dumbbell Step-Up

CORE

Captain's Chair Leg Raise

Lying Leg Raise

Hanging Leg Raise

Crunch

Weighted Sit-Up

Plank

Abdominal Rollout

Dumbbell Weighted Crunch

Dumbbell Weighted Sit-Up

Dumbbell Leg Raise

ARMS

Dumbbell Curl

Dumbbell Hammer Curl

Dumbbell Triceps Kickback

Dumbbell Lying Triceps Extension (Skullcrusher)

SHOULDERS

Seated Dumbbell Press

Dumbbell Side Lateral Raise

Dumbbell Rear Lateral Raise

CHEST

Dumbbell Bench Press

Incline Dumbbell Bench Press

Dumbbell Fly

Dumbbell Pullover

Dumbbell Floor Press

BACK

Dumbbell Deadlift

One-Arm Dumbbell Row

Band-Supported Chin-Up

Inverted Row

And as far as workouts go, here's a training phase to get you started:

FIVE-DAY ROUTINE

WORKOUT 1

LOWER BODY (LEGS AND GLUTES)

Goblet Squat: Warm-up and 3 hard sets

Dumbbell Lunge (In-Place): 3 hard sets

Dumbbell Romanian Deadlift: 3 hard sets

Dumbbell Hip Thrust: 3 hard sets

WORKOUT 2

PUSH AND CORE

Dumbbell Bench Press: Warm-up and 3 hard sets

Seated Dumbbell Press: 3 hard sets

Dumbbell Side Lateral Raise: 3 hard sets

Crunch: 3 hard sets

WORKOUT 3

PULL

Dumbbell Deadlift: Warm-up and 3 hard sets

One-Arm Dumbbell Row: 3 hard sets

Band-Supported Chin-Up: 3 hard sets

Dumbbell Curl: 3 hard sets

WORKOUT 4

UPPER BODY AND CORE

Seated Dumbbell Press: Warm-up and 3 hard sets
Dumbbell Rear Lateral Raise: 3 hard sets
Seated Triceps Press: 3 hard sets
Lying Leg Raise: 3 hard sets

WORKOUT 5

LOWER BODY (LEGS AND GLUTES)

Goblet Squat: Warm-up and 3 hard sets
Dumbbell Step-Up: 3 hard sets
Dumbbell Romanian Deadlift: 3 hard sets
Dumbbell Hip Thrust: 3 hard sets

FOUR-DAY ROUTINE

WORKOUT 1

LOWER BODY (LEGS AND GLUTES)

Goblet Squat: Warm-up and 3 hard sets
Dumbbell Lunge (In-Place): 3 hard sets
Dumbbell Romanian Deadlift: 3 hard sets
Dumbbell Hip Thrust: 3 hard sets

WORKOUT2

UPPER BODY AND CORE

Dumbbell Bench Press: Warm-up and 3 hard sets
Dumbbell Side Lateral Raise: 3 hard sets
Seated Triceps Press: 3 hard sets
Crunch: 3 hard sets

WORKOUT 3

PULL

Dumbbell Deadlift: Warm-up and 3 hard sets
One-Arm Dumbbell Row: 3 hard sets
Band-Supported Chin-Up: 3 hard sets
Dumbbell Curl: 3 hard sets

WORKOUT 4

LOWER BODY (LEGS AND GLUTES)

Goblet Squat: Warm-up and 3 hard sets
Dumbbell Step-Up: 3 hard sets
Dumbbell Romanian Deadlift: 3 hard sets
Dumbbell Hip Thrust: 3 hard sets

THREE-DAY ROUTINE

WORKOUT 1

LOWER BODY (LEGS AND GLUTES)

Goblet Squat: Warm-up and 3 hard sets
Dumbbell Lunge (In-Place): 3 hard sets
Dumbbell Romanian Deadlift: 3 hard sets
Dumbbell Hip Thrust: 3 hard sets

WORKOUT 2

UPPER BODY AND CORE

Dumbbell Bench Press: Warm-up and 3 hard sets
Dumbbell Side Lateral Raise: 3 hard sets
Seated Triceps Press: 3 hard sets
Crunch: 3 hard sets

WORKOUT 3

LOWER BODY AND PULL (LEGS AND BACK)

Dumbbell Squat: Warm-up and 3 hard sets

Dumbbell Deadlift: Warm-up and 3 hard sets

One-Arm Dumbbell Row: 3 hard sets

Band-Supported Chin-Up: 3 hard sets

Dumbbell Curl: 3 hard sets

36

WOULD YOU DO ME A FAVOR?

"Taking joy in living is a woman's best cosmetic."
—ROSALIND RUSSELL

Thank you for reading *Thinner Leaner Stronger*. I hope you'll use what you've learned to look, feel, and live better than you ever have before.

I have a small favor to ask.

Would you mind taking a minute to write a blurb on Amazon about this book? I check all my reviews and love to get honest feedback. That's the real pay for my work—knowing that I'm helping people.

To leave me a review, you can:

1. Pull up Amazon on your web browser, search for "thinner leaner stronger," click on the book, and scroll down and click on the "Write a customer review" button.

2. Visit www.thinnerleanerstronger.com/review and you'll be automatically forwarded to Amazon to leave a review.

Thanks again, and I look forward to reading your feedback!

FREE BONUS
MATERIAL

WORKOUTS, MEAL PLANS, AND MORE!

Thank you for reading *Thinner Leaner Stronger*.

I hope you've found it insightful, inspiring, and practical, and I hope it helps you build that lean, sculpted, and strong body you really desire.

I want to make sure that you get as much value from this book as possible, so I've put together a number of additional free resources to help you, including:

• A savable, shareable, printable reference guide with all of this book's key takeaways, checklists, and action items.

• Links to form demonstration videos for all *Thinner Leaner Stronger* exercises.

• An entire year's worth of *Thinner Leaner Stronger* workouts neatly laid out and provided in several formats, including PDF, Excel, and Google Sheets.

If you'd prefer the workouts in a digital or hardcopy book, check out *The Year One Challenge for Women* (www.thinnerleanerstronger.com/challenge).

• 10 *Thinner Leaner Stronger* meal plans that make losing fat and gaining lean muscle as simple as possible.

• A list of my favorite tools for getting and staying motivated and on track inside and outside of the gym.

• And more.

To get instant access to all of those free bonuses (plus a few additional surprise gifts), go here now:

www.thinnerleanerstronger.com/bonus

Also, if you have any questions or run into any difficulties, just shoot me an e-mail at mike@muscleforlife.com and I'll do my best to help!

DO YOU WANT ONE-ON-ONE COACHING?

Why do you want to get fit?

Sure, there's the obvious—great biceps, butts, and abs are kind of neat—but methinks it goes deeper than that.

What are the "benefits of the benefits" you're after?

Do you want to wear the clothes you really want to wear? And look fantastic when you take them off?

Do you want to be a better role model for your family and friends and promote healthy living?

Do you want more intimacy in your relationships and better sex?

Do you want more confidence and self-esteem?

Do you want to be able to play with your kids without getting winded?

Do you want to jump out of bed every morning with more energy, enthusiasm, and vitality?

Or maybe you just want to stop stressing over what you see in the mirror every day and finally be comfortable in your own skin?

Whatever your reasons are, I want you to know this:

My reason for doing everything I do is to help you make your reasons a reality.

The real pay for my work isn't dollars and cents or even seeing people with leaner and more muscular bodies. It's the way I'm helping them change their lives for the better. That's priceless.

That's why I continue to write books and articles and record podcasts and videos, and why I'm always trying to push my work to the next level.

That's also why I offer a VIP one-on-one coaching service, which I'm extremely proud of.

In just a few short years, we've worked with over 450 men and women of all ages and circumstances and helped them do a lot more than lose a bunch of fat and gain a bunch of strength and muscle.

- We've helped them skyrocket their grades and productivity.

- We've helped them achieve promotions at work.

- We've helped them rekindle their love lives and even save their marriages.

- We've helped them break food, drug, and alcohol addictions.

- We've helped them form deeper bonds with friends and family.

- We've helped them reverse and resolve health conditions and ditch medications.

- And so much more ...

One of our clients, Esther (30), is a perfect example of what you can accomplish when experts do all the thinking for you and make your dieting and training paint-by-numbers simple.

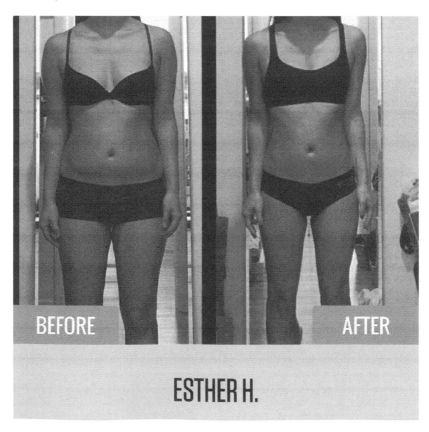

BEFORE   AFTER

ESTHER H.

As you can see, she dramatically improved her body composition, but she also gained a tremendous amount of strength.

For instance, when she started with us, she was deadlifting just the bar, and by the end of her 90-day coaching experience, she was close to her body weight for reps.

I'm also really proud of Chandler (55), who dropped nearly 14 pounds, 6 percent body fat, and two dress sizes in just three months:

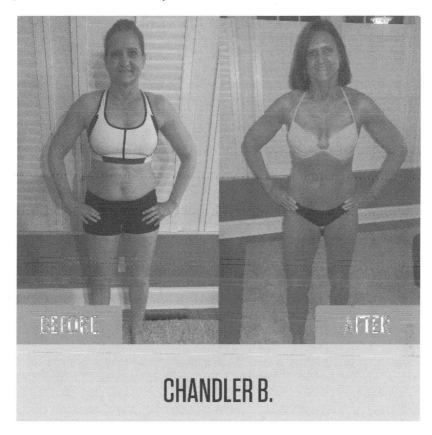

CHANDLER B.

"It took a couple of weeks to kick in," she told me afterward, "but when it did, I saw progress every week, both in my body composition and the weight I was lifting."

Cassandra (38) also killed it, reducing her waist size by five inches and weight by 25 pounds in 12 weeks. Since a picture is worth a thousand words and all that:

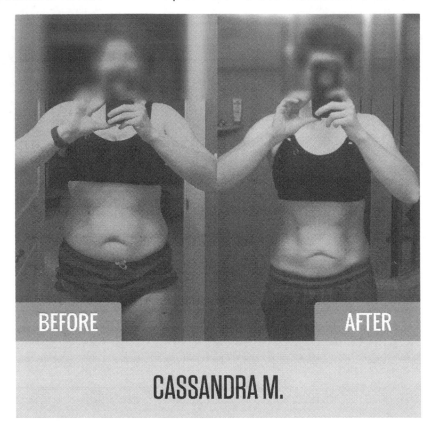

"I'm definitely more confident and feeling better about myself," she said afterward. "I'm feeling just better overall. I definitely have more energy and determination."

Now, what about YOU?

Do you want to make this the year you finally get super fit?

Are you ready to transform YOUR body and life?

If so, you need to visit the following URL and schedule your free consultation call to see if my coaching service is right for you:

Go here now: www.muscleforlife.com/coaching

You have to hurry, though, because my coaches are always in high demand and availability is always limited.

This will NOT be a high-pressure sales call, by the way. It's a friendly chat to learn where you're at, where you've been, and where you want to go, and then determine whether the service is right for you.

You should also know that this service comes with a very simple money-back guarantee:

Either you love the experience and are thrilled with your results, or you get every penny you've paid back.

That's how much confidence I have in my team's ability to help you get great results.

So, take the first step in your journey to a fitter, happier, and healthier you. Go to www.muscleforlife.com/coaching and schedule your call now.

OTHER BOOKS BY MICHAEL MATTHEWS

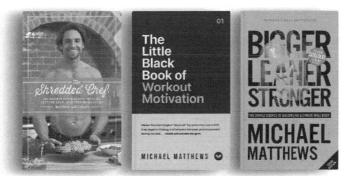

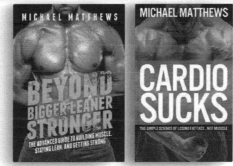

The Shredded Chef: 125 Recipes for Building Muscle, Getting Lean, and Staying Healthy

The Little Black Book of Workout Motivation

Bigger Leaner Stronger: The Simple Science of Building the Ultimate Male Body

Beyond Bigger Leaner Stronger: The Advanced Guide to Building Muscle, Staying Lean, and Getting Strong

Cardio Sucks: The Simple Science of Losing Fat Fast ... Not Muscle

REFERENCES

CHAPTER 5

WHAT MOST WOMEN WILL NEVER KNOW ABOUT GETTING FIT
– PART 1

1.   Bianconi E, Piovesan A, Facchin F, et al. An estimation of the number of cells in the human body. Ann Hum Biol. 2013;40(6):463-471. doi:10.3109/03014460.2013.807878.

CHAPTER 7

THE 10 ABSOLUTE WORST FAT LOSS MYTHS AND MISTAKES

1.   Park M. Twinkie diet helps nutrition professor lose 27 pounds. CNN Website. http://www.cnn.com/2010/HEALTH/11/08/twinkie.diet.professor/index.html. November 8, 2010. Accessed August 15, 2018.

2.   Peterson H. A teacher who lost 56 pounds eating only McDonald's is starring in a documentary to show kids about 'healthy' eating. Business Insider Website. https://www.businessinsider.com/how-to-lose-weight-eating-only-mcdonalds-2015-10. October 13, 2015. Accessed August 15, 2018.

3.   Innes E. Fitness fanatic claims to be in the best shape of his life despite only eating MCDONALD'S for a month. Daily Mail Website. http://www.dailymail.co.uk/health/article-2643936/Fitness-fanatic-claims-best-shape-life-despite-ONLY-eating-McDonalds.html. May 30, 2014. Accessed August 15, 2018.

4.   Romieu I, Dossus L, Barquera S, et al. Energy balance and obesity: what are the main drivers? *Cancer Causes Control.* 2017;28(3):247-258. doi:10.1007/s10552-017-0869-z.

5.   Lean MEJ, Astrup A, Roberts SB. Making progress on the global crisis of obesity and weight management. *BMJ.* 2018;361:k2538. doi:10.1136/BMJ.K2538.

6.   Johnston CS, Tjonn SL, Swan PD, White A, Hutchins H, Sears B. Ketogenic low-carbohydrate diets have no metabolic advantage over nonketogenic low-carbohydrate diets. *Am J Clin Nutr.* 2006;83(5):1055-1061. doi:10.1093/ajcn/83.5.1055.

7.   Phillips SA, Jurva JW, Syed AQ, et al. Benefit of Low-Fat Over Low-Carbohydrate Diet on Endothelial Health in Obesity. *Hypertension.* 2008;51(2):376-382. doi:10.1161/HYPERTENSIONAHA.107.101824.

8.   Sacks FM, Bray GA, Carey VJ, et al. Comparison of Weight-Loss Diets with Different Compositions of Fat, Protein, and Carbohydrates. *N Engl J Med.* 2009;360(9):859-873. doi:10.1056/NEJMoa0804748.

9.   Gardner CD, Trepanowski JF, Del Gobbo LC, et al. Effect of Low-Fat vs Low-Carbohydrate Diet on 12-Month Weight Loss in Overweight Adults and the Association With Genotype Pattern or Insulin Secretion. *JAMA.* 2018;319(7):667. doi:10.1001/jama.2018.0245.

10.   Surwit RS, Feinglos MN, McCaskill CC, et al. Metabolic and behavioral effects of a high-sucrose diet during weight loss. *Am J Clin Nutr.* 1997;65(4):908-915. doi:10.1093/ajcn/65.4.908.

11.   West J, de Looy A. Weight loss in overweight subjects following low-sucrose or sucrose-containing diets. *Int J Obes.* 2001;25(8):1122-1128. doi:10.1038/sj.ijo.0801652.

12. Cook A, Pryer J, Shetty P. The problem of accuracy in dietary surveys. Analysis of the over 65 UK National Diet and Nutrition Survey. *J Epidemiol Community Health*. 2000;54(8):611-616.

13. Buhl KM, Gallagher D, Hoy K, Matthews DE, Heymsfield SB. Unexplained Disturbance in Body Weight Regulation. *J Am Diet Assoc*. 1995;95(12):1393-1400. doi:10.1016/S0002-8223(95)00367-3.

14. Urban LE, Dallal GE, Robinson LM, Ausman LM, Saltzman E, Roberts SB. The Accuracy of Stated Energy Contents of Reduced-Energy, Commercially Prepared Foods. *J Am Diet Assoc*. 2010;110(1):116-123. doi:10.1016/j.jada.2009.10.003.

15. CFR - Code of Federal Regulations Title 21. U.S. Food & Drug Administration Website. https://www.accessdata.fda.gov/scripts/cdrh/cfdocs/cfcfr/CFRSearch.cfm?fr=101.9. April 1, 2017. Accessed August 15, 2018.

16. Horton TJ, Drougas H, Brachey A, Reed GW, Peters JC, Hill JO. Fat and carbohydrate overfeeding in humans: different effects on energy storage. *Am J Clin Nutr*. 1995;62(1):19-29. doi:10.1093/ajcn/62.1.19.

17. Westerterp-Plantenga MS, Nieuwenhuizen A, Tomé D, Soenen S, Westerterp KR. Dietary Protein, Weight Loss, and Weight Maintenance. *Annu Rev Nutr*. 2009;29(1):21-41. doi:10.1146/annurev-nutr-080508-141056.

18. Horton TJ, Drougas H, Brachey A, Reed GW, Peters JC, Hill JO. Fat and carbohydrate overfeeding in humans: different effects on energy storage. *Am J Clin Nutr*. 1995;62(1):19-29. doi:10.1093/ajcn/62.1.19; Leaf A, Antonio J. The Effects of Overfeeding on Body Composition: The Role of Macronutrient Composition - A Narrative Review. *Int J Exerc Sci*. 2017;10(8):1275-1296.

19. Siler SQ, Neese RA, Hellerstein MK. De novo lipogenesis, lipid kinetics, and whole-body lipid balances in humans after acute alcohol consumption. *Am J Clin Nutr*. 1999;70(5):928-936. doi:10.1093/ajcn/70.5.928; Shelmet JJ, Reichard GA, Skutches CL, Hoeldtke RD, Owen OE, Boden G. Ethanol causes acute inhibition of carbohydrate, fat, and protein oxidation and insulin resistance. *J Clin Invest*. 1988;81(4):1137-1145. doi:10.1172/JCI113428.

20. Stallknecht B, Dela F, Helge JW. Are blood flow and lipolysis in subcutaneous adipose tissue influenced by contractions in adjacent muscles in humans? *Am J Physiol Metab*. 2007;292(2):E394-E399. doi:10.1152/ajpendo.00215.2006.

21. Kostek MA, Pescatello LS, Seip RL, et al. Subcutaneous Fat Alterations Resulting from an Upper-Body Resistance Training Program. *Med Sci Sport Exerc*. 2007;39(7):1177-1185. doi:10.1249/mss.0b0138058a5cb.

22. Vispute SS, Smith JD, LeCheminant JD, Hurley KS. The Effect of Abdominal Exercise on Abdominal Fat. *J Strength Cond Res*. 2011;25(9):2559-2564. doi:10.1519/JSC.0b013e3181fb4a46.

23. Leibel RL, Rosenbaum M, Hirsch J. Changes in Energy Expenditure Resulting from Altered Body Weight. *N Engl J Med*. 1995;332(10):621-628. doi:10.1056/NEJM199503093321001; Camps SG, Verhoef SP, Westerterp KR. Weight loss, weight maintenance, and adaptive thermogenesis. *Am J Clin Nutr*. 2013;97(5):990-994. doi:10.3945/ajcn.112.050310; Zinchenko A. Metabolic Damage: do Negative Metabolic Adaptations During Underfeeding Persist After Refeeding in Non-Obese Populations? *Med Res Arch*. 2016;4(8). doi:10.18103/mra.v4i8.908.

24. Bryner RW, Ullrich IH, Sauers J, et al. Effects of resistance vs. aerobic training combined with an 800 calorie liquid diet on lean body mass and resting metabolic rate. *J Am Coll Nutr*. 1999;18(2):115-121.

25. University of Minnesota. Laboratory of Physiological Hygiene., Keys A, Simonson E, Sturgeon Skinner A, Wells SM, University of Minnesota. Laboratory of Physiological Hygiene. *The Biology of Human Starvation*. University of Minnesota Press; 1950.

26. Zinchenko A. Metabolic Damage: do Negative Metabolic Adaptations During Underfeeding Persist After Refeeding in Non-Obese Populations? *Med Res Arch*. 2016;4(8). doi:10.18103/mra.v4i8.908.

27. Bellisle F, McDevitt R, Prentice AM. Meal frequency and energy balance. *Br J Nutr*. 1997;77 Suppl 1:S57-70.

28. Cameron JD, Cyr M-J, Doucet É. Increased meal frequency does not promote greater weight loss in subjects who were prescribed an 8-week equi-energetic energy-restricted diet. *Br J Nutr*. 2009;103(8):1. doi:10.1017/S0007114509992984.

29. Leidy HJ, Tang M, Armstrong CLH, Martin CB, Campbell WW. The Effects of Consuming Frequent, Higher Protein Meals on Appetite and Satiety During Weight Loss in Overweight/Obese Men. *Obesity*. 2011;19(4):818-824. doi:10.1038/oby.2010.203.

30. Leidy HJ, Armstrong CLH, Tang M, Mattes RD, Campbell WW. The Influence of Higher Protein Intake and Greater Eating Frequency on Appetite Control in Overweight and Obese Men. *Obesity*. 2010;18(9):1725-1732. doi:10.1038/oby.2010.45.

31. Leidy HJ, Campbell WW. The Effect of Eating Frequency on Appetite Control and Food Intake: Brief Synopsis of Controlled Feeding Studies. *J Nutr.* 2011;141(1):154-157. doi:10.3945/jn.109.114389.

32. Ballor DL, Katch VL, Becque MD, Marks CR. Resistance weight training during caloric restriction enhances lean body weight maintenance. *Am J Clin Nutr.* 1988;47(1):19-25. doi:10.1093/ajcn/47.1.19.

33. Bryner RW, Ullrich IH, Sauers J, et al. Effects of resistance vs. aerobic training combined with an 800 calorie liquid diet on lean body mass and resting metabolic rate. *J Am Coll Nutr.* 1999;18(2):115-121.

34. Walberg JL. Aerobic exercise and resistance weight-training during weight reduction. Implications for obese persons and athletes. *Sports Med.* 1989;7(6):343-356; Stiegler P, Cunliffe A. The role of diet and exercise for the maintenance of fat-free mass and resting metabolic rate during weight loss. *Sports Med.* 2006;36(3):239-262; Ballor DL, Katch VL, Becque MD, Marks CR. Resistance weight training during caloric restriction enhances lean body weight maintenance. *Am J Clin Nutr.* 1988;47(1):19-25. doi:10.1093/ajcn/47.1.19.

35. Sawyer BJ, Bhammar DM, Angadi SS, et al. Predictors of Fat Mass Changes in Response to Aerobic Exercise Training in Women. *J Strength Cond Res.* 2015;29(2):297-304. doi:10.1519/JSC.0000000000000726.

36. Melanson EL, Keadle SK, Donnelly JE, Braun B, King NA. Resistance to Exercise-Induced Weight Loss. *Med Sci Sport Exerc.* 2013;45(8):1600-1609. doi:10.1249/MSS.0b013e31828ba942.

37. Thomas DM, Bouchard C, Church T, et al. Why do individuals not lose more weight from an exercise intervention at a defined dose? An energy balance analysis. *Obes Rev.* 2012;13(10):835-847. doi:10.1111/j.1467-789X.2012.01012.x.

38. Geliebter A, Maher MM, Gerace L, Gutin B, Heymsfield SB, Hashim SA. Effects of strength or aerobic training on body composition, resting metabolic rate, and peak oxygen consumption in obese dieting subjects. *Am J Clin Nutr.* 1997;66(3):557-563. doi:10.1093/ajcn/66.3.557.

39. Willis LH, Slentz CA, Bateman LA, et al. Effects of aerobic and/or resistance training on body mass and fat mass in overweight or obese adults. *J Appl Physiol.* 2012;113(12):1831-1837. doi:10.1152/japplphysiol.01370.2011.

CHAPTER 8

THE 10 ABSOLUTE WORST MUSCLE-BUILDING MYTHS AND MISTAKES

1. Bozsik F, Whisenhunt BL, Hudson DL, Bennett B, Lundgren JD. Thin Is In? Think Again: The Rising Importance of Muscularity in the Thin Ideal Female Body. *Sex Roles.* January 2018:1-7. doi:10.1007/s11199-017-0886-0.

2. Keogh JWL, Winwood PW. The Epidemiology of Injuries Across the Weight-Training Sports. *Sport Med.* 2017;47(3):479-501. doi:10.1007/s40279-016-0575-0.

3. Spinks AB, McClure RJ. Quantifying the risk of sports injury: a systematic review of activity-specific rates for children under 16 years of age. *Br J Sports Med.* 2007;41(9):548-57; discussion 557. doi:10.1136/bjsm.2006.033605; Moore IS, Ranson C, Mathema P. Injury Risk in International Rugby Union: Three-Year Injury Surveillance of the Welsh National Team. Orthop J Sport Med. 2015;3(7):2325967115596194. doi:10.1177/2325967115596194; Videbæk S, Bueno AM, Nielsen RO, Rasmussen S. Incidence of Running-Related Injuries Per 1000 h of running in Different Types of Runners: A Systematic Review and Meta-Analysis. Sports Med. 2015;45(7):1017-1026. doi:10.1007/s40279-015-0333-8.

4. Kjaer M. Role of Extracellular Matrix in Adaptation of Tendon and Skeletal Muscle to Mechanical Loading. *Physiol Rev.* 2004;84(2):649-698. doi:10.1152/physrev.00031.2003.

5. Willis LH, Slentz CA, Bateman LA, et al. Effects of aerobic and/or resistance training on body mass and fat mass in overweight or obese adults. *J Appl Physiol.* 2012;113(12):1831-1837. doi:10.1152/japplphysiol.01370.2011.

6. Umpierre D, Stein R. Hemodynamic and vascular effects of resistance training: implications for cardiovascular disease. *Arq Bras Cardiol.* 2007;89(4):256-262.

7. Church DD, Hoffman JR, Mangine GT, et al. Comparison of high-intensity vs. high-volume resistance training on the BDNF response to exercise. *J Appl Physiol.* 2016;121(1):123-128. doi:10.1152/japplphysiol.00233.2016.

8. Westcott WL. Resistance Training is Medicine. *Curr Sports Med Rep.* 2012;11(4):209-216. doi:10.1249/JSR.0b013e31825dabb8.

9.   Guadalupe-Grau A, Fuentes T, Guerra B, Calbet JAL. Exercise and bone mass in adults. *Sports Med.* 2009;39(6):439-468.

10. Russo CR, MD. The effects of exercise on bone. Basic concepts and implications for the prevention of fractures. *Clin Cases Miner Bone Metab.* 2009;6(3):223-228.

11. Pratley R, Nicklas B, Rubin M, et al. Strength training increases resting metabolic rate and norepinephrine levels in healthy 50- to 65-yr-old men. *J Appl Physiol.* 1994;76(1):133-137. doi:10.1152/jappl.1994.76.1.133.

12. Simão R, Lemos A, Salles B, et al. The Influence of Strength, Flexibility, and Simultaneous Training on Flexibility and Strength Gains. *J Strength Cond Res.* 2011;25(5):1333-1338. doi:10.1519/JSC.0b013e3181da85bf.

13. Testosterone. MedlinePlus Medical Encyclopedia. https://medlineplus.gov/ency/article/003707.htm. August 14, 2018. Accessed August 17, 2018.

14. Velders M, Diel P. How Sex Hormones Promote Skeletal Muscle Regeneration. *Sport Med.* 2013;43(11):1089-1100. doi:10.1007/s40279-013-0081-6; Hansen M, Kjaer M. Influence of Sex and Estrogen on Musculotendinous Protein Turnover at Rest and After Exercise. Exerc Sport Sci Rev. 2014;42(4):183-192. doi:10.1249/JES.0000000000000026.

15. Van den Berg G, Veldhuis JD, Frölich M, Roelfsema F. An amplitude-specific divergence in the pulsatile mode of growth hormone (GH) secretion underlies the gender difference in mean GH concentrations in men and premenopausal women. *J Clin Endocrinol Metab.* 1996;81(7):2460-2467. doi:10.1210/jcem.81.7.8675561.

16. Walts CT, Hanson ED, Delmonico MJ, Yao L, Wang MQ, Hurley BF. Do sex or race differences influence strength training effects on muscle or fat? *Med Sci Sports Exerc.* 2008;40(4):669-676. doi:10.1249/MSS.0b013e318161aa82; Roth SM, Ivey FM, Martel GF, et al. Muscle size responses to strength training in young and older men and women. *J Am Geriatr Soc.* 2001;49(11):1428-1433; Healy ML, Gibney J, Pentecost C, Wheeler MJ, Sonksen PH. Endocrine profiles in 693 elite athletes in the postcompetition setting. *Clin Endocrinol (Oxf).* 2014;81(2):294-305. doi:10.1111/cen.12445.

17. Goldberg AL, Etlinger JD, Goldspink DF, Jablecki C. Mechanism of work-induced hypertrophy of skeletal muscle. *Med Sci Sports.* 1975;7(3):185-198.

18. Schwanbeck S, Chilibeck PD, Binsted G. A Comparison of Free Weight Squat to Smith Machine Squat Using Electromyography. *J Strength Cond Res.* 2009;23(9):2588-2591. doi:10.1519/JSC.0b013e3181b1b181.

19. Schick EE, Coburn JW, Brown LE, et al. A Comparison of Muscle Activation Between a Smith Machine and Free Weight Bench Press. *J Strength Cond Res.* 2010;24(3):779-784. doi:10.1519/JSC.0b013e3181cc2237.

20. Escamilla RF, Fleisig GS, Zheng N, et al. Effects of technique variations on knee biomechanics during the squat and leg press. *Med Sci Sports Exerc.* 2001;33(9):1552-1566.

21. Kraemer W, Fry A, Warren B, et al. Acute Hormonal Responses in Elite Junior Weightlifters. *Int J Sports Med.* 1992;13(02):103-109. doi:10.1055/s-2007-1021240.

22. Phillips SM, Van Loon LJC. Dietary protein for athletes: From requirements to optimum adaptation. *J Sports Sci.* 2011;29(sup1):S29-S38. doi:10.1080/02640414.2011.619204.

23. Tarnopolsky MA, Atkinson SA, MacDougall JD, Chesley A, Phillips S, Schwarcz HP. Evaluation of protein requirements for trained strength athletes. *J Appl Physiol.* 1992;73(5):1986-1995. doi:10.1152/jappl.1992.73.5.1986; Lemon PW, Tarnopolsky MA, MacDougall JD, Atkinson SA. Protein requirements and muscle mass/strength changes during intensive training in novice bodybuilders. *J Appl Physiol.* 1992;73(2):767-775. doi:10.1152/jappl.1992.73.2.767; Lemon PWR. Dietary protein requirements in athletes. *J Nutr Biochem.* 1997;8(2):52-60. doi:10.1016/S0955-2863(97)00007-7.

24. Murach KA, Bagley JR. Skeletal Muscle Hypertrophy with Concurrent Exercise Training: Contrary Evidence for an Interference Effect. *Sport Med.* 2016;46(8):1029-1039. doi:10.1007/s40279-016-0496-y.

25. Jones TW, Howatson G, Russell M, French DN. Performance and Neuromuscular Adaptations Following Differing Ratios of Concurrent Strength and Endurance Training. *J Strength Cond Res.* 2013;27(12):3342-3351. doi:10.1519/JSC.0b013e3181b2cf39.

CHAPTER 9

THE 3 LITTLE BIG THINGS ABOUT RAPID FAT LOSS

1.   Kersten S. Mechanisms of nutritional and hormonal regulation of lipogenesis. *EMBO Rep.* 2001;2(4):282-286. doi:10.1093/embo-reports/kve07.

2.   Leaf A, Antonio J. The Effects of Overfeeding on Body Composition: The Role of Macronutrient Composition - A Narrative Review. *Int J Exerc Sci.* 2017;10(8):1275-1296.

3.   Pal S, Ellis V. The acute effects of four protein meals on insulin, glucose, appetite and energy intake in lean men. *Br J Nutr.* 2010;104(08):1241-1248. doi:10.1017/S0007114510001911.

4.   Salehi A, Gunnerud U, Muhammed SJ, et al. The insulinogenic effect of whey protein is partially mediated by a direct effect of amino acids and GIP on β-cells. *Nutr Metab (Lond).* 2012;9(1):48. doi:10.1186/1743-7075-9-48; Holt SH, Miller JC, Petocz P. An insulin index of foods: the insulin demand generated by 1000-kJ portions of common foods. *Am J Clin Nutr.* 1997;66(5):1264-1276. doi:10.1093/ajcn/66.5.1264.

5.   Pal S, Ellis V. The acute effects of four protein meals on insulin, glucose, appetite and energy intake in lean men. *Br J Nutr.* 2010;104(08):1241-1248. doi:10.1017/S0007114510001911.

6.   Evans K, Clark ML, Frayn KN. Effects of an oral and intravenous fat load on adipose tissue and forearm lipid metabolism. *Am J Physiol.* 1999;276(2 Pt 1):E241-8; Wajchenberg BL. Subcutaneous and Visceral Adipose Tissue: Their Relation to the Metabolic Syndrome. *Endocr Rev.* 2000;21(6):697-738. doi:10.1210/edrv.21.6.0415.

7.   Meijssen S, Cabezas MC, Ballieux CGM, Derksen RJ, Bilecen S, Erkelens DW. Insulin Mediated Inhibition of Hormone Sensitive Lipase Activity *in Vivo* in Relation to Endogenous Catecholamines in Healthy Subjects. *J Clin Endocrinol Metab.* 2001;86(9):4193-4197. doi:10.1210/jcem.86.9.7794.

8.   Tomiyama AJ, Mann T, Vinas D, Hunger JM, Dejager J, Taylor SE. Low calorie dieting increases cortisol. *Psychosom Med.* 2010;72(4):357-364. doi:10.1097/PSY.0b013e3181d9523c.

9.   Hall KD, Bemis T, Brychta R, et al. Calorie for Calorie, Dietary Fat Restriction Results in More Body Fat Loss than Carbohydrate Restriction in People with Obesity. *Cell Metab.* 2015;22(3):427-436. doi:10.1016/j.cmet.2015.07.021; Friedl KE, Moore RJ, Martinez-Lopez LE, et al. Lower limit of body fat in healthy active men. *J Appl Physiol.* 1994;77(2):933-940. doi:10.1152/jappl.1994.77.2.933.

10.   Helms ER, Zinn C, Rowlands DS, Naidoo R, Cronin J. High-Protein, Low-Fat, Short-Term Diet Results in Less Stress and Fatigue than Moderate-Protein, Moderate-Fat Diet during Weight Loss in Male Weightlifters: A Pilot Study. *Int J Sport Nutr Exerc Metab.* 2015;25(2):163-170. doi:10.1123/ijsnem.2014-0056; Soenen S, Bonomi AG, Lemmens SGT, et al. Relatively high-protein or 'low-carb' energy-restricted diets for body weight loss and body weight maintenance? *Physiol Behav.* 2012;107(3):374-380. doi:10.1016/j.physbeh.2012.08.004; Sacks FM, Bray GA, Carey VJ, et al. Comparison of Weight-Loss Diets with Different Compositions of Fat, Protein, and Carbohydrates. *N Engl J Med.* 2009;360(9):859-873. doi:10.1056/NEJMoa0804748.

11.   Evans EM, Mojtahedi MC, Thorpe MP, Valentine RJ, Kris-Etherton PM, Layman DK. Effects of protein intake and gender on body composition changes: a randomized clinical weight loss trial. *Nutr Metab (Lond).* 2012;9(1):55. doi:10.1186/1743-7075-9-55.

12.   Helms ER, Aragon AA, Fitschen PJ. Evidence-based recommendations for natural bodybuilding contest preparation: nutrition and supplementation. *J Int Soc Sports Nutr.* 2014;11(1):20. doi:10.1186/1550-2783-11-20.

13.   Westerterp KR. Diet induced thermogenesis. *Nutr Metab (Lond).* 2004;1(1):5. doi:10.1186/1743-7075-1-5.

14.   Paddon-Jones D, Westman E, Mattes RD, Wolfe RR, Astrup A, Westerterp-Plantenga M. Protein, weight management, and satiety. *Am J Clin Nutr.* 2008;87(5):1558S-1561S. doi:10.1093/ajcn/87.5.1558S.

15.   Campbell WW, Tang M. Protein intake, weight loss, and bone mineral density in postmenopausal women. *J Gerontol A Biol Sci Med Sci.* 2010;65(10):1115-1122. doi:10.1093/gerona/glq083.

16.   Helms ER, Aragon AA, Fitschen PJ. Evidence-based recommendations for natural bodybuilding contest preparation: nutrition and supplementation. *J Int Soc Sports Nutr.* 2014;11(1):20. doi:10.1186/1550-2783-11-20.

17.   Phillips SM, Van Loon LJC. Dietary protein for athletes: From requirements to optimum adaptation. *J Sports Sci.* 2011;29(sup1):S29-S38. doi:10.1080/02640414.2011.619204.

18.   Krieger JW, Sitren HS, Daniels MJ, Langkamp-Henken B. Effects of variation in protein and carbohydrate intake on body mass and composition during energy restriction: a meta-regression. *Am J Clin Nutr.* 2006;83(2):260-274. doi:10.1093/ajcn/83.2.260.

19. Metter EJ, Talbot LA, Schrager M, Conwit R. Skeletal muscle strength as a predictor of all-cause mortality in healthy men. *J Gerontol A Biol Sci Med Sci.* 2002;57(10):B359-65.

20. Johnson RK, Appel LJ, Brands M, et al. Dietary Sugars Intake and Cardiovascular Health: A Scientific Statement From the American Heart Association. *Circulation.* 2009;120(11):1011-1020. doi:10.1161/CIRCULATIONAHA.109.192627; Brownell KD, Farley T, Willett WC, et al. The Public Health and Economic Benefits of Taxing Sugar-Sweetened Beverages. *N Engl J Med.* 2009;361(16):1599-1605. doi:10.1056/NEJMhpr0905723.

21. Siri-Tarino PW, Sun Q, Hu FB, Krauss RM. Meta-analysis of prospective cohort studies evaluating the association of saturated fat with cardiovascular disease. *Am J Clin Nutr.* 2010;91(3):535-546. doi:10.3945/ajcn.2009.27725.

22. Pedersen JI, James PT, Brouwer IA, et al. The importance of reducing SFA to limit CHD. *Br J Nutr.* 2011;106(07):961-963. doi:10.1017/S000711451100506X; Kromhout D, Geleijnse JM, Menotti A, Jacobs DR. The confusion about dietary fatty acids recommendations for CHD prevention. *Br J Nutr.* 2011;106(05):627-632. doi:10.1017/S0007114511002236.

23. Schwingshackl L, Hoffmann G. Monounsaturated fatty acids, olive oil and health status: a systematic review and meta-analysis of cohort studies. *Lipids Health Dis.* 2014;13(1):154. doi:10.1186/1476-511X-13-154; Sofi F, Abbate R, Gensini GF, Casini A. Accruing evidence on benefits of adherence to the Mediterranean diet on health: an updated systematic review and meta-analysis. *Am J Clin Nutr.* 2010;92(5):1189-1196. doi:10.3945/ajcn.2010.29673.

24. Bloomer RJ, Larson DE, Fisher-Wellman KH, Galpin AJ, Schilling BK. Effect of eicosapentaenoic and docosahexaenoic acid on resting and exercise-induced inflammatory and oxidative stress biomarkers: a randomized, placebo controlled, cross-over study. *Lipids Health Dis.* 2009;8(1):36. doi:10.1186/1476-511X-8-36.

25. Sublette ME, Ellis SP, Geant AL, Mann JJ. Meta-Analysis of the Effects of Eicosapentaenoic Acid (EPA) in Clinical Trials in Depression. *J Clin Psychiatry.* 2011;72(12):1577-1584. doi:10.4088/JCP.10m06634.

26. Smith GI, Atherton P, Reeds DN, et al. Omega-3 polyunsaturated fatty acids augment the muscle protein anabolic response to hyperinsulinaemia–hyperaminoacidaemia in healthy young and middle-aged men and women. *Clin Sci.* 2011;121(6):267-278. doi:10.1042/CS20100597.

27. Muldoon MF, Ryan CM, Sheu L, Yao JK, Conklin SM, Manuck SB. Serum Phospholipid Docosahexaenonic Acid Is Associated with Cognitive Functioning during Middle Adulthood. *J Nutr.* 2010;140(4):848-853. doi:10.3945/jn.109.119578.

28. Couet C, Delarue J, Ritz P, Antoine JM, Lamisse F. Effect of dietary fish oil on body fat mass and basal fat oxidation in healthy adults. *Int J Obes Relat Metab Disord.* 1997;21(8):637-643.

29. Johnson GH, Fritsche K. Effect of Dietary Linoleic Acid on Markers of Inflammation in Healthy Persons: A Systematic Review of Randomized Controlled Trials. *J Acad Nutr Diet.* 2012;112(7):1029-1041.e15. doi:10.1016/j.jand.2012.03.029.

30. Willett WC. The role of dietary n-6 fatty acids in the prevention of cardiovascular disease. *J Cardiovasc Med.* 2007;8(Suppl 1):S42-S45. doi:10.2459/01.JCM.0000289275.72556.13.

31. Zazpe I, Beunza JJ, Bes-Rastrollo M, et al. Egg consumption and risk of cardiovascular disease in the SUN Project. *Eur J Clin Nutr.* 2011;65(6):676-682. doi:10.1038/ejcn.2011.30; Micha R, Wallace SK, Mozaffarian D. Red and Processed Meat Consumption and Risk of Incident Coronary Heart Disease, Stroke, and Diabetes Mellitus: A Systematic Review and Meta-Analysis. *Circulation.* 2010;121(21):2271-2283. doi:10.1161/CIRCULATIONAHA.109.924977.

32. Baigent C, Keech A, Kearney PM, et al. Efficacy and safety of cholesterol-lowering treatment: prospective meta-analysis of data from 90 056 participants in 14 randomised trials of statins. *Lancet.* 2005;366(9493):1267-1278. doi:10.1016/S0140-6736(05)67394-1.

33. Pedersen JI, James PT, Brouwer IA, et al. The importance of reducing SFA to limit CHD. *Br J Nutr.* 2011;106(07):961-963. doi:10.1017/S000711451100506X; Kromhout D, Geleijnse JM, Menotti A, Jacobs DR. The confusion about dietary fatty acids recommendations for CHD prevention. *Br J Nutr.* 2011;106(05):627-632. doi:10.1017/S0007114511002236.

CHAPTER 10

THE 3 LITTLE BIG THINGS ABOUT BUILDING LEAN MUSCLE

1.   Schoenfeld BJ. The Mechanisms of Muscle Hypertrophy and Their Application to Resistance Training. *J Strength Cond Res.* 2010;24(10):2857-2872. doi:10.1519/JSC.0b013e3181e840f3.

2.   Goldberg AL, Etlinger JD, Goldspink DF, Jablecki C. Mechanism of work-induced hypertrophy of skeletal muscle. *Med Sci Sports.* 1975;7(3):185-198.

3.   Vandenburgh HH. Motion into mass: how does tension stimulate muscle growth? *Med Sci Sports Exerc.* 1987;19(5 Suppl):S142-9; Hornberger TA, Chien S. Mechanical stimuli and nutrients regulate rapamycin-sensitive signaling through distinct mechanisms in skeletal muscle. *J Cell Biochem.* 2006;97(6):1207-1216. doi:10.1002/jcb.20671; Schoenfeld BJ. The Mechanisms of Muscle Hypertrophy and Their Application to Resistance Training. *J Strength Cond Res.* 2010;24(10):2857-2872. doi:10.1519/JSC.0b013e3181e840f3; Hoppeler H, Klossner S, Flück M. Gene expression in working skeletal muscle. *Adv Exp Med Biol.* 2007;618:245-254.

4.   Campos G, Luecke T, Wendeln H, et al. Muscular adaptations in response to three different resistance-training regimens: specificity of repetition maximum training zones. *Eur J Appl Physiol.* 2002;88(1-2):50-60. doi:10.1007/s00421-002-0681-6.

5.   Schoenfeld BJ, Grgic J, Ogborn D, Krieger JW. Strength and Hypertrophy Adaptations Between Low- vs. High-Load Resistance Training. *J Strength Cond Res.* 2017;31(12):3508-3523. doi:10.1519/JSC.0000000000002200.

6.   Matthews M. Research Review: What's the Best Rep Range for Building Muscle? Muscle for Life Website. June 27, 2018. Accessed August 22, 2018.

7.   Chargé SBP, Rudnicki MA. Cellular and Molecular Regulation of Muscle Regeneration. *Physiol Rev.* 2004;84(1):209-238. doi:10.1152/physrev.00019.2003.

8.   Kumar V, Atherton P, Smith K, Rennie MJ. Human muscle protein synthesis and breakdown during and after exercise. *J Appl Physiol.* 2009;106(6):2026-2039. doi:10.1152/japplphysiol.91481.2008.

9.   Patel SR, Zhu X, Storfer-Isser A, et al. Sleep duration and biomarkers of inflammation. *Sleep.* 2009;32(2):200-204.

10.   Dattilo M, Antunes HKM, Medeiros A, et al. Paradoxical sleep deprivation induces muscle atrophy. *Muscle Nerve.* 2012;45(3):431-433. doi:10.1002/mus.22322.

11.   Nedeltcheva A V., Kilkus JM, Imperial J, Schoeller DA, Penev PD. Insufficient Sleep Undermines Dietary Efforts to Reduce Adiposity. *Ann Intern Med.* 2010;153(7):435. doi:10.7326/0003-4819-153-7-201010050-00006.

12.   Reilly T, Piercy M. The effect of partial sleep deprivation on weight-lifting performance. *Ergonomics.* 1994;37(1):107-115. doi:10.1080/00140139408963628.

13.   Fullagar HHK, Skorski S, Duffield R, Hammes D, Coutts AJ, Meyer T. Sleep and Athletic Performance: The Effects of Sleep Loss on Exercise Performance, and Physiological and Cognitive Responses to Exercise. *Sport Med.* 2015;45(2):161-186. doi:10.1007/s40279-014-0260-0; Fullagar HHK, Duffield R, Skorski S, Coutts AJ, Julian R, Meyer T. Sleep and Recovery in Team Sport: Current Sleep-Related Issues Facing Professional Team-Sport Athletes. *Int J Sports Physiol Perform.* 2015;10(8):950-957. doi:10.1123/ijspp.2014-0565.

14.   Helms ER, Aragon AA, Fitschen PJ. Evidence-based recommendations for natural bodybuilding contest preparation: nutrition and supplementation. *J Int Soc Sports Nutr.* 2014;11(1):20. doi:10.1186/1550-2783-11-20.

15.   Bosse JD, Dixon BM. Dietary protein to maximize resistance training: a review and examination of protein spread and change theories. *J Int Soc Sports Nutr.* 2012;9(1):42. doi:10.1186/1550-2783-9-42.

16.   Burke LM, Hawley JA, Wong SHS, Jeukendrup AE. Carbohydrates for training and competition. *J Sports Sci.* 2011;29(sup1):S17-S27. doi:10.1080/02640414.2011.585473; Creer A, Gallagher P, Slivka D, Jemiolo B, Fink W, Trappe S. Influence of muscle glycogen availability on ERK1/2 and Akt signaling after resistance exercise in human skeletal muscle. *J Appl Physiol.* 2005;99(3):950-956. doi:10.1152/japplphysiol.00110.2005.

17.   Lane AR, Duke JW, Hackney AC. Influence of dietary carbohydrate intake on the free testosterone: cortisol ratio responses to short-term intensive exercise training. *Eur J Appl Physiol.* 2010;108(6):1125-1131. doi:10.1007/s00421-009-1220-5.

18.   Benjamin L, Blanpied P, Lamont L. Dietary carbohydrate and protein manipulation and exercise recovery in novice weight-lifters. *Journal of Exercise Physiology.* 2009;12(6):33-39; Howarth KR, Phillips SM, MacDonald

MJ, Richards D, Moreau NA, Gibala MJ. Effect of glycogen availability on human skeletal muscle protein turnover during exercise and recovery. *J Appl Physiol*. 2010;109(2):431-438. doi:10.1152/japplphysiol.00108.2009.

19. Dorgan JF, Judd JT, Longcope C, et al. Effects of dietary fat and fiber on plasma and urine androgens and estrogens in men: a controlled feeding study. *Am J Clin Nutr*. 1996;64(6):850-855. doi:10.1093/ajcn/64.6.850; Hämäläinen E, Adlercreutz H, Puska P, Pietinen P. Diet and serum sex hormones in healthy men. *J Steroid Biochem*. 1984;20(1):459-464; West DWD, Phillips SM. Associations of exercise-induced hormone profiles and gains in strength and hypertrophy in a large cohort after weight training. *Eur J Appl Physiol*. 2012;112(7):2693-2702. doi:10.1007/s00421-011-2246-z; Storer TW, Magliano L, Woodhouse L, et al. Testosterone Dose-Dependently Increases Maximal Voluntary Strength and Leg Power, but Does Not Affect Fatigability or Specific Tension. *J Clin Endocrinol Metab*. 2003;88(4):1478-1485. doi:10.1210/jc.2002-021231; Hartgens F, Kuipers H. Effects of androgenic-anabolic steroids in athletes. *Sports Med*. 2004;34(8):513-554.

CHAPTER 12

THE ANATOMY OF WILLPOWER

1. American Psychological Association. APA: Americans Report Willpower and Stress as Key Obstacles to Meeting Health-Related Resolutions. American Psychological Association Website. http://www.apa.org/news/press/releases/2010/03/lifestyle-changes.aspx. March 29, 2010. Accessed September 9, 2018.

2. Duckworth AL, Seligman MEP. Self-Discipline Outdoes IQ In Predicting Academic Performance of Adolescents. *Psychol Sci*. 2005;16(12):939-944. doi:10.1111/j.1467-9280.2005.01641.x; Tangney JP, Baumeister RF, Boone AL. High Self-Control Predicts Good Adjustment, Less Pathology, Better Grades, and Interpersonal Success. *J Pers*. 2004;72(2):271-324. doi:10.1111/j.0022-3506.2004.00263.x; Kirkpatrick SA, Locke EA. Leadership: do traits matter? *Acad Manag Perspect*. 1991;5(2):48-60. doi:10.5465/ame.1991.4274679.

3. Tucker JS, Kressin NR, Spiro A, Ruscio J. Intrapersonal Characteristics and the Timing of Divorce: A Prospective Investigation. *J Soc Pers Relat*. 1998;15(2):211-225. doi:10.1177/0265407598152005; Kern ML, Friedman HS. Do conscientious individuals live longer? A quantitative review. *Heal Psychol*. 2008;27(5):505-512. doi:10.1037/0278-6133.27.5.505.

4. Berridge KC. The debate over dopamine's role in reward: the case for incentive salience. *Psychopharmacology (Berl)*. 2007;191(3):391-431. doi:10.1007/s00213-006-0578-x.

5. Wang XT, Dvorak RD. Sweet Future: Fluctuating Blood Glucose Levels Affect Future Discounting. *Psychol Sci*. 2010;21(2):183-188. doi:10.1177/0956797609358096.

6. Berridge KC. Wanting and Liking: Observations from the Neuroscience and Psychology Laboratory. *Inquiry (Oslo)*. 2009;52(4):378. doi:10.1080/00201740903087359.

7. Berridge KC. The debate over dopamine's role in reward: the case for incentive salience. *Psychopharmacology (Berl)*. 2007;191(3):391-431. doi:10.1007/s00213-006-0578-x.

8. Kash TL, Nobis WP, Matthews RT, Winder DG. Dopamine enhances fast excitatory synaptic transmission in the extended amygdala by a CRF-R1-dependent process. *J Neurosci*. 2008;28(51):13856-13865. doi:10.1523/JNEUROSCI.4715-08.2008.

9. Knutson B, Wimmer GE, Kuhnen CM, Winkielman P. Nucleus accumbens activation mediates the influence of reward cues on financial risk taking. *Neuroreport*. 2008;19(5):509-513. doi:10.1097/WNR.0b013e-3282f85c01.

10. Briers B, Pandelaere M, Dewitte S, Warlop L. Hungry for Money: The Desire for Caloric Resources Increases the Desire for Financial Resources and Vice Versa. *Psychol Sci*. 2006;17(11):939-943. doi:10.1111/j.1467-9280.2006.01808.x.

11. Koepp MJ, Gunn RN, Lawrence AD, et al. Evidence for striatal dopamine release during a video game. *Nature*. 1998;393(6682):266-268. doi:10.1038/30498.

CHAPTER 13

13 EASY WAYS TO BOOST YOUR WILLPOWER AND SELF-CONTROL

1.   Neal DT, Wood W, Drolet A. How do people adhere to goals when willpower is low? The profits (and pitfalls) of strong habits. *J Pers Soc Psychol.* 2013;104(6):959-975. doi:10.1037/a0032626.

2.   American Psychological Association. Stress in America: Are Teens Adopting Adults' Stress Habits? American Psychological Association Website. https://www.apa.org/news/press/releases/stress/2013/stress-report.pdf. February 11, 2014. Accessed August 21, 2018.

3.   Childs E, O'Connor S, de Wit H. Bidirectional Interactions Between Acute Psychosocial Stress and Acute Intravenous Alcohol in Healthy Men. *Alcohol Clin Exp Res.* 2011;35(10):1794-1803. doi:10.1111/j.1530-0277.2011.01522.x; Reinecke L, Hartmann T, Eden A. The Guilty Couch Potato: The Role of Ego Depletion in Reducing Recovery Through Media Use. *J Commun.* 2014;64(4):569-589. doi:10.1111/jcom.12107.

4.   Wang XT, Dvorak RD. Sweet Future: Fluctuating Blood Glucose Levels Affect Future Discounting. *Psychol Sci.* 2010;21(2):183-188. doi:10.1177/0956797609358096.

5.   Gailliot MT, Baumeister RF, DeWall CN, et al. Self-control relies on glucose as a limited energy source: Willpower is more than a metaphor. *J Pers Soc Psychol.* 2007;92(2):325-336. doi:10.1037/0022-3514.92.2.325; DeWall CN, Deckman T, Gailliot MT, Bushman BJ. Sweetened blood cools hot tempers: physiological self-control and aggression. *Aggress Behav.* 2011;37(1):73-80. doi:10.1002/ab.20366; Gailliot MT, Michelle Peruche B, Plant EA, Baumeister RF. Stereotypes and prejudice in the blood: Sucrose drinks reduce prejudice and stereotyping. *J Exp Soc Psychol.* 2009;45(1):288-290. doi:10.1016/J.JESP.2008.09.003; DeWall CN, Baumeister RF, Gailliot MT, Maner JK. Depletion Makes the Heart Grow Less Helpful: Helping as a Function of Self-Regulatory Energy and Genetic Relatedness. *Personal Soc Psychol Bull.* 2008;34(12):1653-1662. doi:10.1177/0146167208323981.

6.   Thayer JF, Hansen AL, Saus-Rose E, Johnsen BH. Heart Rate Variability, Prefrontal Neural Function, and Cognitive Performance: The Neurovisceral Integration Perspective on Self-regulation, Adaptation, and Health. *Ann Behav Med.* 2009;37(2):141-153. doi:10.1007/s12160-009-9101-z.

7.   Segerstrom SC, Nes LS. Heart Rate Variability Reflects Self-Regulatory Strength, Effort, and Fatigue. *Psychol Sci.* 2007;18(3):275-281. doi:10.1111/j.1467-9280.2007.01888.x; Taylor CB. Depression, heart rate related variables and cardiovascular disease. *Int J Psychophysiol.* 2010;78(1):80-88. doi:10.1016/j.ijpsycho.2010.04.006.

8.   Song H-S, Lehrer PM. The Effects of Specific Respiratory Rates on Heart Rate and Heart Rate Variability. *Appl Psychophysiol Biofeedback.* 2003;28(1):13-23. doi:10.1023/A:1022312815649; Zucker TL, Samuelson KW, Muench F, Greenberg MA, Gevirtz RN. The Effects of Respiratory Sinus Arrhythmia Biofeedback on Heart Rate Variability and Posttraumatic Stress Disorder Symptoms: A Pilot Study. *Appl Psychophysiol Biofeedback.* 2009;34(2):135-143. doi:10.1007/s10484-009-9085-2; Martarelli D, Cocchioni M, Scuri S, Pompei P. Diaphragmatic Breathing Reduces Exercise-Induced Oxidative Stress. *Evidence-Based Complement Altern Med.* 2011;2011:1-10. doi:10.1093/ecam/nep169.

9.   Kiecolt-Glaser JK, Christian L, Preston H, et al. Stress, Inflammation, and Yoga Practice. *Psychosom Med.* 2010;72(2):113-121. doi:10.1097/PSY.0b013e3181cb9377; Herbert B. The Relaxation Response. New York, NY: HarperCollins; 1975.

10.   Chang K-M, Shen C-W. Aromatherapy benefits autonomic nervous system regulation for elementary school faculty in taiwan. *Evid Based Complement Alternat Med.* 2011;2011:946537. doi:10.1155/2011/946537.

11.   Garner B, Phillips LJ, Schmidt H-M, et al. Pilot Study Evaluating the Effect of Massage Therapy on Stress, Anxiety and Aggression in a Young Adult Psychiatric Inpatient Unit. *Aust New Zeal J Psychiatry.* 2008;42(5):414-422. doi:10.1080/00048670801961131; Jensen AM, Ramasamy A, Hotek J, Roel B, Riffe D. The Benefits of Giving a Massage on the Mental State of Massage Therapists: A Randomized, Controlled Trial. *J Altern Complement Med.* 2012;18(12):1142-1146. doi:10.1089/acm.2011.0643.

12.   Cherkin DC, Sherman KJ, Kahn J, et al. A Comparison of the Effects of 2 Types of Massage and Usual Care on Chronic Low Back Pain. *Ann Intern Med.* 2011;155(1):1-9. doi:10.7326/0003-4819-155-1-201107050-00002; Field T, Ironson G, Scafidi F, et al. Massage therapy reduces anxiety and enhances EEG pattern of alertness and math computations. *Int J Neurosci.* 1996;86(3-4):197-205; Field TM, Sunshine W, Hernandez-Reif M, et al. Massage Therapy Effects on Depression and Somatic Symptoms in Chronic Fatigue Syndrome. *J*

Chronic Fatigue Syndr. 1997;3(3):43-51. doi:10.1300/J092v03n03_03; Rapaport MH, Schettler P, Bresee C. A Preliminary Study of the Effects of a Single Session of Swedish Massage on Hypothalamic–Pituitary–Adrenal and Immune Function in Normal Individuals. *J Altern Complement Med.* 2010;16(10):1079-1088. doi:10.1089/acm.2009.0634.

13.   Burleson MH, Trevathan WR, Todd M. In the Mood for Love or Vice Versa? Exploring the Relations Among Sexual Activity, Physical Affection, Affect, and Stress in the Daily Lives of Mid-Aged Women. *Arch Sex Behav.* 2007;36(3):357-368. doi:10.1007/s10508-006-9071-1.

14.   Meltzer AL, Makhanova A, Hicks LL, French JE, McNulty JK, Bradbury TN. Quantifying the Sexual Afterglow: The Lingering Benefits of Sex and Their Implications for Pair-Bonded Relationships. *Psychol Sci.* 2017;28(5):587-598. doi:10.1177/0956797617691361.

15.   Liu H, Waite LJ, Shen S, Wang DH. Is Sex Good for Your Health? A National Study on Partnered Sexuality and Cardiovascular Risk among Older Men and Women. *J Health Soc Behav.* 2016;57(3):276-296. doi:10.1177/0022146516661597.

16.   Meltzer AL, Makhanova A, Hicks LL, French JE, McNulty JK, Bradbury TN. Quantifying the Sexual Afterglow: The Lingering Benefits of Sex and Their Implications for Pair-Bonded Relationships. *Psychol Sci.* 2017;28(5):587-598. doi:10.1177/0956797617691361; Burleson MH, Trevathan WR, Todd M. In the Mood for Love or Vice Versa? Exploring the Relations Among Sexual Activity, Physical Affection, Affect, and Stress in the Daily Lives of Mid-Aged Women. *Arch Sex Behav.* 2007;36(3):357-368. doi:10.1007/s10508-006-9071-1; Brody S. Blood pressure reactivity to stress is better for people who recently had penile–vaginal intercourse than for people who had other or no sexual activity. *Biol Psychol.* 2006;71(2):214-222. doi:10.1016/j.biopsycho.2005.03.005.

17.   Keller A, Litzelman K, Wisk LE, et al. Does the perception that stress affects health matter? The association with health and mortality. *Heal Psychol.* 2012;31(5):677-684. doi:10.1037/a0026743.

18.   Troy AS, Wilhelm FH, Shallcross AJ, Mauss IB. Seeing the silver lining: Cognitive reappraisal ability moderates the relationship between stress and depressive symptoms. *Emotion.* 2010;10(6):783-795. doi:10.1037/a0020262.

19.   Brennan AR, Arnsten AFT. Neuronal Mechanisms Underlying Attention Deficit Hyperactivity Disorder. *Ann N Y Acad Sci.* 2008;1129(1):236-245. doi:10.1196/annals.1417.007.

20.   Figueiro MG, Wood B, Plitnick B, Rea MS. The impact of light from computer monitors on melatonin levels in college students. *Neuro Endocrinol Lett.* 2011;32(2):158-163; Gooley JJ, Chamberlain K, Smith KA, et al. Exposure to Room Light before Bedtime Suppresses Melatonin Onset and Shortens Melatonin Duration in Humans. *J Clin Endocrinol Metab.* 2011;96(3):E463-E472. doi:10.1210/jc.2010-2098.

21.   Reiter RJ, Tan D-X, Korkmaz A, et al. Light at night, chronodisruption, melatonin suppression, and cancer risk: a review. *Crit Rev Oncog.* 2007;13(4):303-328; Reiter RJ, Tan D-X, Korkmaz A, Ma S. Obesity and metabolic syndrome: Association with chronodisruption, sleep deprivation, and melatonin suppression. *Ann Med.* 2012;44(6):564-577. doi:10.3109/07853890.2011.586365; Dominguez-Rodriguez A, Abreu-Gonzalez P, Sanchez-Sanchez JJ, Kaski JC, Reiter RJ. Melatonin and circadian biology in human cardiovascular disease. *J Pineal Res.* 2010;49(1):no-no. doi:10.1111/j.1600-079X.2010.00773.x.

22.   McIntyre IM, Norman TR, Burrows GD, Armstrong SM. Human melatonin suppression by light is intensity dependent. *J Pineal Res.* 1989;6(2):149-156.

23.   Brainard GC, Hanifin JP, Greeson JM, et al. Action spectrum for melatonin regulation in humans: evidence for a novel circadian photoreceptor. *J Neurosci.* 2001;21(16):6405-6412. doi:10.1523/JNEUROSCI.21-16-06405.2001.

24.   Kimberly B, James R. P. Amber Lenses To Block Blue Light And Improve Sleep: A Randomized Trial. *Chronobiol Int.* 2009;26(8):1602-1612. doi:10.3109/07420520903523719.

25.   Thomée S, Härenstam A, Hagberg M. Mobile phone use and stress, sleep disturbances, and symptoms of depression among young adults - a prospective cohort study. *BMC Public Health.* 2011;11(1):66. doi:10.1186/1471-2458-11-66; Lepp A, Barkley JE, Karpinski AC. The relationship between cell phone use, academic performance, anxiety, and Satisfaction with Life in college students. *Comput Human Behav.* 2014;31:343-350. doi:10.1016/J.CHB.2013.10.049.

26.   Thomée S, Härenstam A, Hagberg M. Mobile phone use and stress, sleep disturbances, and symptoms of depression among young adults - a prospective cohort study. *BMC Public Health.* 2011;11(1):66. doi:10.1186/1471-2458-11-66.

27.   Jenkins JS. The Mozart effect. J R Soc Med. 2001;94(4):170-172; Jensen KL. The effects of selected classical music on self-disclosure. *J Music Ther.* 2001;38(1):2-27; Chafin S, Roy M, Gerin W, Christenfeld N. Music can facilitate blood pressure recovery from stress. *Br J Health Psychol.* 2004;9(3):393-403. doi:10.1348/1359107041557020; Siedliecki SL, Good M. Effect of music on power, pain, depression and disability. *J Adv Nurs.* 2006;54(5):553-562. doi:10.1111/j.1365-2648.2006.03860.x; Hanser SB, Thompson LW. Effects of a music therapy strategy on depressed older adults. *J Gerontol.* 1994;49(6):P265-9; Scheufele PM. Effects of Progressive Relaxation and Classical Music on Measurements of Attention, Relaxation, and Stress Responses. *J Behav Med.* 2000;23(2):207-228. doi:10.1023/A:1005542121935.

28.   Hozawa A, Kuriyama S, Nakaya N, et al. Green tea consumption is associated with lower psychological distress in a general population: the Ohsaki Cohort 2006 Study. *Am J Clin Nutr.* 2009;90(5):1390-1396. doi:10.3945/ajcn.2009.28214.

29.   Brody S, Preut R, Schommer K, Schürmeyer TH. A randomized controlled trial of high dose ascorbic acid for reduction of blood pressure, cortisol, and subjective responses to psychological stress. *Psychopharmacology (Berl).* 2002;159(3):319-324. doi:10.1007/s00213-001-0929-6.

30.   Aspinall P, Mavros P, Coyne R, Roe J. The urban brain: analysing outdoor physical activity with mobile EEG. *Br J Sports Med.* 2015;49(4):272-276. doi:10.1136/bjsports-2012-091877.

31.   Faulkner SH, Jackson S, Fatania G, Leicht CA. The effect of passive heating on heat shock protein 70 and interleukin-6: A possible treatment tool for metabolic diseases? *Temperature.* 2017;4(3):292-304. doi:10.1080/23328940.2017.1288688.

32.   Mandel N, Smeesters D. The Sweet Escape: Effects of Mortality Salience on Consumption Quantities for High- and Low-Self-Esteem Consumers. *J Consum Res.* 2008;35(2):309-323. doi:10.1086/587626; Mandel N, Heine SJ. Terror Management and Marketing: He Who Dies With the Most Toys Wins. *ACR North Am Adv.* 1999;NA-26; Burke BL, Martens A, Faucher EH. Two Decades of Terror Management Theory: A Meta-Analysis of Mortality Salience Research. *Personal Soc Psychol Rev.* 2010;14(2):155-195. doi:10.1177/1088868309352321.

33.   Van Rensburg KJ, Taylor A, Hodgson T. The effects of acute exercise on attentional bias towards smoking-related stimuli during temporary abstinence from smoking. *Addiction.* 2009;104(11):1910-1917. doi:10.1111/j.1360-0443.2009.02692.x; Hansen AL, Johnsen BH, Sollers JJ, Stenvik K, Thayer JF. Heart rate variability and its relation to prefrontal cognitive function: the effects of training and detraining. *Eur J Appl Physiol.* 2004;93(3):263-272. doi:10.1007/s00421-004-1208-0; Nabkasorn C, Miyai N, Sootmongkol A, et al. Effects of physical exercise on depression, neuroendocrine stress hormones and physiological fitness in adolescent females with depressive symptoms. *Eur J Public Health.* 2006;16(2):179-184. doi:10.1093/eurpub/cki159; Hillman CH, Erickson KI, Kramer AF. Be smart, exercise your heart: exercise effects on brain and cognition. *Nat Rev Neurosci.* 2008;9(1):58-65. doi:10.1038/nrn2298.

34.   Barton J, Pretty J. What is the Best Dose of Nature and Green Exercise for Improving Mental Health? A Multi-Study Analysis. *Environ Sci Technol.* 2010;44(10):3947-3955. doi:10.1021/es903183r.

35.   Dhabhar FS. Enhancing versus Suppressive Effects of Stress on Immune Function: Implications for Immunoprotection and Immunopathology. *Neuroimmunomodulation.* 2009;16(5):300-317. doi:10.1159/000216188; Rosenberger PH, Ickovics JR, Epel E, et al. Surgical Stress-Induced Immune Cell Redistribution Profiles Predict Short-Term and Long-Term Postsurgical Recovery. *J Bone Jt Surgery-American Vol.* 2009;91(12):2783-2794. doi:10.2106/JBJS.H.00989.

36.   Frenck RW, Blackburn EH, Shannon KM, et al. The rate of telomere sequence loss in human leukocytes varies with age. *Proc Natl Acad Sci USA.* 1998;95(10):5607-5610. doi:10.1073/pnas.95.10.5607; Epel E, Lin J, Wilhelm F, et al. Cell aging in relation to stress arousal and cardiovascular disease risk factors. *Psychoneuroendocrinology.* 2006;31(3):277-287. doi:10.1016/j.psyneuen.2005.08.011; Irie M, Asami S, Nagata S, Miyata M, Kasai H. Psychological Mediation of a Type of Oxidative DNA Damage, 8-Hydroxydeoxyguanosine, in Peripheral Blood Leukocytes of Non-Smoking and Non-Drinking Workers. *Psychother Psychosom.* 2002;71(2):90-96. doi:10.1159/000049351.

37.   Dusek JA, Otu HH, Wohlhueter AL, et al. Genomic Counter-Stress Changes Induced by the Relaxation Response. Awadalla P, ed. *PLoS One.* 2008;3(7):e2576. doi:10.1371/journal.pone.0002576.

38.   Muise A, Schimmack U, Impett EA. Sexual Frequency Predicts Greater Well-Being, But More is Not Always Better. *Soc Psychol Personal Sci.* 2016;7(4):295-302. doi:10.1177/1948550615616462.

CHAPTER 14

USE IT OR LOSE IT: HOW TO TRAIN YOUR WILLPOWER

1.   Baumeister RF, Heatherton TF, Tice DM. Losing Control: How and Why People Fail at Self-Regulation. San Diego, CA: Academic Press; 1994.

2.   *Ibid.*

3.   Muraven M, Baumeister RF, Tice DM. Longitudinal Improvement of Self-Regulation Through Practice: Building Self-Control Strength Through Repeated Exercise. *J Soc Psychol.* 1999;139(4):446-457. doi:10.1080/00224549909598404; Muraven M. Building Self-Control Strength: Practicing Self-Control Leads to Improved Self-Control Performance. *J Exp Soc Psychol.* 2010;46(2):465-468. doi:10.1016/j.jesp.2009.12.011; Oaten M, Cheng K. Improvements in self-control from financial monitoring. *J Econ Psychol.* 2007;28(4):487-501. doi:10.1016/j.joep.2006.11.003; Baumeister RF, Gailliot M, DeWall CN, Oaten M. Self-Regulation and Personality: How Interventions Increase Regulatory Success, and How Depletion Moderates the Effects of Traits on Behavior. *J Pers.* 2006;74(6):1773-1802. doi:10.1111/j.1467-6494.2006.00428.x.

4.   Segerstrom SC, Hardy JK, Evans DR, Winters NF. Pause and plan: Self-regulation and the heart. In: *How Motivation Affects Cardiovascular Response: Mechanisms and Applications.* Washington: American Psychological Association; 2012;181-198. doi:10.1037/13090-009.

5.   Oaten M, Cheng K. Longitudinal gains in self-regulation from regular physical exercise. *Br J Health Psychol.* 2006;11(4):717-733. doi:10.1348/135910706X96481.

6.   Goldin P, Ramel W, Gross J. Mindfulness Meditation Training and Self-Referential Processing in Social Anxiety Disorder: Behavioral and Neural Effects. *J Cogn Psychother.* 2009;23(3):242-257. doi:10.1891/0889-8391.23.3.242; Goldin PR, Gross JJ. Effects of mindfulness-based stress reduction (MBSR) on emotion regulation in social anxiety disorder. *Emotion.* 2010;10(1):83-91. doi:10.1037/a0018441.

7.   Markowitz LJ, Borton JLS. Suppression of negative self-referent and neutral thoughts: a preliminary investigation. *Behav Cogn Psychother.* 2002;30(03):271-277. doi:10.1017/S135246580200303X; Hofmann SG, Heering S, Sawyer AT, Asnaani A. How to handle anxiety: The effects of reappraisal, acceptance, and suppression strategies on anxious arousal. *Behav Res Ther.* 2009;47(5):389-394. doi:10.1016/J.BRAT.2009.02.010; Wegner DM, Zanakos S. Chronic Thought Suppression. *J Pers.* 1994;62(4):615-640. doi:10.1111/j.1467-6494.1994.tb00311.x; Muris P, Merckelbach H, Horselenberg R. Individual differences in thought suppression. The White Bear Suppression Inventory: Factor structure, reliability, validity and correlates. *Behav Res Ther.* 1996;34(5-6):501-513. doi:10.1016/0005-7967(96)00005-8; Wegner DM, Erber R, Zanakos S. Ironic processes in the mental control of mood and mood-related thought. *J Pers Soc Psychol.* 1993;65(6):1093-1104. doi:10.1037/0022-3514.65.6.1093; Erskine JAK, Georgiou GJ. Effects of thought suppression on eating behaviour in restrained and non-restrained eaters. *Appetite.* 2010;54(3):499-503. doi:10.1016/j.appet.2010.02.001.

8.   Barnes RD, Tantleff-Dunn S. Food for thought: Examining the relationship between food thought suppression and weight-related outcomes. *Eat Behav.* 2010;11(3):175-179. doi:10.1016/j.eatbeh.2010.03.001.

9.   Bowen S, Marlatt A. Surfing the urge: Brief mindfulness-based intervention for college student smokers. *Psychol Addict Behav.* 2009;23(4):666-671. doi:10.1037/a0017127.

10.   Berns GS, McClure SM, Pagnoni G, Montague PR, Cohen JD. Predictability modulates human brain response to reward. *J Neurosci.* 2001;21(8):2793-2798. doi:10.1523/jneurosci.4246-06.2007.

11.   Kalenscher T, Pennartz CMA. Is a bird in the hand worth two in the future? The neuroeconomics of intertemporal decision-making. *Prog Neurobiol.* 2008;84(3):284-315. doi:10.1016/j.pneurobio.2007.11.004.

12.   Kahneman D, Tversky A. Prospect Theory: An Analysis of Decision under Risk. *Econometrica.* 1979;47(2):263. doi:10.2307/1914185.

13.   Weber EU, Johnson EJ, Milch KF, Chang H, Brodscholl JC, Goldstein DG. Asymmetric Discounting in Intertemporal Choice. *Psychol Sci.* 2007;18(6):516-523. doi:10.1111/j.1467-9280.2007.01932.x.

14.   Crockett MJ, Braams BR, Clark L, Tobler PN, Robbins TW, Kalenscher T. Restricting Temptations: Neural Mechanisms of Precommitment. *Neuron.* 2013;79(2):391-401. doi:10.1016/j.neuron.2013.05.028.

15.   Centers for Disease Control and Prevention. Only 1 in 10 Adults Get Enough Fruits or Vegetables. Centers for Disease Control and Prevention Website. https://www.cdc.gov/media/releases/2017/p1116-fruit-vege-

table-consumption.html. November 16, 2017. Accessed August 20, 2018; Centers for Disease Control and Prevention. One in five adults meet overall physical activity guidelines. Centers for Disease Control and Prevention Website. https://www.cdc.gov/media/releases/2013/p0502-physical-activity.html. May 2, 2013. Accessed August 20, 2018.

16.   Statista. U.S. - average fast food consumption per week | Survey 2016. Statista Website. https://www.statista.com/statistics/561297/us-average-fast-food-consumption-per-week/. 2016. Accessed August 20, 2018; Centers for Disease Control and Prevention. Dietary guidelines for americans 2015 and related NHANES updates. Centers for Disease Control and Prevention Website. https://www.cdc.gov/nchs/data/bsc/bscpres_ahluwalia_may_2016.pdf. 2015. Accessed August 20, 2018; Williams O. One in three people would rather do housework than exercise, survey reveals. Daily Mail Website. http://www.dailymail.co.uk/news/article-2323912/One-people-housework-exercise-survey-reveals.html. May 13, 2013. Accessed August 20, 2018.

17.   Centola D. The spread of behavior in an online social network experiment. *Science*. 2010;329(5996):1194-1197. doi:10.1126/science.1185231.

18.   Wagner DD, Dal Cin S, Sargent JD, Kelley WM, Heatherton TF. Spontaneous action representation in smokers when watching movie characters smoke. *J Neurosci*. 2011;31(3):894-898. doi:10.1523/JNEUROSCI.5174-10.2011.

19.   Fowler JH, Christakis NA. Estimating peer effects on health in social networks: A response to Cohen-Cole and Fletcher; and Trogdon, Nonnemaker, and Pais. *J Health Econ*. 2008;27(5):1400-1405. doi:10.1016/j.jhealeco.2008.07.001; Christakis NA, Fowler JH. The Spread of Obesity in a Large Social Network over 32 Years. *N Engl J Med*. 2007;357(4):370-379. doi:10.1056/NEJMsa066082.

20.   McCabe DL, Treviño LK, Butterfield KD. Honor codes and other contextual influences on academic integrity: A replication and extension to modified honor code settings. *Res High Educ*. 2002;43(3):357-378. doi:10.1023/A:1014893102151.

21.   Wenzel M. Misperceptions of social norms about tax compliance: From theory to intervention. *J Econ Psychol*. 2005;26(6):862-883. doi:10.1016/J.JOEP.2005.02.002.

22.   Rosenquist JN, Murabito J, Fowler JH, Christakis NA. The spread of alcohol consumption behavior in a large social network. *Ann Intern Med*. 2010;152(7):426-433, W141. doi:10.7326/0003-4819-152-7-201004060-00007.

23.   Christakis NA, Fowler JH. The Collective Dynamics of Smoking in a Large Social Network. *N Engl J Med*. 2008;358(21):2249-2258. doi:10.1056/NEJMsa0706154.

24.   Cacioppo JT, Fowler JH, Christakis NA. Alone in the crowd: the structure and spread of loneliness in a large social network. *J Pers Soc Psychol*. 2009;97(6):977-991. doi:10.1037/a0016076.

25.   Keizer K, Lindenberg S, Steg L. The Spreading of Disorder. *Science (80-)*. 2008;322(5908):1681-1685. doi:10.1126/science.1161405.

26.   Fowler JH, Christakis NA. Dynamic spread of happiness in a large social network: longitudinal analysis over 20 years in the Framingham Heart Study. *BMJ*. 2008;337:a2338. doi:10.1136/BMJ.A2338; Aarts H, Gollwitzer PM, Hassin RR. Goal Contagion: Perceiving Is for Pursuing. *J Pers Soc Psychol*. 2004;87(1):23-37. doi:10.1037/0022-3514.87.1.23.

27.   VanDellen MR, Hoyle RH. Regulatory Accessibility and Social Influences on State Self-Control. *Personal Soc Psychol Bull*. 2010;36(2):251-263. doi:10.1177/0146167209356302.

28.   Fishbach A, Yaacov T. Implicit and Explicit Counteractive Self-Control. In: Handbook of Motivation Science. New York, NY: Guilford; 2008:281-294.

29.   Mukhopadhyay A, Johar GV. Indulgence as self-reward for prior shopping restraint: A justification-based mechanism. *J Consum Psychol*. 2009;19(3):334-345. doi:10.1016/j.jcps.2009.02.016; Sachdeva S, Iliev R, Medin DL. Sinning Saints and Saintly Sinners. *Psychol Sci*. 2009;20(4):523-528. doi:10.1111/j.1467-9280.2009.02326.x; Khan U, Dhar R. Licensing Effect in Consumer Choice. *J Mark Res*. 2006;43(2):259-266. doi:10.1509/jmkr.43.2.259.

30.   Wilcox K, Vallen B, Block L, Fitzsimons GJ. Vicarious Goal Fulfillment: When the Mere Presence of a Healthy Option Leads to an Ironically Indulgent Decision. *J Consum Res*. 2009;36(3):380-393. doi:10.1086/599219.

31.   *Ibid*.

32.   Khan U, Dhar R. Where there is a way, is there a will? The effect of future choices on self-control. *J Exp Psychol Gen*. 2007;136(2):277-288. doi:10.1037/0096-3445.136.2.277.

33. Khan U, Dhar R. Licensing Effect in Consumer Choice. *J Mark Res*. 2006;43(2):259-266. doi:10.1509/jmkr.43.2.259.

34. *Ibid*.

35. Ersner-Hershfield H, Wimmer GE, Knutson B. Saving for the future self: Neural measures of future self-continuity predict temporal discounting. *Soc Cogn Affect Neurosci*. 2009;4(1):85-92. doi:10.1093/scan/nsn042.

36. Peters J, Büchel C. Episodic Future Thinking Reduces Reward Delay Discounting through an Enhancement of Prefrontal-Mediotemporal Interactions. *Neuron*. 2010;66(1):138-148. doi:10.1016/j.neuron.2010.03.026; Murru EC, Martin Ginis KA. Imagining the possibilities: the effects of a possible selves intervention on self-regulatory efficacy and exercise behavior. *J Sport Exerc Psychol*. 2010;32(4):537-554; Schippers MC, Scheepers AWA, Peterson JB. A scalable goal-setting intervention closes both the gender and ethnic minority achievement gap. *Palgrave Commun*. 2015;1(1):15014. doi:10.1057/palcomms.2015.14.

37. Polivy J, Herman CP. Dieting and binging. A causal analysis. *Am Psychol*. 1985;40(2):193-201.

38. Wohl MJA, Pychyl TA, Bennett SH. I forgive myself, now I can study: How self-forgiveness for procrastinating can reduce future procrastination. *Pers Individ Dif*. 2010;48(7):803-808. doi:10.1016/j.paid.2010.01.029; Leary MR, Tate EB, Adams CE, Batts Allen A, Hancock J. Self-compassion and reactions to unpleasant self-relevant events: The implications of treating oneself kindly. J Pers Soc Psychol. 2007;92(5):887-904. doi:10.1037/0022-3514.92.5.887; Allen AB, Leary MR. Self-Compassion, Stress, and Coping. Soc Personal Psychol Compass. 2010;4(2):107-118. doi:10.1111/j.1751-9004.2009.00246.x.

39. Fishbach A, Dhar R. Goals as Excuses or Guides: The Liberating Effect of Perceived Goal Progress on Choice. *J Consum Res*. 2005;32(3):370-377. doi:10.1086/497518.

40. Fishbach A, Dhar R, Zhang Y. Subgoals as substitutes or complements: The role of goal accessibility. *J Pers Soc Psychol*. 2006;91(2):232-242. doi:10.1037/0022-3514.91.2.232.

CHAPTER 15

FINDING YOUR BIGGEST FITNESS WHYS

1. Cascio CN, O'Donnell MB, Tinney FJ, et al. Self-affirmation activates brain systems associated with self-related processing and reward and is reinforced by future orientation. *Soc Cogn Affect Neurosci*. 2016;11(4):621-629. doi:10.1093/scan/nsv136; Harris PS, Harris PR, Miles E. Self-affirmation improves performance on tasks related to executive functioning. *J Exp Soc Psychol*. 2017;70:281-285. doi:10.1016/J.JESP.2016.11.011.

CHAPTER 16

WELCOME TO THE WONDERFUL WORLD OF FLEXIBLE DIETING

1. Slavin JL. Dietary fiber: classification, chemical analyses, and food sources. *J Am Diet Assoc*. 1987;87(9):1164-1171; Stephen AM, Cummings JH. Mechanism of action of dietary fibre in the human colon. *Nature*. 1980;284(5753):283-284.

2. Rabassa AA, Rogers AI. The role of short-chain fatty acid metabolism in colonic disorders. *Am J Gastroenterol*. 1992;87(4):419-423.

3. Medical College of Georgia. Scientists Learn More About How Roughage Keeps You 'Regular'. Science Daily Website. https://www.sciencedaily.com/releases/2006/08/060823093156.htm. August 23, 3006. Accessed August 18, 2018.

4. Park Y, Subar AF, Hollenbeck A, Schatzkin A. Dietary Fiber Intake and Mortality in the NIH-AARP Diet and Health Study. *Arch Intern Med*. 2011;171(12):1061-1068. doi:10.1001/archinternmed.2011.18; McRae MP. Dietary Fiber Intake and Type 2 Diabetes Mellitus: An Umbrella Review of Meta-analyses. *J Chiropr Med*. 2018;17(1):44-53. doi:10.1016/j.jcm.2017.11.002.

5.   Dahl WJ, Stewart ML. Position of the Academy of Nutrition and Dietetics: Health Implications of Dietary Fiber. *J Acad Nutr Diet.* 2015;115(11):1861-1870. doi:10.1016/j.jand.2015.09.003.

CHAPTER 17

THE EASIEST WAY TO CALCULATE YOUR CALORIES AND MACROS

1.   Mifflin MD, St Jeor ST, Hill LA, Scott BJ, Daugherty SA, Koh YO. A new predictive equation for resting energy expenditure in healthy individuals. *Am J Clin Nutr.* 1990;51(2):241-247. doi:10.1093/ajcn/51.2.241.

2.   Tappy L. Thermic effect of food and sympathetic nervous system activity in humans. *Reprod Nutr Dev.* 1996;36(4):391-397.

3.   Westerterp KR. Diet induced thermogenesis. *Nutr Metab (Lond).* 2004;1(1):5. doi:10.1186/1743-7075-1-5.

4.   Barr S, Wright J. Postprandial energy expenditure in whole-food and processed-food meals: implications for daily energy expenditure. *Food Nutr Res.* 2010;54(1):5144. doi:10.3402/fnr.v54i0.5144.

5.   De Jonge L, Bray GA. The thermic effect of food and obesity: a critical review. *Obes Res.* 1997;5(6):622-631.

6.   Bouchard C, Tremblay A, Nadeau A, et al. Genetic effect in resting and exercise metabolic rates. *Metabolism.* 1989;38(4):364-370.

7.   Pesta DH, Samuel VT. A high-protein diet for reducing body fat: mechanisms and possible caveats. *Nutr Metab (Lond).* 2014;11(1):53. doi:10.1186/1743-7075-11-53; Hall KD, Bemis T, Brychta R, et al. Calorie for Calorie, Dietary Fat Restriction Results in More Body Fat Loss than Carbohydrate Restriction in People with Obesity. *Cell Metab.* 2015;22(3):427-436. doi:10.1016/j.cmet.2015.07.021.

8.   Van Remoortel H, Giavedoni S, Raste Y, et al. Validity of activity monitors in health and chronic disease: a systematic review. *Int J Behav Nutr Phys Act.* 2012;9(1):84. doi:10.1186/1479-5868-9-84.

9.   Cruz J, Brooks D, Marques A. Accuracy of piezoelectric pedometer and accelerometer step counts. *J Sports Med Phys Fitness.* 2017;57(4):426-433. doi:10.23736/S0022-4707.16.06177-X.

10.   Evenson KR, Goto MM, Furberg RD. Systematic review of the validity and reliability of consumer-wearable activity trackers. *Int J Behav Nutr Phys Act.* 2015;12:159. doi:10.1186/s12966-015-0314-1.

11.   Konharn K, Eungpinichpong W, Promdee K, et al. Validity and Reliability of Smartphone Applications for the Assessment of Walking and Running in Normal-weight and Overweight/Obese Young Adults. *J Phys Act Heal.* 2016;13(12):1333-1340. doi:10.1123/jpah.2015-0544; Hiilloskorpi HK, Pasanen ME, Fogelholm MG, Laukkanen RM, Mänttäri AT. Use of Heart Rate to Predict Energy Expenditure from Low to High Activity Levels. *Int J Sports Med.* 2003;24(5):332-336. doi:10.1055/s-2003-40701.

12.   University of California San Francisco. UCSF Human Performance Center featured on Good Morning America. University of California San Francisco Website. https://www.ucsf.edu/news/2010/02/3569/ucsf-human-performance-center-featured-good-morning-america. Accessed August 20, 2018.

13.   Thomas DM, Bouchard C, Church T, et al. Why do individuals not lose more weight from an exercise intervention at a defined dose? An energy balance analysis. *Obes Rev.* 2012;13(10):835-847. doi:10.1111/j.1467-789X.2012.01012.x.

14.   Huovinen HT, Hulmi JJ, Isolehto J, et al. Body Composition and Power Performance Improved After Weight Reduction in Male Athletes Without Hampering Hormonal Balance. *J Strength Cond Res.* 2015;29(1):29-36. doi:10.1519/JSC.0000000000000619.

15.   Demling RH, DeSanti L. Effect of a Hypocaloric Diet, Increased Protein Intake and Resistance Training on Lean Mass Gains and Fat Mass Loss in Overweight Police Officers. Ann Nutr Metab. 2000;44(1):21-29. doi:10.1159/000012817.

16.   Donnelly JE, Sharp T, Houmard J, et al. Muscle hypertrophy with large-scale weight loss and resistance training. *Am J Clin Nutr.* 1993;58(4):561-565. doi:10.1093/ajcn/58.4.561.

17.   Zito CI, Qin H, Blenis J, Bennett AM. SHP-2 Regulates Cell Growth by Controlling the mTOR/S6 Kinase 1 Pathway. *J Biol Chem.* 2007;282(10):6946-6953. doi:10.1074/jbc.M608338200; Cangemi R, Friedmann AJ, Holloszy JO, Fontana L. Long-term effects of calorie restriction on serum sex-hormone concentrations in

men. *Aging Cell*. 2010;9(2):236-242. doi:10.1111/j.1474-9726.2010.00553.x; Tomiyama AJ, Mann T, Vinas D, Hunger JM, DeJager J, Taylor SE. Low Calorie Dieting Increases Cortisol. *Psychosom Med*. 2010;72(4):357-364. doi:10.1097/PSY.0b013e3181d9523c; Papadopoulou S. Impact of Energy Intake and Balance on the Athletic Performance and Health of Top Female Volleyball Athletes. *Medicina Sportiva*. 2015;11(1):2477-2481.

18.   Dyck DJ, Heigenhauser GJF, Bruce CR. The role of adipokines as regulators of skeletal muscle fatty acid metabolism and insulin sensitivity. *Acta Physiol*. 2006;186(1):5-16. doi:10.1111/j.1748-1716.2005.01502.x.

19.   Zhang J, Hupfeld CJ, Taylor SS, Olefsky JM, Tsien RY. Insulin disrupts β-adrenergic signalling to protein kinase A in adipocytes. *Nature*. 2005;437(7058):569-573. doi:10.1038/nature04140; Shanik MH, Xu Y, Skrha J, Dankner R, Zick Y, Roth J. Insulin Resistance and Hyperinsulinemia: Is hyperinsulinemia the cart or the horse? *Diabetes Care*. 2008;31(Supplement 2):S262-S268. doi:10.2337/dc08-s264; Wang X, Hu Z, Hu J, Du J, Mitch WE. Insulin Resistance Accelerates Muscle Protein Degradation: Activation of the Ubiquitin-Proteasome Pathway by Defects in Muscle Cell Signaling. *Endocrinology*. 2006;147(9):4160-4168. doi:10.1210/en.2006-0251.

20.   Helms ER, Zinn C, Rowlands DS, Naidoo R, Cronin J. High-Protein, Low-Fat, Short-Term Diet Results in Less Stress and Fatigue than Moderate-Protein, Moderate-Fat Diet during Weight Loss in Male Weightlifters: A Pilot Study. *Int J Sport Nutr Exerc Metab*. 2015;25(2):163-170. doi:10.1123/ijsnem.2014-0056.

21.   Helms ER, Aragon AA, Fitschen PJ. Evidence-based recommendations for natural bodybuilding contest preparation: nutrition and supplementation. *J Int Soc Sports Nutr*. 2014;11(1):20. doi:10.1186/1550-2783-11-20.

22.   Sacks FM, Bray GA, Carey VJ, et al. Comparison of Weight-Loss Diets with Different Compositions of Fat, Protein, and Carbohydrates. *N Engl J Med*. 2009;360(9):859-873. doi:10.1056/NEJMoa0804748.

23.   Naude CE, Schoonees A, Senekal M, Young T, Garner P, Volmink J. Low Carbohydrate versus Isoenergetic Balanced Diets for Reducing Weight and Cardiovascular Risk: A Systematic Review and Meta-Analysis. Cameron DW, ed. *PLoS One*. 2014;9(7):e100652. doi:10.1371/journal.pone.0100652.

24.   Mumford SL, Chavarro JE, Zhang C, et al. Dietary fat intake and reproductive hormone concentrations and ovulation in regularly menstruating women. *Am J Clin Nutr*. 2016;103(3):868-877. doi:10.3945/ajcn.115.119321.

CHAPTER 18

THE TRUTH ABOUT PREWORKOUT AND POSTWORKOUT NUTRITION

1.   Biolo G, Tipton KD, Klein S, Wolfe RR. An abundant supply of amino acids enhances the metabolic effect of exercise on muscle protein. *Am J Physiol Metab*. 1997;273(1):E122-E129. doi:10.1152/ajpendo.1997.273.1.E122.

2.   Kumar V, Atherton P, Smith K, Rennie MJ. Human muscle protein synthesis and breakdown during and after exercise. *J Appl Physiol*. 2009;106(6):2026-2039. doi:10.1152/japplphysiol.91481.2008.

3.   Cribb PJ, Hayes A. Effects of Supplement Timing and Resistance Exercise on Skeletal Muscle Hypertrophy. *Med Sci Sport Exerc*. 2006;38(11):1918-1925. doi:10.1249/01.mss.0000233790.08788.3e; Wycherley TP, Noakes M, Clifton PM, Cleanthous X, Keogh JB, Brinkworth GD. Timing of protein ingestion relative to resistance exercise training does not influence body composition, energy expenditure, glycaemic control or cardiometabolic risk factors in a hypocaloric, high protein diet in patients with type 2 diabetes. *Diabetes, Obes Metab*. 2010;12(12):1097-1105. doi:10.1111/j.1463-1326.2010.01307.x.

4.   Burk A, Timpmann S, Medijainen L, Vähi M, Ööpik V. Time-divided ingestion pattern of casein-based protein supplement stimulates an increase in fat-free body mass during resistance training in young untrained men. *Nutr Res*. 2009;29(6):405-413. doi:10.1016/j.nutres.2009.03.008.

5.   Jeukendrup AE, Killer SC. The Myths Surrounding Pre-Exercise Carbohydrate Feeding. *Ann Nutr Metab*. 2010;57(s2):18-25. doi:10.1159/000322698; Hargreaves M, Hawley JA, Jeukendrup A. Pre-exercise carbohydrate and fat ingestion: effects on metabolism and performance. *J Sports Sci*. 2004;22(1):31-38. doi:10.1080/0264041031000140536.

6.   Haff GG, Lehmkuhl MJ, McCoy LB, Stone MH. Carbohydrate supplementation and resistance training. *J strength Cond Res*. 2003;17(1):187-196.

7.   Knuiman P, Hopman MTE, Mensink M. Glycogen availability and skeletal muscle adaptations with endurance and resistance exercise. *Nutr Metab (Lond)*. 2015;12(1):59. doi:10.1186/s12986-015-0055-9.

8.   Cribb PJ, Hayes A. Effects of Supplement Timing and Resistance Exercise on Skeletal Muscle Hypertrophy. *Med Sci Sport Exerc.* 2006;38(11):1918-1925. doi:10.1249/01.mss.0000233790.08788.3e; Haff GG, Lehmkuhl MJ, McCoy LB, Stone MH. Carbohydrate supplementation and resistance training. *J strength Cond Res.* 2003;17(1):187-196.

9.   Hargreaves M, Hawley JA, Jeukendrup A. Pre-exercise carbohydrate and fat ingestion: effects on metabolism and performance. *J Sports Sci.* 2004;22(1):31-38. doi:10.1080/0264041031000140536.

10.   Breen L, Churchward-Venne TA. Leucine: a nutrient "trigger" for muscle anabolism, but what more? *J Physiol.* 2012;590(9):2065-2066. doi:10.1113/jphysiol.2012.230631.

11.   Gelfand RA, Barrett EJ. Effect of physiologic hyperinsulinemia on skeletal muscle protein synthesis and breakdown in man. *J Clin Invest.* 1987;80(1):1-6. doi:10.1172/JCI113033.

12.   Biolo G, Tipton KD, Klein S, Wolfe RR. An abundant supply of amino acids enhances the metabolic effect of exercise on muscle protein. *Am J Physiol Metab.* 1997;273(1):E122-E129. doi:10.1152/ajpendo.1997.273.1.E122.

13.   Hamer HM, Wall BT, Kiskini A, et al. Carbohydrate co-ingestion with protein does not further augment post-prandial muscle protein accretion in older men. *Nutr Metab (Lond).* 2013;10(1):15. doi:10.1186/1743-7075-10-15; Staples AW, Burd NA, West DWD, et al. Carbohydrate Does Not Augment Exercise-Induced Protein Accretion versus Protein Alone. *Med Sci Sport Exerc.* 2011;43(7):1154-1161. doi:10.1249/MSS.0b013e31820751cb.

14.   Greenhaff PL, Karagounis LG, Peirce N, et al. Disassociation between the effects of amino acids and insulin on signaling, ubiquitin ligases, and protein turnover in human muscle. *Am J Physiol Metab.* 2008;295(3):E595-E604. doi:10.1152/ajpendo.90411.2008; Van Loon LJ, Saris WH, Verhagen H, Wagenmakers AJ. Plasma insulin responses after ingestion of different amino acid or protein mixtures with carbohydrate. *Am J Clin Nutr.* 2000;72(1):96-105. doi:10.1093/ajcn/72.1.96.

15.   Kersten S. Mechanisms of nutritional and hormonal regulation of lipogenesis. *EMBO Rep.* 2001;2(4):282-286. doi:10.1093/embo-reports/kve071; Denne SC, Liechty EA, Liu YM, Brechtel G, Baron AD. Proteolysis in skeletal muscle and whole body in response to euglycemic hyperinsulinemia in normal adults. *Am J Physiol Metab.* 1991;261(6):E809-E814. doi:10.1152/ajpendo.1991.261.6.E809.

16.   Jentjens R, Jeukendrup A. Determinants of post-exercise glycogen synthesis during short-term recovery. *Sports Med.* 2003;33(2):117-144.

17.   Ivy J. Glycogen Resynthesis After Exercise: Effect of Carbohydrate Intake. *Int J Sports Med.* 1998;19(S 2):S142-S145. doi:10.1055/s-2007-971981.

18.   Moghaddam E, Vogt JA, Wolever TMS. The Effects of Fat and Protein on Glycemic Responses in Non-diabetic Humans Vary with Waist Circumference, Fasting Plasma Insulin, and Dietary Fiber Intake. *J Nutr.* 2006;136(10):2506-2511. doi:10.1093/jn/136.10.2506.

19.   Burke LM, Collier GR, Beasley SK, et al. Effect of coingestion of fat and protein with carbohydrate feedings on muscle glycogen storage. *J Appl Physiol.* 1995;78(6):2187-2192. doi:10.1152/jappl.1995.78.6.2187; Roy BD, Tarnopolsky MA. Influence of differing macronutrient intakes on muscle glycogen resynthesis after resistance exercise. *J Appl Physiol.* 1998;84(3):890-896. doi:10.1152/jappl.1998.84.3.890; Elliot TA, Cree MG, Sanford AP, Wolfe RR, Tipton KD. Milk Ingestion Stimulates Net Muscle Protein Synthesis following Resistance Exercise. *Med Sci Sport Exerc.* 2006;38(4):667-674. doi:10.1249/01.mss.0000210190.64458.25.

CHAPTER 19

HOW TO MAKE MEAL PLANS THAT REALLY WORK

1.   Wansink B, Sobal J. Mindless Eating. *Environ Behav.* 2007;39(1):106-123. doi:10.1177/0013916506295573.

2.   Urban LE, Weber JL, Heyman MB, et al. Energy Contents of Frequently Ordered Restaurant Meals and Comparison with Human Energy Requirements and US Department of Agriculture Database Information: A Multisite Randomized Study. *J Acad Nutr Diet.* 2016;116(4):590-598.e6. doi:10.1016/j.jand.2015.11.009.

3.   Yeomans MR. Alcohol, appetite and energy balance: Is alcohol intake a risk factor for obesity? *Physiol Behav.* 2010;100(1):82-89. doi:10.1016/j.physbeh.2010.01.012.

4.   Gruchow HW, Sobocinski KA, Barboriak JJ, Scheller JG. Alcohol consumption, nutrient intake and relative body weight among US adults. *Am J Clin Nutr*. 1985;42(2):289-295. doi:10.1093/ajcn/42.2.289.

5.   Flechtner-Mors M, Biesalski HK, Jenkinson CP, Adler G, Ditschuneit HH. Effects of moderate consumption of white wine on weight loss in overweight and obese subjects. *Int J Obes*. 2004;28(11):1420-1426.
doi:10.1038/sj.ijo.0802786.

6.   Kokavec A. Is decreased appetite for food a physiological consequence of alcohol consumption? *Appetite*. 2008;51(2):233-243. doi:10.1016/j.appet.2008.03.011; McCarty MF. Does regular ethanol consumption
promote insulin sensitivity and leanness by stimulating AMP-activated protein kinase? *Med Hypotheses*.
2001;57(3):405-407. doi:10.1054/mehy.2001.1404; Ukropcova B, McNeil M, Sereda O, et al. Dynamic changes in fat oxidation in human primary myocytes mirror metabolic characteristics of the donor. *J Clin Invest*.
2005;115(7):1934-1941. doi:10.1172/JCI24332.

7.   Siler SQ, Neese RA, Hellerstein MK. De novo lipogenesis, lipid kinetics, and whole-body lipid balances
in humans after acute alcohol consumption. *Am J Clin Nutr*. 1999;70(5):928-936. doi:10.1093/ajcn/70.5.928.

8.   Mattes RD, Campbell WW. Effects of Food Form and Timing of Ingestion on Appetite and Energy Intake
in Lean Young Adults and in Young Adults with Obesity. *J Am Diet Assoc*. 2009;109(3):430-437. doi:10.1016/j.
jada.2008.11.031.

9.   *Ibid*; Malik VS, Schulze MB, Hu FB. Intake of sugar-sweetened beverages and weight gain: a systematic
review. *Am J Clin Nutr*. 2006;84(2):274-288. doi:10.1093/ajcn/84.1.274.

CHAPTER 20

HOW TO "CHEAT" ON YOUR DIET WITHOUT RUINING IT

1.   DiNicolantonio JJ, O'Keefe JH, Wilson W. Subclinical magnesium deficiency: a principal driver of cardiovascular disease and a public health crisis. *Open Hear*. 2018;5(1):e000668. doi:10.1136/openhrt-2017-000668;
Kulie T, Groff A, Redmer J, Hounshell J, Schrager S. Vitamin D: an evidence-based review. *J Am Board Fam
Med*. 2009;22(6):698-706. doi:10.3122/jabfm.2009.06.090037; Miller JL. Iron deficiency anemia: a common
and curable disease. *Cold Spring Harb Perspect Med*. 2013;3(7). doi:10.1101/cshperspect.a011866.

2.   Urban LE, Weber JL, Heyman MB, et al. Energy Contents of Frequently Ordered Restaurant Meals and
Comparison with Human Energy Requirements and US Department of Agriculture Database Information: A
Multisite Randomized Study. *J Acad Nutr Diet*. 2016;116(4):590-598.e6. doi:10.1016/j.jand.2015.11.009.

3.   Center for Science in the Public Interest. Xtreme Eating 2014. Center for Science in the Public Interest
Website. https://cspinet.org/eating-healthy/foods-avoid/xtreme2014. Accessed August 22, 2018.

4.   An R. Fast-food and full-service restaurant consumption and daily energy and nutrient intakes in US
adults. *Eur J Clin Nutr*. 2016;70(1):97-103. doi:10.1038/ejcn.2015.104.

5.   Horton TJ, Drougas H, Brachey A, Reed GW, Peters JC, Hill JO. Fat and carbohydrate overfeeding in
humans: different effects on energy storage. *Am J Clin Nutr*. 1995;62(1):19-29. doi:10.1093/ajcn/62.1.19.

6.   Hellerstein MK. No common energy currency: de novo lipogenesis as the road less traveled. *Am J Clin
Nutr*. 2001;74(6):707-708. doi:10.1093/ajcn/74.6.707.

7.   Acheson KJ, Schutz Y, Bessard T, Anantharaman K, Flatt JP, Jéquier E. Glycogen storage capacity and
de novo lipogenesis during massive carbohydrate overfeeding in man. *Am J Clin Nutr*. 1988;48(2):240-247.
doi:10.1093/ajcn/48.2.240.

8.   Aarsland A, Chinkes D, Wolfe RR. Contributions of de novo synthesis of fatty acids to total VLDL-tri-
glyceride secretion during prolonged hyperglycemia/hyperinsulinemia in normal man. *J Clin Invest*.
1996;98(9):2008-2017. doi:10.1172/JCI119005.

9.   Acheson KJ, Flatt JP, Jéquier E. Glycogen synthesis versus lipogenesis after a 500 gram carbohydrate
meal in man. *Metabolism*. 1982;31(12):1234-1240.

10.   Horton TJ, Drougas H, Brachey A, Reed GW, Peters JC, Hill JO. Fat and carbohydrate overfeeding in
humans: different effects on energy storage. *Am J Clin Nutr*. 1995;62(1):19-29. doi:10.1093/ajcn/62.1.19.

11.   Hall KD, Bemis T, Brychta R, et al. Calorie for Calorie, Dietary Fat Restriction Results in More Body Fat Loss than Carbohydrate Restriction in People with Obesity. *Cell Metab.* 2015;22(3):427-436. doi:10.1016/j.cmet.2015.07.021; Rolls BJ. Carbohydrates, fats, and satiety. *Am J Clin Nutr.* 1995;61(4):960S-967S. doi:10.1093/ajcn/61.4.960S; Bludell JE, Lawton CL, Cotton JR, Macdiarmid JI. Control of Human Appetite: Implications for The Intake of Dietary Fat. *Annu Rev Nutr.* 1996;16(1):285-319. doi:10.1146/annurev.nu.16.070196.001441.

12.   Schwarz J-M, Linfoot P, Dare D, Aghajanian K. Hepatic de novo lipogenesis in normoinsulinemic and hyperinsulinemic subjects consuming high-fat, low-carbohydrate and low-fat, high-carbohydrate isoenergetic diets. *Am J Clin Nutr.* 2003;77(1):43-50. doi:10.1093/ajcn/77.1.43.

13.   Jéquier E. Leptin signaling, adiposity, and energy balance. *Ann N Y Acad Sci.* 2002;967:379-388.

14.   Park H-K, Ahima RS. Physiology of leptin: energy homeostasis, neuroendocrine function and metabolism. *Metabolism.* 2015;64(1):24-34. doi:10.1016/j.metabol.2014.08.004.

15.   Olson BR, Cartledge T, Sebring N, Defensor R, Nieman L. Short-term fasting affects luteinizing hormone secretory dynamics but not reproductive function in normal-weight sedentary women. *J Clin Endocrinol Metab.* 1995;80(4):1187-1193. doi:10.1210/jcem.80.4.7714088.

16.   Dirlewanger M, di Vetta V, Guenat E, et al. Effects of short-term carbohydrate or fat overfeeding on energy expenditure and plasma leptin concentrations in healthy female subjects. *Int J Obes Relat Metab Disord.* 2000;24(11):1413-1418.

CHAPTER 21

THE ULTIMATE WORKOUT PLAN FOR WOMEN
– STRENGTH TRAINING

1.   Schoenfeld BJ. The Mechanisms of Muscle Hypertrophy and Their Application to Resistance Training. *J Strength Cond Res.* 2010;24(10):2857-2872. doi:10.1519/JSC.0b013e3181e840f3.

2.   Souza-Junior TP, Willardson JM, Bloomer R, et al. Strength and hypertrophy responses to constant and decreasing rest intervals in trained men using creatine supplementation. *J Int Soc Sports Nutr.* 2011;8(1):17. doi:10.1186/1550-2783-8-17.

3.   Radaelli R, Fleck SJ, Leite T, et al. Dose-Response of 1, 3, and 5 Sets of Resistance Exercise on Strength, Local Muscular Endurance, and Hypertrophy. *J Strength Cond Res.* 2015;29(5):1349-1358. doi:10.1519/JSC.0000000000000758; Robbins DW, Marshall PW, McEwen M. The Effect of Training Volume on Lower-Body Strength. *J Strength Cond Res.* 2012;26(1):34-39. doi:10.1519/JSC.0b013e31821d5cc4.

4.   De Salles BF, Simão R, Miranda F, da Silva Novaes J, Lemos A, Willardson JM. Rest Interval between Sets in Strength Training. *Sport Med.* 2009;39(9):765-777. doi:10.2165/11315230-000000000-00000.

5.   Willardson JM, Burkett LN. The Effect of Different Rest Intervals Between Sets on Volume Components and Strength Gains. J Strength Cond Res. 2008;22(1):146-152. doi:10.1519/JSC.0b013e31815f912d.

6.   Robbins DW, Marshall PW, McEwen M. The Effect of Training Volume on Lower-Body Strength. *J Strength Cond Res.* 2012;26(1):34-39. doi:10.1519/JSC.0b013e31821d5cc4.

7.   Gomes GK, Franco CM, Nunes PRP, Orsatti FL. High-frequency resistance training is not more effective than low-frequency resistance training in increasing muscle mass and strength in well-trained men. *J Strength Cond Res.* February 2018:1. doi:10.1519/JSC.0000000000002559; Colquhoun RJ, Gai CM, Aguilar D, et al. Training Volume, Not Frequency, Indicative of Maximal Strength Adaptations to Resistance Training. *J Strength Cond Res.* 2018;32(5):1207-1213. doi:10.1519/JSC.0000000000002414.

8.   Kreher JB, Schwartz JB. Overtraining syndrome: a practical guide. *Sports Health.* 2012;4(2):128-138. doi:10.1177/1941738111434406.

9.   Halson SL, Jeukendrup AE. Does overtraining exist? An analysis of overreaching and overtraining research. *Sports Med.* 2004;34(14):967-981.

10.   Kreher JB. Diagnosis and prevention of overtraining syndrome: an opinion on education strategies. *Open access J Sport Med.* 2016;7:115-122. doi:10.2147/OAJSM.S91657.

11.   Finn HT, Brennan SL, Gonano BM, et al. Muscle Activation Does Not Increase After a Fatigue Plateau Is Reached During 8 Sets of Resistance Exercise in Trained Individuals. *J Strength Cond Res*. 2014;28(5):1226-1234. doi:10.1097/JSC.0000000000000226; Hooper DR, Szivak TK, Comstock BA, et al. Effects of Fatigue From Resistance Training on Barbell Back Squat Biomechanics. *J Strength Cond Res*. 2014;28(4):1127-1134. doi:10.1097/JSC.0000000000000237.

12.   Rozzi SL, Lephart SM, Fu FH. Effects of muscular fatigue on knee joint laxity and neuromuscular characteristics of male and female athletes. *J Athl Train*. 1999;34(2):106-114.

13.   Headley SA, Henry K, Nindl BC, Thompson BA, Kraemer WJ, Jones MT. Effects of Lifting Tempo on One Repetition Maximum and Hormonal Responses to a Bench Press Protocol. *J Strength Cond Res*. 2011;25(2):406-413. doi:10.1519/JSC.0b013e3181bf053b.

14.   Radaelli R, Fleck SJ, Leite T, et al. Dose-Response of 1, 3, and 5 Sets of Resistance Exercise on Strength, Local Muscular Endurance, and Hypertrophy. *J Strength Cond Res*. 2015;29(5):1349-1358. doi:10.1519/JSC.0000000000000758.

15.   Hatfield DL, Kraemer WJ, Spiering BA, et al. The Impact of Velocity of Movement on Performance Factors in Resistance Exercise. *J Strength Cond Res*. 2006;20(4):760. doi:10.1519/R-155552.1; Goldberg AL, Etlinger JD, Goldspink DF, Jablecki C. Mechanism of work-induced hypertrophy of skeletal muscle. *Med Sci Sports*. 1975;7(3):185-198.

16.   Munn J, Herbert RD, Hancock MJ, Gandevia SC. Resistance training for strength: effect of number of sets and contraction speed. *Med Sci Sports Exerc*. 2005;37(9):1622-1626.

17.   Neils CM, Udermann BE, Brice GA, Winchester JB, McGuigan MR. Influence of Contraction Velocity in Untrained Individuals Over the Initial Early Phase of Resistance Training. *J Strength Cond Res*. 2005;19(4):883. doi:10.1519/R-15794.1.

18.   Kim E, Dear A, Ferguson SL, Seo D, Bemben MG. Effects of 4 Weeks of Traditional Resistance Training vs. Superslow Strength Training on Early Phase Adaptations in Strength, Flexibility, and Aerobic Capacity in College-Aged Women. *J Strength Cond Res*. 2011;25(11):3006-3013. doi:10.1519/JSC.0b013e318212e3a2.

19.   Woods K, Bishop P, Jones E. Warm-up and stretching in the prevention of muscular injury. *Sports Med*. 2007;37(12):1089-1099.

20.   Fradkin AJ, Gabbe BJ, Cameron PA. Does warming up prevent injury in sport? *J Sci Med Sport*. 2006;9(3):214-220. doi:10.1016/j.jsams.2006.03.026.

21.   Gabriel DA, Kamen G, Frost G. Neural adaptations to resistive exercise: mechanisms and recommendations for training practices. *Sports Med*. 2006;36(2):133-149.

22.   Fradkin AJ, Zazryn TR, Smoliga JM. Effects of warming-up on physical performance: a systematic review with meta-analysis. *J strength Cond Res*. 2010;24(1):140-148. doi:10.1519/JSC.0b013e3181c643a0.

23.   Decostre V, Bianco P, Lombardi V, Piazzesi G. Effect of temperature on the working stroke of muscle myosin. *Proc Natl Acad Sci*. 2005;102(39):13927-13932. doi:10.1073/pnas.0506795102.

24.   Lebon F, Collet C, Guillot A. Benefits of Motor Imagery Training on Muscle Strength. *J Strength Cond Res*. 2010;24(6):1680-1687. doi:10.1519/JSC.0b013e3181d8e936.

25.   Kujala UM, Kvist M, Osterman K. Knee injuries in athletes. Review of exertion injuries and retrospective study of outpatient sports clinic material. *Sports Med*. 3(6):447-460; Maffulli N, Longo UG, Gougoulias N, Caine D, Denaro V. Sport injuries: a review of outcomes. *Br Med Bull*. 2011;97(1):47-80. doi:10.1093/bmb/ldq026.

CHAPTER 22

THE ULTIMATE WORKOUT PLAN FOR WOMEN – CARDIO

1.   Macpherson REK, Hazell TJ, Olver TD, Paterson DH, Lemon PWR. Run Sprint Interval Training Improves Aerobic Performance but Not Maximal Cardiac Output. *Med Sci Sport Exerc*. 2011;43(1):115-122. doi:10.1249/MSS.0b013e3181e5eacd.

2.   Boutcher SH. High-Intensity Intermittent Exercise and Fat Loss. *J Obes*. 2011;2011:1-10. doi:10.1155/2011/868305.

3.   Trapp EG, Chisholm DJ, Freund J, Boutcher SH. The effects of high-intensity intermittent exercise training on fat loss and fasting insulin levels of young women. *Int J Obes.* 2008;32(4):684-691. doi:10.1038/sj.ijo.0803781.

4.   Boutcher SH. High-Intensity Intermittent Exercise and Fat Loss. *J Obes.* 2011;2011:1-10. doi:10.1155/2011/868305.

5.   Gergley JC. Comparison of Two Lower-Body Modes of Endurance Training on Lower-Body Strength Development While Concurrently Training. *J Strength Cond Res.* 2009;23(3):979-987. doi:10.1519/JSC.0b013e3181a0629d.

6.   Spencer MR, Gastin PB. Energy system contribution during 200- to 1500-m running in highly trained athletes. *Med Sci Sports Exerc.* 2001;33(1):157-162.

7.   Lindsay FH, Hawley JA, Myburgh KH, Schomer HH, Noakes TD, Dennis SC. Improved athletic performance in highly trained cyclists after interval training. *Med Sci Sports Exerc.* 1996;28(11):1427-1434; Weston AR, Myburgh KH, Lindsay FH, Dennis SC, Noakes TD, Hawley JA. Skeletal muscle buffering capacity and endurance performance after high-intensity interval training by well-trained cyclists. *Eur J Appl Physiol Occup Physiol.* 1997;75(1):7-13; Westgarth-Taylor C, Hawley JA, Rickard S, Myburgh KH, Noakes TD, Dennis SC. Metabolic and performance adaptations to interval training in endurance-trained cyclists. *Eur J Appl Physiol.* 1997;75(4):298-304. doi:10.1007/s004210050164.

8.   Stepto NK, Hawley JA, Dennis SC, Hopkins WG. Effects of different interval-training programs on cycling time-trial performance. *Med Sci Sports Exerc.* 1999;31(5):736-741; Laursen PB, Blanchard MA, Jenkins DG. Acute high-intensity interval training improves Tvent and peak power output in highly trained males. *Can J Appl Physiol.* 2002;27(4):336-348.

9.   Billat L V. Interval training for performance: a scientific and empirical practice. Special recommendations for middle- and long-distance running. Part I: aerobic interval training. *Sports Med.* 2001;31(1):13-31.

10.   Wilkin LD, Cheryl A, Haddock BL. Energy Expenditure Comparison Between Walking and Running in Average Fitness Individuals. *J Strength Cond Res.* 2012;26(4):1039-1044. doi:10.1519/JSC.0b013e31822e592c.

11.   Park BJ, Tsunetsugu Y, Kasetani T, Kagawa T, Miyazaki Y. The physiological effects of Shinrin-yoku (taking in the forest atmosphere or forest bathing): evidence from field experiments in 24 forests across Japan. *Environ Health Prev Med.* 2010;15(1):18-26. doi:10.1007/s12199-009-0086-9.

12.   Wilson JM, Marin PJ, Rhea MR, Wilson SMC, Loenneke JP, Anderson JC. Concurrent Training: a meta-analysis examining interference of aerobic and resistance exercises. *J Strength Cond Res.* 2012;26(8):2293-2307. doi:10.1519/JSC.0b013e31823a3e2d; Bell G, Petersen S, Wessel J, Bagnall K, Quinney H. Physiological Adaptations to Concurrent Endurance Training and Low Velocity Resistance Training. *Int J Sports Med.* 1991;12(04):384-390. doi:10.1055/s-2007-1024699.

13.   Gergley JC. Comparison of Two Lower-Body Modes of Endurance Training on Lower-Body Strength Development While Concurrently Training. *J Strength Cond Res.* 2009;23(3):979-987. doi:10.1519/JSC.0b013e3181a0629d.

14.   Scott C. Misconceptions about Aerobic and Anaerobic Energy Expenditure. *J Int Soc Sports Nutr.* 2005;2(2):32-37. doi:10.1186/1550-2783-2-2-32.

15.   Van Loon LJ, Greenhaff PL, Constantin-Teodosiu D, Saris WH, Wagenmakers AJ. The effects of increasing exercise intensity on muscle fuel utilisation in humans. *J Physiol.* 2001;536(Pt 1):295-304. doi:10.1111/J.1469-7793.2001.00295.X.

16.   Brown SP, Clemons JM, He Q, Liu S. Prediction of the oxygen cost of the deadlift exercise. *J Sports Sci.* 1994;12(4):371-375. doi:10.1080/02640419408732183.

CHAPTER 23

THE BEST EXERCISES FOR BUILDING YOUR BEST BODY EVER

1.   Grob K, Ackland T, Kuster MS, Manestar M, Filgueira L. A newly discovered muscle: The tensor of the vastus intermedius. *Clin Anat.* 2016;29(2):256-263. doi:10.1002/ca.22680.

2.   Holcomb WR, Rubley MD, Lee HJ, Guadagnoli MA. Effect of Hamstring-Emphasized Resistance Training on Hamstring:Quadriceps Strength Ratios. *J Strength Cond Res.* 2007;21(1):41. doi:10.1519/R-18795.1; Arendt E,

Dick R. Knee Injury Patterns Among Men and Women in Collegiate Basketball and Soccer. *Am J Sports Med*. 1995;23(6):694-701. doi:10.1177/036354659502300611.

3.   Yavuz HU, Erdağ D, Amca AM, Aritan S. Kinematic and EMG activities during front and back squat variations in maximum loads. *J Sports Sci*. 2015;33(10):1058-1066. doi:10.1080/02640414.2014.984240.

4.   Bressel E, Willardson JM, Thompson B, Fontana FE. Effect of instruction, surface stability, and load intensity on trunk muscle activity. *J Electromyogr Kinesiol*. 2009;19(6):e500-e504. doi:10.1016/j.jelekin.2008.10.006.

5.   Trebs AA, Brandenburg JP, Pitney WA. An Electromyography Analysis of 3 Muscles Surrounding the Shoulder Joint During the Performance of a Chest Press Exercise at Several Angles. *J Strength Cond Res*. 2010;24(7):1925-1930. doi:10.1519/JSC.0b013e3181ddfae7.

6.   Chilibeck PD, Calder AW, Sale DG, Webber CE. A comparison of strength and muscle mass increases during resistance training in young women. *Eur J Appl Physiol Occup Physiol*. 1998;77(1-2):170-175.

CHAPTER 24

THE DEFINITIVE GUIDE TO THE "BIG THREE"

1.   Pinto RS, Gomes N, Radaelli R, Botton CE, Brown LE, Bottaro M. Effect of Range of Motion on Muscle Strength and Thickness. *J Strength Cond Res*. 2012;26(8):2140-2145. doi:10.1519/JSC.0b013e31823a3b15.

2.   Chandler TJ, Wilson GD, Stone MH. The effect of the squat exercise on knee stability. *Med Sci Sports Exerc*. 1989;21(3):299-303; Magni NE, McNair PJ, Rice DA. The effects of resistance training on muscle strength, joint pain, and hand function in individuals with hand osteoarthritis: a systematic review and meta-analysis. *Arthritis Res Ther*. 2017;19(1):131. doi:10.1186/s13075-017-1348-3; Susko AM, Fitzgerald GK. The pain-relieving qualities of exercise in knee osteoarthritis. *Open access Rheumatol Res Rev*. 2013;5:81-91. doi:10.2147/OARRR.S53974.

3.   Steiner ME, Grana WA, Chillag K, Schelberg-Karnes E. The effect of exercise on anterior-posterior knee laxity. *Am J Sports Med*. 1986;14(1):24-29. doi:10.1177/036354658601400105.

4.   Solomonow M, Baratta R, Zhou BH, et al. The synergistic action of the anterior cruciate ligament and thigh muscles in maintaining joint stability. *Am J Sports Med*. 1987;15(3):207-213. doi:10.1177/036354658701500302.

5.   Schoenfeld BJ. Squatting Kinematics and Kinetics and Their Application to Exercise Performance. *J Strength Cond Res*. 2010;24(12):3497-3506. doi:10.1519/JSC.0b013e3181bac2d7.

6.   Ariel BG. Biomechanical analysis of the knee joint during deep knee bends with heavy load. In: *Biomechanics IV*. London: Macmillan Education UK; 1974:44-52. doi:10.1007/978-1-349-02612-8_7.

7.   Myer GD, Kushner AM, Brent JL, et al. The back squat: A proposed assessment of functional deficits and technical factors that limit performance. *Strength Cond J*. 2014;36(6):4-27. doi:10.1519/SSC.0000000000000103.

8.   Schwanbeck S, Chilibeck PD, Binsted G. A Comparison of Free Weight Squat to Smith Machine Squat Using Electromyography. *J Strength Cond Res*. 2009;23(9):2588-2591. doi:10.1519/JSC.0b013e3181b1b181.

9.   Kay AD, Blazevich AJ. Effect of Acute Static Stretch on Maximal Muscle Performance. *Med Sci Sport Exerc*. 2012;44(1):154-164. doi:10.1249/MSS.0b013e318225cb27.

10.   Blanchard TW, Smith C, Grenier SG. In a dynamic lifting task, the relationship between cross-sectional abdominal muscle thickness and the corresponding muscle activity is affected by the combined use of a weightlifting belt and the Valsalva maneuver. *J Electromyogr Kinesiol*. 2016;28:99-103. doi:10.1016/j.jelekin.2016.03.006.

11.   Hackett DA, Chow C-M. The Valsalva Maneuver. *J Strength Cond Res*. 2013;27(8):2338-2345. doi:10.1519/JSC.0b013e31827de07d; Fleck SJ, Dean LS. Resistance-training experience and the pressor response during resistance exercise. *J Appl Physiol*. 1987;63(1):116-120. doi:10.1152/jappl.1987.63.1.116.

12.   Colado JC, Pablos C, Chulvi-Medrano I, Garcia-Masso X, Flandez J, Behm DG. The Progression of Paraspinal Muscle Recruitment Intensity in Localized and Global Strength Training Exercises Is Not Based on Instability Alone. *Arch Phys Med Rehabil*. 2011;92(11):1875-1883. doi:10.1016/j.apmr.2011.05.015.

13.   Cholewicki J, McGill SM. Lumbar posterior ligament involvement during extremely heavy lifts estimated from fluoroscopic measurements. *J Biomech*. 1992;25(1):17-28.

14.   Beggs LA. Comparison of muscle activation and kinematics during the deadlift using a double-pronated and overhand/underhand grip. *University of Kentucky Master's Theses*. 2011.

15.   Green CM, Comfort P. The Affect of Grip Width on Bench Press Performance and Risk of Injury. *Strength Cond J*. 2007;29(5):10-14. doi:10.1519/00126548-200710000-00001.

16.   Duffey MJ, Challis JH. Vertical and Lateral Forces Applied to the Bar during the Bench Press in Novice Lifters. *J Strength Cond Res*. 2011;25(9):2442-2447. doi:10.1519/JSC.0b013e3182281939; Madsen N, McLaughlin T. Kinematic factors influencing performance and injury risk in the bench press exercise. *Med Sci Sports Exerc*. 1984;16(4):376-381.

17.   Duffey MJ, Challis JH. Vertical and Lateral Forces Applied to the Bar during the Bench Press in Novice Lifters. *J Strength Cond Res*. 2011;25(9):2442-2447. doi:10.1519/JSC.0b013e3182281939.

CHAPTER 25

THE GREAT SUPPLEMENT HOAX

1.   O'Connor A. New York Attorney General Targets Supplements at Major Retailers. New York Times Website. https://well.blogs.nytimes.com/2015/02/03/new-york-attorney-general-targets-supplements-at-major-retailers/. February 3, 2015. Accessed August 23, 2018.

2.   Morrell A. Lawsuits Say Protein Powders Lack Protein, Ripping Off Athletes. Forbes Website. https://www.forbes.com/sites/alexmorrell/2015/03/12/lawsuits-say-protein-powders-lack-protein-ripping-off-athletes/#14fbd4467729. March 12, 2015. Accessed August 23, 2018.

3.   Young A. Popular sports supplements contain meth-like compound. USA Today Website. https://www.usatoday.com/story/news/nation/2013/10/14/tests-of-supplements-craze-and-detonate-find-methamphetamine-like-compound/2968041/. October 14, 2013. Accessed August 23, 2018.

4.   Young A. Sports supplement designer has history of risky products. USA Today Website. https://www.usatoday.com/story/news/nation/2013/07/25/bodybuilding-supplement-designer-matt-cahill-usa-today-investigation/2568815/. July 25, 2014. Accessed August 23, 2018.

5.   Young A. Firm in outbreak probe has history of run-ins with FDA. USA Today Website. https://www.usatoday.com/story/news/nation/2013/10/24/usplabs-has-history-of-fda-run-ins-ceo-with-criminal-history/3179113/. October 24, 2013. Accessed August 23, 2018; U.S. Food & Drug Administration. DMAA in Products Marketed as Dietary Supplements. U.S. Food & Drug Administration Website. https://www.fda.gov/food/dietarysupplements/productsingredients/ucm346576.htm. August 7, 2018. Accessed August 23, 2018; U.S. Food & Drug Administration. Public Notification: Oxy ELITE Pro Super Thermogenic contains hidden drug ingredient. U.S. Food & Drug Administration Website. https://www.fda.gov/drugs/resourcesforyou/consumers/buyingusingmedicinesafely/medicationhealthfraud/ucm436017.htm. February 28, 2015. Accessed August 23, 2018; National Institutes of Health. Drug Record: OxyELITE Pro. National Institutes of Health LiverTox Website. https://livertox.nih.gov/OxyELITEPro.htm. July 5, 2018. Accessed August 23, 2018.

6.   United States Department of Justice. USPlabs and Corporate Officers Indicted. United States Department of Justice Website. https://www.justice.gov/usao-ndtx/pr/usplabs-and-corporate-officers-indicted. November 17, 2015. Accessed August 23, 2018.

7.   Wilson JM, Lowery RP, Joy JM, et al. The effects of 12 weeks of beta-hydroxy-beta-methylbutyrate free acid supplementation on muscle mass, strength, and power in resistance-trained individuals: a randomized, double-blind, placebo-controlled study. *Eur J Appl Physiol*. 2014;114(6):1217-1227. doi:10.1007/s00421-014-2854-5.

8.   Bhasin S, Storer TW, Berman N, et al. The Effects of Supraphysiologic Doses of Testosterone on Muscle Size and Strength in Normal Men. *N Engl J Med*. 1996;335(1):1-7. doi:10.1056/NEJM199607043350101.

9.   Panton LB, Rathmacher JA, Baier S, Nissen S. Nutritional supplementation of the leucine metabolite beta-hydroxy-beta-methylbutyrate (hmb) during resistance training. *Nutrition*. 2000;16(9):734-739; Nissen SL, Sharp RL. Effect of dietary supplements on lean mass and strength gains with resistance exercise: a meta-analysis. *J Appl Physiol*. 2003;94(2):651-659. doi:10.1152/japplphysiol.00755.2002.

10. Thomson JS, Watson PE, Rowlands DS. Effects of Nine Weeks of β-Hydroxy-β- Methylbutyrate Supplementation on Strength and Body Composition in Resistance Trained Men. *J Strength Cond Res.* 2009;23(3):827-835. doi:10.1519/JSC.0b013e3181a00d47.

11. Slater G, Jenkins D, Logan P, et al. Beta-hydroxy-beta-methylbutyrate (HMB) supplementation does not affect changes in strength or body composition during resistance training in trained men. *Int J Sport Nutr Exerc Metab.* 2001;11(3):384-396.

12. Kreider RB, Ferreira M, Wilson M, Almada AL. Effects of Calcium β-Hydroxy-β-methylbutyrate (HMB) Supplementation During Resistance-Training on Markers of Catabolism, Body Composition and Strength. *Int J Sports Med.* 1999;20(8):503-509. doi:10.1055/s-1999-8835.

13. Rowlands DS, Thomson JS. Effects of β-Hydroxy-β-Methylbutyrate Supplementation During Resistance Training on Strength, Body Composition, and Muscle Damage in Trained and Untrained Young Men: A Meta-Analysis. *J Strength Cond Res.* 2009;23(3):836-846. doi:10.1519/JSC.0b013e3181a00c80.

CHAPTER 26

THE SMART SUPPLEMENT BUYER'S GUIDE

1. Branch JD. Effect of creatine supplementation on body composition and performance: a meta-analysis. *Int J Sport Nutr Exerc Metab.* 2003;13(2):198-226; Hobson RM, Saunders B, Ball G, Harris RC, Sale C. Effects of β-alanine supplementation on exercise performance: a meta analysis. *Amino Acids.* 2012;43(1):25-37. doi:10.1007/s00726-011-1200-z; Pérez-Guisado J, Jakeman PM. Citrulline Malate Enhances Athletic Anaerobic Performance and Relieves Muscle Soreness. *J Strength Cond Res.* 2010;24(5):1215-1222. doi:10.1519/JSC.0b013e3181cb28e0; Haaz S, Fontaine KR, Cutter G, Limdi N, Perumean-Chaney S, Allison DB. Citrus aurantium and synephrine alkaloids in the treatment of overweight and obesity: an update. *Obes Rev.* 2006;7(1):79-88. doi:10.1111/j.1467-789X.2006.00195.x; Ostojic SM. Yohimbine: The Effects on Body Composition and Exercise Performance in Soccer Players. *Res Sport Med.* 2006;14(4):289-299. doi:10.1080/15438620600987106; Morris MC, Sacks F, Rosner B. Does fish oil lower blood pressure? A meta-analysis of controlled trials. *Circulation.* 1993;88(2):523-533; Serban M-C, Sahebkar A, Dragan S, et al. A systematic review and meta-analysis of the impact of Spirulina supplementation on plasma lipid concentrations. *Clin Nutr.* 2016;35(4):842-851. doi:10.1016/j.clnu.2015.09.007; Dawson-Hughes B, Mithal A, Bonjour J-P, et al. IOF position statement: vitamin D recommendations for older adults. *Osteoporos Int.* 2010;21(7):1151-1154. doi:10.1007/s00198-010-1285-3.

2. Wolfe RR. Branched-chain amino acids and muscle protein synthesis in humans: myth or reality? *J Int Soc Sports Nutr.* 2017;14(1):30. doi:10.1186/s12970-017-0184-9.

3. Heymsfield SB, Allison DB, Vasselli JR, Pietrobelli A, Greenfield D, Nunez C. Garcinia cambogia (hydroxycitric acid) as a potential antiobesity agent: a randomized controlled trial. *JAMA.* 1998;280(18):1596-1600; Kim J-E, Jeon S-M, Park KH, et al. Does Glycine max leaves or Garcinia Cambogia promote weight-loss or lower plasma cholesterol in overweight individuals: a randomized control trial. *Nutr J.* 2011;10(1):94. doi:10.1186/1475-2891-10-94; Mattes RD, Bormann L. Effects of (-)-hydroxycitric acid on appetitive variables. *Physiol Behav.* 71(1-2):87-94.

4. Rogerson S, Riches CJ, Jennings C, Weatherby RP, Meir RA, Marshall-Gradisnik SM. The Effect of Five Weeks of Tribulus terrestris Supplementation on Muscle Strength and Body Composition During Preseason Training in Elite Rugby League Players. *J Strength Cond Res.* 2007;21(2):348. doi:10.1519/R-18395.1; Neychev VK, Mitev VI. The aphrodisiac herb Tribulus terrestris does not influence the androgen production in young men. *J Ethnopharmacol.* 2005;101(1-3):319-323. doi:10.1016/j.jep.2005.05.017; Saudan C, Baume N, Emery C, Strahm E, Saugy M. Short term impact of Tribulus terrestris intake on doping control analysis of endogenous steroids. *Forensic Sci Int.* 2008;178(1):e7-e10. doi:10.1016/j.forsciint.2008.01.003.

5. Piper JD, Piper PW. Benzoate and Sorbate Salts: A Systematic Review of the Potential Hazards of These Invaluable Preservatives and the Expanding Spectrum of Clinical Uses for Sodium Benzoate. *Compr Rev Food Sci Food Saf.* 2017;16(5):868-880. doi:10.1111/1541-4337.12284; Potera C. The artificial food dye blues. *Environ Health Perspect.* 2010;118(10):A428. doi:10.1289/ehp.118-a428; Brown RJ, de Banate MA, Rother KI. Artificial sweeteners: a systematic review of metabolic effects in youth. *Int J Pediatr Obes.* 2010;5(4):305-312. doi:10.3109/17477160903497027.

6.   Norton LE, Wilson GJ, Layman DK, Moulton CJ, Garlick PJ. Leucine content of dietary proteins is a determinant of postprandial skeletal muscle protein synthesis in adult rats. *Nutr Metab (Lond)*. 2012;9(1):67. doi:10.1186/1743-7075-9-67.

7.   Boirie Y, Dangin M, Gachon P, Vasson MP, Maubois JL, Beaufrère B. Slow and fast dietary proteins differently modulate postprandial protein accretion. *Proc Natl Acad Sci USA*. 1997;94(26):14930-14935.

8.   Dangin M, Boirie Y, Garcia-Rodenas C, et al. The digestion rate of protein is an independent regulating factor of postprandial protein retention. *Am J Physiol Metab*. 2001;280(2):E340-E348. doi:10.1152/ajpendo.2001.280.2.E340.

9.   Manninen AH. Protein hydrolysates in sports and exercise: a brief review. *J Sports Sci Med*. 2004;3(2):60-63; Potier M, Tomé D. Comparison of digestibility and quality of intact proteins with their respective hydrolysates. *J AOAC Int*. 91(4):1002-1005.

10.   Hoffman JR, Falvo MJ. Protein - Which is Best? *J Sports Sci Med*. 2004;3(3):118-130; Miller PE, Alexander DD, Perez V. Effects of Whey Protein and Resistance Exercise on Body Composition: A Meta-Analysis of Randomized Controlled Trials. *J Am Coll Nutr*. 2014;33(2):163-175. doi:10.1080/07315724.2013.875365.

11.   Hoffman JR, Falvo MJ. Protein - Which is Best? *J Sports Sci Med*. 2004;3(3):118-130.

12.   Boirie Y, Dangin M, Gachon P, Vasson MP, Maubois JL, Beaufrère B. Slow and fast dietary proteins differently modulate postprandial protein accretion. *Proc Natl Acad Sci USA*. 1997;94(26):14930-14935. doi:10.1073/PNAS.94.26.14930.

13.   Tipton KD, Elliott TA, Cree MG, Wolf SE, Sanford AP, Wolfe RR. Ingestion of casein and whey proteins result in muscle anabolism after resistance exercise. *Med Sci Sports Exerc*. 2004;36(12):2073-2081; West DW, Burd NA, Coffey VG, et al. Rapid aminoacidemia enhances myofibrillar protein synthesis and anabolic intramuscular signaling responses after resistance exercise. *Am J Clin Nutr*. 2011;94(3):795-803. doi:10.3945/ajcn.111.013722.

14.   Boirie Y, Dangin M, Gachon P, Vasson MP, Maubois JL, Beaufrère B. Slow and fast dietary proteins differently modulate postprandial protein accretion. *Proc Natl Acad Sci USA*. 1997;94(26):14930-14935.

15.   Res PT, Groen B, Pennings B, et al. Protein Ingestion before Sleep Improves Postexercise Overnight Recovery. *Med Sci Sport Exerc*. 2012;44(8):1560-1569. doi:10.1249/MSS.0b013e31824cc363.

16.   Boirie Y, Dangin M, Gachon P, Vasson MP, Maubois JL, Beaufrère B. Slow and fast dietary proteins differently modulate postprandial protein accretion. *Proc Natl Acad Sci USA*. 1997;94(26):14930-14935.

17.   Hoffman JR, Falvo MJ. Protein - Which is Best? *J Sports Sci Med*. 2004;3(3):118-130.

18.   Matsuoka R, Shirouchi B, Umegatani M, et al. Dietary egg-white protein increases body protein mass and reduces body fat mass through an acceleration of hepatic β-oxidation in rats. *Br J Nutr*. 2017;118(06):423-430. doi:10.1017/S0007114517002306.

19.   Van Vliet S, Shy EL, Abou Sawan S, et al. Consumption of whole eggs promotes greater stimulation of postexercise muscle protein synthesis than consumption of isonitrogenous amounts of egg whites in young men. *Am J Clin Nutr*. 2017;106(6):1401-1412. doi:10.3945/ajcn.117.159855.

20.   Tang JE, Moore DR, Kujbida GW, Tarnopolsky MA, Phillips SM. Ingestion of whey hydrolysate, casein, or soy protein isolate: effects on mixed muscle protein synthesis at rest and following resistance exercise in young men. *J Appl Physiol*. 2009;107(3):987-992. doi:10.1152/japplphysiol.00076.2009.

21.   Chavarro JE, Toth TL, Sadio SM, Hauser R. Soy food and isoflavone intake in relation to semen quality parameters among men from an infertility clinic. *Hum Reprod*. 2008;23(11):2584-2590. doi:10.1093/humrep/den243; Liu B, Qin L, Liu A, Shi Y, Wang P. [Equol-producing phenotype and in relation to serum sex hormones among healthy adults in Beijing]. *Wei Sheng Yan Jiu*. 2011;40(6):727-731.

22.   Beaton LK, McVeigh BL, Dillingham BL, Lampe JW, Duncan AM. Soy protein isolates of varying isoflavone content do not adversely affect semen quality in healthy young men. *Fertil Steril*. 2010;94(5):1717-1722. doi:10.1016/j.fertnstert.2009.08.055; Messina M. Soybean isoflavone exposure does not have feminizing effects on men: a critical examination of the clinical evidence. *Fertil Steril*. 2010;93(7):2095-2104. doi:10.1016/j.fertnstert.2010.03.002; Hamilton-Reeves JM, Vazquez G, Duval SJ, Phipps WR, Kurzer MS, Messina MJ. Clinical studies show no effects of soy protein or isoflavones on reproductive hormones in men: results of a meta-analysis. *Fertil Steril*. 2010;94(3):997-1007. doi:10.1016/j.fertnstert.2009.04.038.

23.   Mobley C, Haun C, Roberson P, et al. Effects of Whey, Soy or Leucine Supplementation with 12 Weeks of Resistance Training on Strength, Body Composition, and Skeletal Muscle and Adipose Tissue Histological Attributes in College-Aged Males. *Nutrients*. 2017;9(9):972. doi:10.3390/nu9090972.

24.   Joy JM, Lowery RP, Wilson JM, et al. The effects of 8 weeks of whey or rice protein supplementation on body composition and exercise performance. *Nutr J*. 2013;12(1):86. doi:10.1186/1475-2891-12-86; Padhye VW, Salunkhe DK. Extraction and characterization of rice proteins. *Cereal Chemistry*. 1979;56(5):389-393; Kalman D. Amino Acid Composition of an Organic Brown Rice Protein Concentrate and Isolate Compared to Soy and Whey Concentrates and Isolates. *Foods*. 2014;3(3):394-402. doi:10.3390/foods3030394.

25.   Mariotti F, Pueyo ME, Tomé D, Bérot S, Benamouzig R, Mahé S. The Influence of the Albumin Fraction on the Bioavailability and Postprandial Utilization of Pea Protein Given Selectively to Humans. *J Nutr*. 2001;131(6):1706-1713. doi:10.1093/jn/131.6.1706.

26.   Babault N, Païzis C, Deley G, et al. Pea proteins oral supplementation promotes muscle thickness gains during resistance training: a double-blind, randomized, Placebo-controlled clinical trial vs. Whey protein. *J Int Soc Sports Nutr*. 2015;12(1):3. doi:10.1186/s12970-014-0064-5.

27.   House JD, Neufeld J, Leson G. Evaluating the Quality of Protein from Hemp Seed (*Cannabis sativa L.*) Products Through the use of the Protein Digestibility-Corrected Amino Acid Score Method. *J Agric Food Chem*. 2010;58(22):11801-11807. doi:10.1021/jf102636b; Wang X-S, Tang C-H, Yang X-Q, Gao W-R. Characterization, amino acid composition and in vitro digestibility of hemp (Cannabis sativa L.) proteins. *Food Chem*. 2008;107(1):11-18. doi:10.1016/J.FOODCHEM.2007.06.064.

28.   Eastoe JE. The amino acid composition of mammalian collagen and gelatin. *Biochem J*. 1955;61(4):589-600; Hulmi JJ, Lockwood CM, Stout JR. Effect of protein/essential amino acids and resistance training on skeletal muscle hypertrophy: A case for whey protein. *Nutr Metab (Lond)*. 2010;7:51. doi:10.1186/1743-7075-7-51.

29.   Kabil O, Vitvitsky V, Banerjee R. Sulfur as a signaling nutrient through hydrogen sulfide. *Annu Rev Nutr*. 2014;34:171-205. doi:10.1146/annurev-nutr-071813-105654.

30.   Kris-Etherton P, Taylor DS, Yu-Poth S, et al. Polyunsaturated fatty acids in the food chain in the United States. *Am J Clin Nutr*. 2000;71(1):179S-188S. doi:10.1093/ajcn/71.1.179S.

31.   Swanson D, Block R, Mousa SA. Omega-3 fatty acids EPA and DHA: health benefits throughout life. *Adv Nutr*. 2012;3(1):1-7. doi:10.3945/an.111.000893; Nkondjock A, Ghadirian P. Intake of specific carotenoids and essential fatty acids and breast cancer risk in Montreal, Canada. *Am J Clin Nutr*. 2004;79(5):857-864. doi:10.1093/ajcn/79.5.857.

32.   Parker G, Gibson NA, Brotchie H, Heruc G, Rees A-M, Hadzi-Pavlovic D. Omega-3 Fatty Acids and Mood Disorders. *Am J Psychiatry*. 2006;163(6):969-978. doi:10.1176/ajp.2006.163.6.969; Logan AC. Omega-3 fatty acids and major depression: a primer for the mental health professional. *Lipids Health Dis*. 2004;3:25. doi:10.1186/1476-511X-3-25; Kiecolt-Glaser JK, Belury MA, Andridge R, Malarkey WB, Glaser R. Omega-3 supplementation lowers inflammation and anxiety in medical students: a randomized controlled trial. *Brain Behav Immun*. 2011;25(8):1725-1734. doi:10.1016/j.bbi.2011.07.229.

33.   Kalmijn S, van Boxtel MPJ, Ocké M, Verschuren WMM, Kromhout D, Launer LJ. Dietary intake of fatty acids and fish in relation to cognitive performance at middle age. *Neurology*. 2004;62(2):275-280.

34.   Goldberg RJ, Katz J. A meta-analysis of the analgesic effects of omega-3 polyunsaturated fatty acid supplementation for inflammatory joint pain. *Pain*. 2007;129(1):210-223. doi:10.1016/j.pain.2007.01.020.

35.   Couet C, Delarue J, Ritz P, Antoine JM, Lamisse F. Effect of dietary fish oil on body fat mass and basal fat oxidation in healthy adults. *Int J Obes Relat Metab Disord*. 1997;21(8):637-643.

36.   Buckley JD, Howe PRC. Anti-obesity effects of long-chain omega-3 polyunsaturated fatty acids. *Obes Rev*. 2009;10(6):648-659. doi:10.1111/j.1467-789X.2009.00584.x.

37.   Smith GI, Atherton P, Reeds DN, et al. Omega-3 polyunsaturated fatty acids augment the muscle protein anabolic response to hyperinsulinaemia–hyperaminoacidaemia in healthy young and middle-aged men and women. *Clin Sci*. 2011;121(6):267-278. doi:10.1042/CS20100597.

38.   Ponnampalam EN, Mann NJ, Sinclair AJ. Effect of feeding systems on omega-3 fatty acids, conjugated linoleic acid and trans fatty acids in Australian beef cuts: potential impact on human health. *Asia Pac J Clin Nutr*. 2006;15(1):21-29.

39.   Poudyal H, Panchal SK, Diwan V, Brown L. Omega-3 fatty acids and metabolic syndrome: Effects and emerging mechanisms of action. *Prog Lipid Res*. 2011;50(4):372-387. doi:10.1016/j.plipres.2011.06.003.

40.   Rosell MS, Lloyd-Wright Z, Appleby PN, Sanders TA, Allen NE, Key TJ. Long-chain n–3 polyunsaturated fatty acids in plasma in British meat-eating, vegetarian, and vegan men. *Am J Clin Nutr*. 2005;82(2):327-334. doi:10.1093/ajcn/82.2.327.

41. Dyerberg J, Madsen P, Møller JM, Aardestrup I, Schmidt EB. Bioavailability of marine n-3 fatty acid formulations. *Prostaglandins, Leukotrienes, and Essential Fatty Acids.* 2010;83(3):137-141. doi:10.1016/j.plefa.2010.06.007.

42. Neubronner J, Schuchardt JP, Kressel G, Merkel M, von Schacky C, Hahn A. Enhanced increase of omega-3 index in response to long-term n-3 fatty acid supplementation from triacylglycerides versus ethyl esters. *Eur J Clin Nutr.* 2011;65(2):247-254. doi:10.1038/ejcn.2010.239.

43. Dyerberg J, Bang HO. Haemostatic function and platelet polyunsaturated fatty acids in Eskimos. *Lancet (London, England).* 1979;2(8140):433-435.

44. WebMD. Lovaza. WebMD Website. https://www.webmd.com/drugs/2/drug-148529/lovaza-oral/details. Accessed August 26, 2018.

45. Dyerberg J, Madsen P, Møller JM, Aardestrup I, Schmidt EB. Bioavailability of marine n-3 fatty acid formulations. *Prostaglandins, Leukotrienes, and Essential Fatty Acids.* 2010;83(3):137-141. doi:10.1016/j.plefa.2010.06.007.

46. Song J-H, Inoue Y, Miyazawa T. Oxidative Stability of Docosahexaenoic Acid-containing Oils in the Form of Phospholipids, Triacylglycerols, and Ethyl Esters. *Biosci Biotechnol Biochem.* 1997;61(12):2085-2088. doi:10.1271/bbb.61.2085.

47. Holick MF. Vitamin D is essential to the modern indoor lifestyle. Science News Website. https://www.sciencenews.org/article/vitamin-d-essential-modern-indoor-lifestyle. October 8, 2010. Accessed August 26, 2018; Holick MF. Vitamin D: evolutionary, physiological and health perspectives. *Curr Drug Targets.* 2011;12(1):4-18.

48. Wacker M, Holick MF. Vitamin D - effects on skeletal and extraskeletal health and the need for supplementation. *Nutrients.* 2013;5(1):111-148. doi:10.3390/nu5010111.

49. Dawson-Hughes B, Mithal A, Bonjour J-P, et al. IOF position statement: vitamin D recommendations for older adults. *Osteoporos Int.* 2010;21(7):1151-1154. doi:10.1007/s00198-010-1285-3; Wang TJ, Pencina MJ, Booth SL, et al. Vitamin D Deficiency and Risk of Cardiovascular Disease. *Circulation.* 2008;117(4):503-511. doi:10.1161/CIRCULATIONAHA.107.706127; Pilz S, Dobnig H, Fischer JE, et al. Low Vitamin D Levels Predict Stroke in Patients Referred to Coronary Angiography. *Stroke.* 2008;39(9):2611-2613. doi:10.1161/STROKEAHA.107.513655; Giovannucci E. Epidemiological Evidence for Vitamin D and Colorectal Cancer. *J Bone Miner Res.* 2007;22(S2):V81-V85. doi:10.1359/jbmr.07s206; Hyppönen E, Läärä E, Reunanen A, Järvelin M-R, Virtanen SM. Intake of vitamin D and risk of type 1 diabetes: a birth-cohort study. *Lancet.* 2001;358(9292):1500-1503. doi:10.1016/S0140-6736(01)06580-1; Munger KL, Levin LI, Hollis BW, Howard NS, Ascherio A. Serum 25-Hydroxyvitamin D Levels and Risk of Multiple Sclerosis. *JAMA.* 2006;296(23):2832. doi:10.1001/jama.296.23.2832; Nnoaham KE, Clarke A. Low serum vitamin D levels and tuberculosis: a systematic review and meta-analysis. *Int J Epidemiol.* 2008;37(1):113-119. doi:10.1093/ije/dym247; Cannell JJ, Vieth R, Umhau JC, et al. Epidemic influenza and vitamin D. *Epidemiol Infect.* 2006;134(06):1129. doi:10.1017/S0950268806007175.

50. Holick MF. Vitamin D: importance in the prevention of cancers, type 1 diabetes, heart disease, and osteoporosis. *Am J Clin Nutr.* 2004;79(3):362-371. doi:10.1093/ajcn/79.3.362.

51. Terushkin V, Bender A, Psaty EL, Engelsen O, Wang SQ, Halpern AC. Estimated equivalency of vitamin D production from natural sun exposure versus oral vitamin D supplementation across seasons at two US latitudes. *J Am Acad Dermatol.* 2010;62(6):929.e1-929.e9. doi:10.1016/j.jaad.2009.07.028.

52. Cordain L, Eaton SB, Sebastian A, et al. Origins and evolution of the Western diet: health implications for the 21st century. *Am J Clin Nutr.* 2005;81(2):341-354. doi:10.1093/ajcn.81.2.341.

53. Blumberg JB, Frei BB, Fulgoni VL, Weaver CM, Zeisel SH, Zeisel SH. Impact of Frequency of Multi-Vitamin/Multi-Mineral Supplement Intake on Nutritional Adequacy and Nutrient Deficiencies in U.S. Adults. *Nutrients.* 2017;9(8). doi:10.3390/nu9080849.

54. Erkkilä AT, Booth SL. Vitamin K intake and atherosclerosis. *Curr Opin Lipidol.* 2008;19(1):39-42. doi:10.1097/MOL.0b013e3282f1c57f; Dawson-Hughes B, Mithal A, Bonjour J-P, et al. IOF position statement: vitamin D recommendations for older adults. *Osteoporos Int.* 2010;21(7):1151-1154. doi:10.1007/s00198-010-1285-3.

55. Schwalfenberg GK. Vitamins K1 and K2: The Emerging Group of Vitamins Required for Human Health. *J Nutr Metab.* 2017;2017:6254836. doi:10.1155/2017/6254836.

56. Miller ER, Pastor-Barriuso R, Dalal D, Riemersma RA, Appel LJ, Guallar E. Meta-analysis: high-dosage vitamin E supplementation may increase all-cause mortality. *Ann Intern Med.* 2005;142(1):37-46.

57.   Onakpoya I, Hung SK, Perry R, Wider B, Ernst E. The Use of *Garcinia* Extract (Hydroxycitric Acid) as a Weight loss Supplement: A Systematic Review and Meta-Analysis of Randomised Clinical Trials. *J Obes.* 2011;2011:1-9. doi:10.1155/2011/509038.

58.   Onakpoya I, Terry R, Ernst E. The Use of Green Coffee Extract as a Weight Loss Supplement: A Systematic Review and Meta-Analysis of Randomised Clinical Trials. *Gastroenterol Res Pract.* 2011;2011:1-6. doi:10.1155/2011/382852.

59.   Watras AC, Buchholz AC, Close RN, Zhang Z, Schoeller DA. The role of conjugated linoleic acid in reducing body fat and preventing holiday weight gain. *Int J Obes.* 2007;31(3):481-487. doi:10.1038/sj.ijo.0803437; Joseph S V., Jacques H, Plourde M, Mitchell PL, McLeod RS, Jones PJH. Conjugated Linoleic Acid Supplementation for 8 Weeks Does Not Affect Body Composition, Lipid Profile, or Safety Biomarkers in Overweight, Hyperlipidemic Men. *J Nutr.* 2011;141(7):1286-1291. doi:10.3945/jn.110.135087; Risérus U, Vessby B, Ärnlöv J, Basu S. Effects of cis-9,trans-11 conjugated linoleic acid supplementation on insulin sensitivity, lipid peroxidation, and proinflammatory markers in obese men. *Am J Clin Nutr.* 2004;80(2):279-283. doi:10.1093/ajcn/80.2.279.

60.   Morimoto C, Satoh Y, Hara M, Inoue S, Tsujita T, Okuda H. Anti-obese action of raspberry ketone. *Life Sci.* 2005;77(2):194-204. doi:10.1016/j.lfs.2004.12.029.

61.   Doherty M, Smith PM. Effects of caffeine ingestion on rating of perceived exertion during and after exercise: a meta-analysis. Scand J Med Sci Sport. 2005;15(2):69-78. doi:10.1111/j.1600-0838.2005.00445.x.

62.   Beck TW, Housh TJ, Schmidt RJ, et al. The Acute Effects of a Caffeine-Containing Supplement on Strength, Muscular Endurance, and Anaerobic Capabilities. *J Strength Cond Res.* 2006;20(3):506. doi:10.1519/18285.1.

63.   Fett CA, Aquino NM, Schantz Junior J, Brandão CF, de Araújo Cavalcanti JD, Fett WC. Performance of muscle strength and fatigue tolerance in young trained women supplemented with caffeine. J Sports Med Phys Fitness. 2018;58(3):249-255. doi:10.23736/S0022-4707.17.06615-4.

64.   Richardson DL, Clarke ND. Effect of Coffee and Caffeine Ingestion on Resistance Exercise Performance. J Strength Cond Res. 2016;30(10):2892-2900. doi:10.1519/JSC.0000000000001382.

65.   Astorino TA, Rohmann RL, Firth K. Effect of caffeine ingestion on one-repetition maximum muscular strength. *Eur J Appl Physiol.* 2007;102(2):127-132. doi:10.1007/s00421-007-0557-x.

66.   Da Silva VL, Messias FR, Zanchi NE, Gerlinger-Romero F, Duncan MJ, Guimarães-Ferreira L. Effects of acute caffeine ingestion on resistance training performance and perceptual responses during repeated sets to failure. J Sports Med Phys Fitness. 2015;55(5):383-389.

67.   Astrup A, Toubro S, Cannon S, Hein P, Breum L, Madsen J. Caffeine: a double blind, placebo controlled study of its thermogenic, metabolic, and cardiovascular effects in healthy volunteers. Am J Clin Nutr. 1990;51(5):759-767. doi:10.1093/ajcn/51.5.759.

68.   Mora-Rodríguez R, Pallarés JG, López-Samanes Á, Ortega JF, Fernández-Elías VE. Caffeine Ingestion Reverses the Circadian Rhythm Effects on Neuromuscular Performance in Highly Resistance-Trained Men. Bacurau RFP, ed. *PLoS One.* 2012;7(4):e33807. doi:10.1371/journal.pone.0033807.

69.   Acheson KJ, Zahorska-Markiewicz B, Pittet P, Anantharaman K, Jéquier E. Caffeine and coffee: their influence on metabolic rate and substrate utilization in normal weight and obese individuals. *Am J Clin Nutr.* 1980;33(5):989-997. doi:10.1093/ajcn/33.5.989; Koot P, Deurenberg P. Comparison of Changes in Energy Expenditure and Body Temperatures after Caffeine Consumption. *Ann Nutr Metab.* 1995;39(3):135-142. doi:10.1159/000177854.

70.   Robertson D, Wade D, Workman R, Woosley RL, Oates JA. Tolerance to the humoral and hemodynamic effects of caffeine in man. *J Clin Invest.* 1981;67(4):1111-1117. doi:10.1172/JCI110124.

71.   Ostojic SM. Yohimbine: The Effects on Body Composition and Exercise Performance in Soccer Players. *Res Sport Med.* 2006;14(4):289-299. doi:10.1080/15438620600987106; McCarty MF. Pre-exercise administration of yohimbine may enhance the efficacy of exercise training as a fat loss strategy by boosting lipolysis. *Med Hypotheses.* 2002;58(6):491-495.

72.   Lefkowitz RJ. Direct binding studies of adrenergic receptors: biochemical, physiologic, and clinical implications. *Ann Intern Med.* 1979;91(3):450-458.

73.   Strosberg AD. Structure, function, and regulation of adrenergic receptors. *Protein Sci.* 1993;2(8):1198-1209. doi:10.1002/pro.5560020802.

74.   Manolopoulos KN, Karpe F, Frayn KN. Marked resistance of femoral adipose tissue blood flow and lipolysis to adrenaline in vivo. *Diabetologia.* 2012;55(11):3029-3037. doi:10.1007/s00125-012-2676-0.

75.   Millan MJ, Newman-Tancredi A, Audinot V, et al. Agonist and antagonist actions of yohimbine as com-pared to fluparoxan at 2-adrenergic receptors (AR)s, serotonin (5-HT)1A, 5-HT1B, 5-HT1D and dopamine D2 and D3 receptors. Significance for the modulation of frontocortical monoaminergic transmission and depres-sive states. *Synapse*. 2000;35(2):79-95. doi:10.1002/(SICI)1098-2396(200002)35:2<79::AID-SYN1>3.0.CO;2-X.

76.   Galitzky J, Taouis M, Berlan M, Rivière D, Garrigues M, Lafontan M. Alpha 2-antagonist compounds and lipid mobilization: evidence for a lipid mobilizing effect of oral yohimbine in healthy male volunteers. *Eur J Clin Invest*. 1988;18(6):587-594.

77.   Nelson BC, Putzbach K, Sharpless KE, Sander LC. Mass Spectrometric Determination of the Predom-inant Adrenergic Protoalkaloids in Bitter Orange (Citrus aurantium). *J Agric Food Chem*. 2007;55(24):9769-9775. doi:10.1021/jf072030s.

78.   Haaz S, Fontaine KR, Cutter G, Limdi N, Perumean-Chaney S, Allison DB. Citrus aurantium and syneph-rine alkaloids in the treatment of overweight and obesity: an update. *Obes Rev*. 2006;7(1):79-88. doi:10.1111/j.1467-789X.2006.00195.x; Gougeon R, Harrigan K, Tremblay J-F, Hedrei P, Lamarche M, Morais JA. Increase in the Thermic Effect of Food in Women by Adrenergic Amines Extracted from Citrus Aurantium. *Obes Res*. 2005;13(7):1187-1194. doi:10.1038/oby.2005.141.

79.   Brown CM, McGrath JC, Midgley JM, et al. Activities of octopamine and synephrine stereoisomers on alpha-adrenoceptors. *Br J Pharmacol*. 1988;93(2):417-429.

80.   Du M, Shen QW, Zhu MJ, Ford SP. Leucine stimulates mammalian target of rapamycin signaling in C2C12 myoblasts in part through inhibition of adenosine monophosphate-activated protein kinase. *J Anim Sci*. 2007;85(4):919-927. doi:10.2527/jas.2006-342; Doi M, Yamaoka I, Fukunaga T, Nakayama M. Isoleucine, a potent plasma glucose-lowering amino acid, stimulates glucose uptake in C2C12 myotubes. *Biochem Biophys Res Commun*. 2003;312(4):1111-1117.

81.   Staten MA, Bier DM, Matthews DE. Regulation of valine metabolism in man: a stable isotope study. *Am J Clin Nutr*. 1984;40(6):1224-1234. doi:10.1093/ajcn/40.6.1224.

82.   Calder PC. Branched-Chain Amino Acids and Immunity. *J Nutr*. 2006;136(1):288S-293S. doi:10.1093/jn/136.1.288S; Meeusen R, Watson P. Amino acids and the brain: do they play a role in "central fatigue"? *Int J Sport Nutr Exerc Metab*. 2007;17 Suppl:S37-46; Howatson G, Hoad M, Goodall S, Tallent J, Bell PG, French DN. Exercise-induced muscle damage is reduced in resistance-trained males by branched chain amino acids: a randomized, double-blind, placebo controlled study. *J Int Soc Sports Nutr*. 2012;9(1):20. doi:10.1186/1550-2783-9-20; Blomstrand E, Eliasson J, Karlsson HKR, Köhnke R. Branched-Chain Amino Acids Activate Key Enzymes in Protein Synthesis after Physical Exercise. *J Nutr*. 2006;136(1):269S-273S. doi:10.1093/jn/136.1.269S.

83.   Mourier A, Bigard A, Kerviler E de, Roger B, Legrand H, Guezennec C. Combined Effects of Caloric Re-striction and Branched-Chain Amino Acid Supplementation on Body Composition and Exercise Performance in Elite Wrestlers. *Int J Sports Med*. 1997;18(01):47-55. doi:10.1055/s-2007-972594.

84.   Hulmi JJ, Lockwood CM, Stout JR. Effect of protein/essential amino acids and resistance training on skel-etal muscle hypertrophy: A case for whey protein. *Nutr Metab (Lond)*. 2010;7(1):51. doi:10.1186/1743-7075-7-51.

85.   Wolfe RR. Branched-chain amino acids and muscle protein synthesis in humans: myth or reality? *J Int Soc Sports Nutr*. 2017;14(1):30. doi:10.1186/s12970-017-0184-9.

86.   Branch JD. Effect of creatine supplementation on body composition and performance: a meta-analysis. *Int J Sport Nutr Exerc Metab*. 2003;13(2):198-226.

87.   Volek JS, Ratamess NA, Rubin MR, et al. The effects of creatine supplementation on muscular perfor-mance and body composition responses to short-term resistance training overreaching. *Eur J Appl Physiol*. 2004;91(5-6):628-637. doi:10.1007/s00421-003-1031-z.

88.   Eckerson JM, Stout JR, Moore GA, et al. Effect of Creatine Phosphate Supplementation on Anaerobic Working Capacity and Body Weight After Two and Six Days of Loading in Men and Women. *J Strength Cond Res*. 2005;19(4):756. doi:10.1519/R-16924.1.

89.   Bassit RA, Pinheiro CH da J, Vitzel KF, Sproesser AJ, Silveira LR, Curi R. Effect of short-term creatine sup-plementation on markers of skeletal muscle damage after strenuous contractile activity. *Eur J Appl Physiol*. 2010;108(5):945-955. doi:10.1007/s00421-009-1305-1.

90.   Groeneveld GJ, Beijer C, Veldink JH, Kalmijn S, Wokke JHJ, van den Berg LH. Few Adverse Effects of Long-Term Creatine Supplementation in a Placebo-Controlled Trial. *Int J Sports Med*. 2005;26(4):307-313. doi:10.1055/s-2004-817917.

91. Darrabie MD, Arciniegas AJL, Mishra R, Bowles DE, Jacobs DO, Santacruz L. AMPK and substrate availability regulate creatine transport in cultured cardiomyocytes. *Am J Physiol Metab*. 2011;300(5):E870-E876. doi:10.1152/ajpendo.00554.2010; Guzun R, Timohhina N, Tepp K, et al. Systems bioenergetics of creatine kinase networks: physiological roles of creatine and phosphocreatine in regulation of cardiac cell function. *Amino Acids*. 2011;40(5):1333-1348. doi:10.1007/s00726-011-0854-x.

92. Safdar A, Yardley NJ, Snow R, Melov S, Tarnopolsky MA. Global and targeted gene expression and protein content in skeletal muscle of young men following short-term creatine monohydrate supplementation. *Physiol Genomics*. 2008;32(2):219-228. doi:10.1152/physiolgenomics.00157.2007.

93. Parise G, Mihic S, MacLennan D, Yarasheski KE, Tarnopolsky MA. Effects of acute creatine monohydrate supplementation on leucine kinetics and mixed-muscle protein synthesis. *J Appl Physiol*. 2001;91(3):1041-1047. doi:10.1152/jappl.2001.91.3.1041; Safdar A, Yardley NJ, Snow R, Melov S, Tarnopolsky MA. Global and targeted gene expression and protein content in skeletal muscle of young men following short-term creatine monohydrate supplementation. *Physiol Genomics*. 2008;32(2):219-228. doi:10.1152/physiolgenomics.00157.2007.

94. Tang F-C, Chan C-C, Kuo P-L. Contribution of creatine to protein homeostasis in athletes after endurance and sprint running. *Eur J Nutr*. 2014;53(1):61-71. doi:10.1007/s00394-013-0498-6.

95. Ament W, Verkerke GJ. Exercise and fatigue. *Sports Med*. 2009;39(5):389-422.

96. Hoffman JR, Landau G, Stout JR, et al. β-Alanine Ingestion increases muscle carnosine content and combat specific performance in soldiers. *Amino Acids*. 2015;47(3):627-636. doi:10.1007/s00726-014-1896-7.

97. Hobson RM, Saunders B, Ball G, Harris RC, Sale C. Effects of β-alanine supplementation on exercise performance: a meta-analysis. *Amino Acids*. 2012;43(1):25-37. doi:10.1007/s00726-011-1200-z.

98. Smith AE, Walter AA, Graef JL, et al. Effects of β-alanine supplementation and high-intensity interval training on endurance performance and body composition in men; a double-blind trial. *J Int Soc Sports Nutr*. 2009;6(1):5. doi:10.1186/1550-2783-6-5; Walter AA, Smith AE, Kendall KL, Stout JR, Cramer JT. Six Weeks of High-Intensity Interval Training With and Without β-Alanine Supplementation for Improving Cardiovascular Fitness in Women. *J Strength Cond Res*. 2010;24(5):1199-1207. doi:10.1519/JSC.0b013e3181d82f8b.

99. Pérez-Guisado J, Jakeman PM. Citrulline Malate Enhances Athletic Anaerobic Performance and Relieves Muscle Soreness. J Strength Cond Res. 2010;24(5):1215-1222. doi:10.1519/JSC.0b013e3181cb28e0.

100. Bendahan D, Mattei JP, Ghattas B, Confort-Gouny S, Le Guern ME, Cozzone PJ. Citrulline/malate promotes aerobic energy production in human exercising muscle. *Br J Sports Med*. 2002;36(4):282-289.

101. Curis E, Crenn P, Cynober L. Citrulline and the gut. *Curr Opin Clin Nutr Metab Care*. 2007;10(5):620-626. doi:10.1097/MCO.0b013e32829fb38d.

102. Paddon-Jones D, Børsheim E, Wolfe RR. Potential ergogenic effects of arginine and creatine supplementation. *J Nutr*. 2004;134(10 Suppl):2888S-2894S; discussion 2895S.

103. Bescós R, Sureda A, Tur JA, Pons A. The Effect of Nitric-Oxide-Related Supplements on Human Performance. *Sport Med*. 2012;42(2):99-117. doi:10.2165/11596860-000000000-00000; Orozco-Gutiérrez JJ, Castillo-Martínez L, Orea-Tejeda A, et al. Effect of L-arginine or L-citrulline oral supplementation on blood pressure and right ventricular function in heart failure patients with preserved ejection fraction. *Cardiol J*. 2010;17(6):612-618; Cormio L, De Siati M, Lorusso F, et al. Oral L-Citrulline Supplementation Improves Erection Hardness in Men With Mild Erectile Dysfunction. *Urology*. 2011;77(1):119-122. doi:10.1016/j.urology.2010.08.028.

104. Wu JL, Wu QP, Huang JM, Chen R, Cai M, Tan JB. Effects of L-malate on physical stamina and activities of enzymes related to the malate-aspartate shuttle in liver of mice. *Physiol Res*. 2007;56(2):213-220.

105. Tang X, Liu J, Dong W, et al. The Cardioprotective Effects of Citric Acid and L-Malic Acid on Myocardial Ischemia/Reperfusion Injury. *Evidence-Based Complement Altern Med*. 2013;2013:1-11. doi:10.1155/2013/820695.

CHAPTER 28

THE THINNER LEANER STRONGER DIET PLAN

1. Wang X, Hu Z, Hu J, Du J, Mitch WE. Insulin Resistance Accelerates Muscle Protein Degradation: Activation of the Ubiquitin-Proteasome Pathway by Defects in Muscle Cell Signaling. *Endocrinology*.

2006;147(9):4160-4168. doi:10.1210/en.2006-0251; Zhang J, Hupfeld CJ, Taylor SS, Olefsky JM, Tsien RY. Insulin disrupts β-adrenergic signalling to protein kinase A in adipocytes. *Nature*. 2005;437(7058):569-573. doi:10.1038/nature04140; Shanik MH, Xu Y, Skrha J, Dankner R, Zick Y, Roth J. Insulin Resistance and Hyperinsulinemia: Is hyperinsulinemia the cart or the horse? *Diabetes Care*. 2008;31(Supplement 2):S262-S268. doi:10.2337/dc08-s264.

2.   Burton-Freeman B. Dietary Fiber and Energy Regulation. *J Nutr*. 2000;130(2):272S-275S. doi:10.1093/jn/130.2.272S; Wooley SC. Physiologic versus cognitive factors in short term food regulation in the obese and nonobese. *Psychosom Med*. 34(1):62-68.

3.   Byrne NM, Sainsbury A, King NA, Hills AP, Wood RE. Intermittent energy restriction improves weight loss efficiency in obese men: the MATADOR study. *Int J Obes (Lond)*. 2018;42(2):129-138. doi:10.1038/ijo.2017.206.

4.   Muckelbauer R, Sarganas G, Grüneis A, Müller-Nordhorn J. Association between water consumption and body weight outcomes: a systematic review. *Am J Clin Nutr*. 2013;98(2):282-299. doi:10.3945/ajcn.112.055061.

5.   Dennis EA, Dengo AL, Comber DL, et al. Water Consumption Increases Weight Loss During a Hypocaloric Diet Intervention in Middle-aged and Older Adults. *Obesity*. 2010;18(2):300-307. doi:10.1038/oby.2009.235.

6.   Boschmann M, Steiniger J, Hille U, et al. Water-Induced Thermogenesis. *J Clin Endocrinol Metab*. 2003;88(12):6015-6019. doi:10.1210/jc.2003-030780; Boschmann M, Steiniger J, Franke G, Birkenfeld AL, Luft FC, Jordan J. Water Drinking Induces Thermogenesis through Osmosensitive Mechanisms. *J Clin Endocrinol Metab*. 2007;92(8):3334-3337. doi:10.1210/jc.2006-1438; Brown CM, Dulloo AG, Montani J-P. Water-Induced Thermogenesis Reconsidered: The Effects of Osmolality and Water Temperature on Energy Expenditure after Drinking. *J Clin Endocrinol Metab*. 2006;91(9):3598-3602. doi:10.1210/jc.2006-0407.

7.   Institute of Medicine. Dietary Reference Intakes: Water, Potassium, Sodium, Chloride, and Sulfate. The National Academy of Sciences Website. http://www.nationalacademies.org/hmd/Reports/2004/Dietary-Reference-Intakes-Water-Potassium-Sodium-Chloride-and-Sulfate.aspx. February 11, 2004. Accessed August 26, 2018.

8.   Convertino VA, Armstrong LE, Coyle EF, et al. American College of Sports Medicine position stand. Exercise and fluid replacement. *Med Sci Sports Exerc*. 1996;28(1):i-vii.

9.   Araki T, Matsushita K, Umeno K, Tsujino A, Toda Y. Effect of physical training on exercise-induced sweating in women. *J Appl Physiol*. 1981;51(6):1526-1532. doi:10.1152/jappl.1981.51.6.1526.

10.   Van Cauter E, Plat L. Physiology of growth hormone secretion during sleep. *J Pediatr*. 1996;128(5 Pt 2):S32-7.

11.   Nedeltcheva A V., Kilkus JM, Imperial J, Schoeller DA, Penev PD. Insufficient Sleep Undermines Dietary Efforts to Reduce Adiposity. *Ann Intern Med*. 2010;153(7):435. doi:10.7326/0003-4819-153-7-201010050-00006.

12.   Yi S, Nakagawa T, Yamamoto S, et al. Short sleep duration in association with CT-scanned abdominal fat areas: the Hitachi Health Study. *Int J Obes*. 2013;37(1):129-134. doi:10.1038/ijo.2012.17.

13.   Jitomir J, Willoughby DS. Cassia Cinnamon for the Attenuation of Glucose Intolerance and Insulin Resistance Resulting from Sleep Loss. *J Med Food*. 2009;12(3):467-472. doi:10.1089/jmf.2008.0128; Zhang J, Hupfeld CJ, Taylor SS, Olefsky JM, Tsien RY. Insulin disrupts β-adrenergic signalling to protein kinase A in adipocytes. *Nature*. 2005;437(7058):569-573. doi:10.1038/nature04140.

14.   National Sleep Foundation. How Much Sleep Do We Really Need? National Sleep Foundation Website. https://sleepfoundation.org/how-sleep-works/how-much-sleep-do-we-really-need. Accessed August 26, 2018.

15.   Mattes RD, Campbell WW. Effects of Food Form and Timing of Ingestion on Appetite and Energy Intake in Lean Young Adults and in Young Adults with Obesity. *J Am Diet Assoc*. 2009;109(3):430-437. doi:10.1016/j.jada.2008.11.031.

16.   Flood-Obbagy JE, Rolls BJ. The effect of fruit in different forms on energy intake and satiety at a meal. *Appetite*. 2009;52(2):416-422. doi:10.1016/j.appet.2008.12.001.

CHAPTER 29

THE THINNER LEANER STRONGER TRAINING PLAN

1.   Schoenfeld BJ, Contreras B, Tiryaki-Sonmez G, Willardson JM, Fontana F. An electromyographic comparison of a modified version of the plank with a long lever and posterior tilt versus the traditional plank exercise. *Sport Biomech.* 2014;13(3):296-306. doi:10.1080/14763141.2014.942355.

2.   Bickel CS, Cross JM, Bamman MM. Exercise Dosing to Retain Resistance Training Adaptations in Young and Older Adults. *Med Sci Sport Exerc.* 2011;43(7):1177-1187. doi:10.1249/MSS.0b013e318207c15d; Izquierdo M, Ibañez J, González-Badillo JJ, et al. Detraining and Tapering Effects on Hormonal Responses and Strength Performance. *J Strength Cond Res.* 2007;21(3):768. doi:10.1519/R-21136.1; Bosquet L, Montpetit J, Arvisais D, Mujika I. Effects of Tapering on Performance. *Med Sci Sport Exerc.* 2007;39(8):1358-1365. doi:10.1249/mss.0b013e31806010e0.

3.   Pritchard HJ, Tod DA, Barnes MJ, Keogh JW, McGuigan MR. Tapering Practices of New Zealand's Elite Raw Powerlifters. *J Strength Cond Res.* 2016;30(7):1796-1804. doi:10.1519/JSC.0000000000001292; Mujika I. The Influence of Training Characteristics and Tapering on the Adaptation in Highly Trained Individuals: A Review. *Int J Sports Med.* 1998;19(07):439-446. doi:10.1055/s-2007-971942; Bickel CS, Cross JM, Bamman MM. Exercise Dosing to Retain Resistance Training Adaptations in Young and Older Adults. *Med Sci Sport Exerc.* 2011;43(7):1177-1187. doi:10.1249/MSS.0b013e318207c15d.

CHAPTER 30

THE THINNER LEANER STRONGER SUPPLEMENTATION PLAN

1.   Kris-Etherton PM, Harris WS, Appel LJ, American Heart Association. Nutrition Committee. Fish consumption, fish oil, omega-3 fatty acids, and cardiovascular disease. *Circulation.* 2002;106(21):2747-2757; Smith GI, Atherton P, Reeds DN, et al. Omega-3 polyunsaturated fatty acids augment the muscle protein anabolic response to hyperinsulinaemia–hyperaminoacidaemia in healthy young and middle-aged men and women. *Clin Sci.* 2011;121(6):267-278. doi:10.1042/CS20100597.

2.   Ross AC, Manson JE, Abrams SA, et al. The 2011 Report on Dietary Reference Intakes for Calcium and Vitamin D from the Institute of Medicine: What Clinicians Need to Know. *J Clin Endocrinol Metab.* 2011;96(1):53-58. doi:10.1210/jc.2010-2704; Heaney RP, Holick MF. Why the IOM recommendations for vitamin D are deficient. *J Bone Miner Res.* 2011;26(3):455-457. doi:10.1002/jbmr.328.

3.   Holick MF, Binkley NC, Bischoff-Ferrari HA, et al. Evaluation, Treatment, and Prevention of Vitamin D Deficiency: an Endocrine Society Clinical Practice Guideline. *J Clin Endocrinol Metab.* 2011;96(7):1911-1930. doi:10.1210/jc.2011-0385.

4.   Weber F. Absorption of fat-soluble vitamins. *Int J Vitam Nutr Res Suppl.* 1983;25:55-65; Iqbal J, Hussain MM. Intestinal lipid absorption. *Am J Physiol Metab.* 2009;296(6):E1183-E1194. doi:10.1152/ajpendo.90899.2008.

5.   McCarty MF. Pre-exercise administration of yohimbine may enhance the efficacy of exercise training as a fat loss strategy by boosting lipolysis. *Med Hypotheses.* 2002;58(6):491-495.

6.   Goldberg MR, Hollister AS, Robertson D. Influence of yohimbine on blood pressure, autonomic reflexes, and plasma catecholamines in humans. *Hypertens (Dallas, Tex 1979).* 5(5):772-778.

7.   Seifert JG, Nelson A, Devonish J, Burke ER, Stohs SJ. Effect of acute administration of an herbal preparation on blood pressure and heart rate in humans. *Int J Med Sci.* 2011;8(3):192-197.

8.   Bemben MG, Lamont HS. Creatine supplementation and exercise performance: recent findings. *Sports Med.* 2005;35(2):107-125.

9.   Ibid.

10.   Steenge GR, Simpson EJ, Greenhaff PL. Protein- and carbohydrate-induced augmentation of whole body creatine retention in humans. *J Appl Physiol.* 2000;89(3):1165-1171. doi:10.1152/jappl.2000.89.3.1165.

11.   Antonio J, Ciccone V. The effects of pre versus post workout supplementation of creatine monohydrate on body composition and strength. *J Int Soc Sports Nutr.* 2013;10(1):36. doi:10.1186/1550-2783-10-36; Candow DG, Vogt E, Johannsmeyer S, Forbes SC, Farthing JP. Strategic creatine supplementation and resistance training in healthy older adults. *Appl Physiol Nutr Metab.* 2015;40(7):689-694. doi:10.1139/apnm-2014-0498.

12.   Glenn JM, Gray M, Jensen A, Stone MS, Vincenzo JL. Acute citrulline-malate supplementation improves maximal strength and anaerobic power in female, masters athletes tennis players. *Eur J Sport Sci.* 2016;16(8):1095-1103. doi:10.1080/17461391.2016.1158321.

CHAPTER 31

THE RIGHT AND WRONG WAYS TO TRACK YOUR PROGRESS

1.   Lebon F, Collet C, Guillot A. Benefits of Motor Imagery Training on Muscle Strength. *J Strength Cond Res.* 2010;24(6):1680-1687. doi:10.1519/JSC.0b013e3181d8e936; Yao WX, Ranganathan VK, Allexandre D, Siemionow V, Yue GH. Kinesthetic imagery training of forceful muscle contractions increases brain signal and muscle strength. *Front Hum Neurosci.* 2013;7:561. doi:10.3389/fnhum.2013.00561.

CHAPTER 32

HOW TO BREAK THROUGH WEIGHT LOSS PLATEAUS

1.   Geliebter A, Maher MM, Gerace L, Gutin B, Heymsfield SB, Hashim SA. Effects of strength or aerobic training on body composition, resting metabolic rate, and peak oxygen consumption in obese dieting subjects. *Am J Clin Nutr.* 1997;66(3):557-563. doi:10.1093/ajcn/66.3.557; Larson-Meyer DE, Redman L, Heilbronn LK, Martin CK, Ravussin E. Caloric Restriction with or without Exercise. *Med Sci Sport Exerc.* 2010;42(1):152-159. doi:10.1249/MSS.0b013e3181ad7f17.

2.   Gleeson M, Blannin AK, Walsh NP, Bishop NC, Clark AM. Effect of low- and high-carbohydrate diets on the plasma glutamine and circulating leukocyte responses to exercise. *Int J Sport Nutr.* 1998;8(1):49-59; Tomiyama AJ, Mann T, Vinas D, Hunger JM, Dejager J, Taylor SE. Low calorie dieting increases cortisol. *Psychosom Med.* 2010;72(4):357-364. doi:10.1097/PSY.0b013e3181d9523c.

CHAPTER 35

FREQUENTLY ASKED QUESTIONS

1.   Kerksick CM, Wilborn CD, Campbell BI, et al. Early-Phase Adaptations to a Split-Body, Linear Periodization Resistance Training Program in College-Aged and Middle-Aged Men. *J Strength Cond Res.* 2009;23(3):962-971. doi:10.1519/JSC.0b013e3181a00baf.

2.   Hunter GR, McCarthy JP, Bamman MM. Effects of resistance training on older adults. *Sports Med.* 2004;34(5):329-348; American College of Sports Medicine Position Stand. Exercise and physical activity for older adults. *Med Sci Sports Exerc.* 1998;30(6):992-1008.

3.   Roberts SB, Dallal GE. Energy requirements and aging. *Public Health Nutr.* 2005;8(7A):1028-1036; Piers LS, Soares MJ, McCormack LM, O'Dea K. Is there evidence for an age-related reduction in metabolic rate? *J Appl Physiol.* 1998;85(6):2196-2204. doi:10.1152/jappl.1998.85.6.2196.

4.   Bosy-Westphal A, Eichhorn C, Kutzner D, Illner K, Heller M, Müller MJ. The Age-Related Decline in Resting Energy Expenditure in Humans Is Due to the Loss of Fat-Free Mass and to Alterations in Its Metabolically Active Components. *J Nutr.* 2003;133(7):2356-2362. doi:10.1093/jn/133.7.2356.

5.   Ziaei S, Sayahi M, Faghihzadeh S. Relationship between reproductive aging, body composition, hormonal status and metabolic syndrome in postmenopausal women. *Climacteric*. 2011;14(6):649-653. doi:10.3 109/13697137.2011.570386.

6.   Ziomkiewicz A, Ellison PT, Lipson SF, Thune I, Jasienska G. Body fat, energy balance and estradiol levels: a study based on hormonal profiles from complete menstrual cycles. *Hum Reprod*. 2008;23(11):2555-2563. doi:10.1093/humrep/den213.

7.   Copeland JL, Chu SY, Tremblay MS. Aging, physical activity, and hormones in women--a review. *J Aging Phys Act*. 2004;12(1):101-116.

8.   Sidhu S, Parikh T, Burman KD. *Endocrine Changes in Obesity*. MDText.com, Inc.; 2000.

9.   Purohit V. Moderate alcohol consumption and estrogen levels in postmenopausal women: a review. *Alcohol Clin Exp Res*. 1998;22(5):994-997.

10.   Ziomkiewicz A, Ellison PT, Lipson SF, Thune I, Jasienska G. Body fat, energy balance and estradiol levels: a study based on hormonal profiles from complete menstrual cycles. *Hum Reprod*. 2008;23(11):2555-2563. doi:10.1093/humrep/den213; Copeland JL, Consitt LA, Tremblay MS. Hormonal Responses to Endurance and Resistance Exercise in Females Aged 19-69 Years. *Journals Gerontol Ser A Biol Sci Med Sci*. 2002;57(4):B158-B165. doi:10.1093/gerona/57.4.B158; Leproult R, Van Cauter E. Role of sleep and sleep loss in hormonal release and metabolism. *Endocr Dev*. 2010;17:11-21. doi:10.1159/000262524.

11.   Fell J, Williams D. The effect of aging on skeletal-muscle recovery from exercise: possible implications for aging athletes. *J Aging Phys Act*. 2008;16(1):97-115; Faulkner JA, Davis CS, Mendias CL, Brooks S V. The aging of elite male athletes: age-related changes in performance and skeletal muscle structure and function. *Clin J Sport Med*. 2008;18(6):501-507. doi:10.1097/JSM.0b013e3181845f1c.

12.   Sherratt MJ. Tissue elasticity and the ageing elastic fibre. *Age (Dordr)*. 2009;31(4):305-325. doi:10.1007/ s11357-009-9103-6.

13.   Faulkner JA, Davis CS, Mendias CL, Brooks S V. The aging of elite male athletes: age-related changes in performance and skeletal muscle structure and function. *Clin J Sport Med*. 2008;18(6):501-507. doi:10.1097/ JSM.0b013e3181845f1c; Lepers R, Stapley PJ. Master Athletes Are Extending the Limits of Human Endurance. *Front Physiol*. 2016;7:613. doi:10.3389/fphys.2016.00613.

14.   Geiker NR, Ritz C, Pedersen SD, Larsen TM, Hill JO, Astrup A. A weight-loss program adapted to the menstrual cycle increases weight loss in healthy, overweight, premenopausal women: a 6-mo randomized controlled trial. *Am J Clin Nutr*. 2016;104(1):15-20. doi:10.3945/ajcn.115.126565.

15.   Evenson KR, Barakat R, Brown WJ, et al. Guidelines for Physical Activity during Pregnancy: Comparisons From Around the World. *Am J Lifestyle Med*. 2014;8(2):102-121. doi:10.1177/1559827613498204.

16.   Kominiarek MA, Rajan P. Nutrition Recommendations in Pregnancy and Lactation. *Med Clin North Am*. 2016;100(6):1199-1215. doi:10.1016/j.mcna.2016.06.004.

17.   Barakat R, Lucia A, Ruiz JR. Resistance exercise training during pregnancy and newborn's birth size: a randomised controlled trial. *Int J Obes*. 2009;33(9):1048-1057. doi:10.1038/ijo.2009.150.

18.   Evenson KR, Barakat R, Brown WJ, et al. Guidelines for Physical Activity during Pregnancy: Comparisons From Around the World. *Am J Lifestyle Med*. 2014;8(2):102-121. doi:10.1177/1559827613498204.

19.   *Ibid*.

20.   Sperstad JB, Tennfjord MK, Hilde G, Ellström-Engh M, Bø K. Diastasis recti abdominis during pregnancy and 12 months after childbirth: prevalence, risk factors and report of lumbopelvic pain. *Br J Sports Med*. 2016;50(17):1092-1096. doi:10.1136/bjsports-2016-096065.

21.   Sharma G, Lobo T, Keller L. Postnatal Exercise Can Reverse Diastasis Recti. *Obstet Gynecol*. 2014;123:171S. doi:10.1097/01.AOG.0000447180.36758.7a.

22.   Schoenfeld BJ. The Mechanisms of Muscle Hypertrophy and Their Application to Resistance Training. *J Strength Cond Res*. 2010;24(10):2857-2872. doi:10.1519/JSC.0b013e3181e840f3.

23.   Flann KL, LaStayo PC, McClain DA, Hazel M, Lindstedt SL. Muscle damage and muscle remodeling: no pain, no gain? *J Exp Biol*. 2011;214(4):674-679. doi:10.1242/jeb.050112.

24.   Park K-S, Lee M-G. Effects of unaccustomed downhill running on muscle damage, oxidative stress, and leukocyte apoptosis. *J Exerc Nutr Biochem*. 2015;19(2):55-63. doi:10.5717/jenb.2015.15050702.

25.   Brandenburg JP, Docherty D. The effects of accentuated eccentric loading on strength, muscle hypertrophy, and neural adaptations in trained individuals. *J strength Cond Res*. 2002;16(1):25-32; Walker S,

Blazevich AJ, Haff GG, Tufano JJ, Newton RU, Häkkinen K. Greater Strength Gains after Training with Accentuated Eccentric than Traditional Isoinertial Loads in Already Strength-Trained Men. *Front Physiol*. 2016;7:149. doi:10.3389/fphys.2016.00149.

26.   Nosaka K, Newton M, Sacco P. Delayed-onset muscle soreness does not reflect the magnitude of eccentric exercise-induced muscle damage. *Scand J Med Sci Sports*. 2002;12(6):337-346.

27.   *Ibid*.

28.   Crameri RM, Aagaard P, Qvortrup K, Langberg H, Olesen J, Kjaer M. Myofibre damage in human skeletal muscle: effects of electrical stimulation *versus* voluntary contraction. *J Physiol*. 2007;583(1):365-380. doi:10.1113/jphysiol.2007.128827.

29.   Chen TC, Nosaka K. Responses of Elbow Flexors to Two Strenuous Eccentric Exercise Bouts Separated by Three Days. *J Strength Cond Res*. 2006;20(1):108. doi:10.1519/R-16634.1.

30.   Bishop NC, Gleeson M. Acute and chronic effects of exercise on markers of mucosal immunity. *Front Biosci (Landmark Ed*. 2009;14:4444-4456.

31.   Murphy EA, Davis JM, Carmichael MD, Gangemi JD, Ghaffar A, Mayer EP. Exercise stress increases susceptibility to influenza infection. *Brain Behav Immun*. 2008;22(8):1152-1155. doi:10.1016/j.bbi.2008.06.004; Martin SA, Pence BD, Woods JA. Exercise and respiratory tract viral infections. *Exerc Sport Sci Rev*. 2009;37(4):157-164. doi:10.1097/JES.0b013e3181b7b57b.

32.   Weidner TG, Cranston T, Schurr T, Kaminsky LA. The effect of exercise training on the severity and duration of a viral upper respiratory illness. *Med Sci Sports Exerc*. 1998;30(11):1578-1583.